Introduction to
HUMAN DEVELOPMENT
and HEALTH ISSUES

LORRAINE BRADT DENNIS, R.N., M.S., Ph.D.

Psychology
Roger Williams College
Bristol, Rhode Island

JOAN HASSOL, R.N., Ed.M.

Coordinator of Education and Training
Norfolk County Sexual Assault Unit
Dedham, Massachusetts

W. B. SAUNDERS COMPANY
Philadelphia   London   Toronto   Mexico City   Rio de Janeiro   Sydney   Tokyo

W. B. Saunders Company: West Washington Square
Philadelphia, PA 19105

1 St. Anne's Road
Eastbourne, East Sussex BN21 3UN, England

1 Goldthorne Avenue
Toronto, Ontario M8Z 5T9, Canada

Apartado 26370—Cedro 512
Mexico 4, D.F., Mexico

Rua Coronel Cabrita, 8
Sao Cristovao Caixa Postal 21176
Rio de Janeiro, Brazil

9 Waltham Street
Artarmon, N.S.W. 2064, Australia

Ichibancho, Central Bldg., 22-1 Ichibancho
Chiyoda-Ku, Tokyo 102, Japan

Library of Congress Cataloging in Publication Data

Dennis, Lorraine Bradt.

Introduction to human development and health issues.

1. Children—Growth.   2. Children—Diseases.   3. Child
development.   4. Pediatric nursing.   I. Hassol,
Joan.   II. Title.

RJ131.D426 1983   613   82–40310
ISBN 0–7216–3030–8

Front cover illustration, courtesy of H. Armstrong Roberts

Introduction to Human Development and Health Issues   ISBN 0-7216-3030-8

Last digit is the print number: 9   8   7   6   5   4   3   2

We, Lorraine and Joan, dedicate this book to our families who taught us more than we can acknowledge about human development.

PREFACE

My intention in presenting this text has been to give an overview of human development, focusing on the psychosocial influences as well as maturation, and pointing up the implications of a theory of development for health service professionals. The text was written with the conviction that men and women of the health services are in a position of particular advantage to carry out the mission of education, which turns a present responsibility into an expanding benefit for the future. An attempt was made to render the information readily accessible to the reader.

The frame of reference is provided here by Erik Erikson's *Eight Ages of Man*, which describes a developmental task for each stage of life that enables a subsequent stage to proceed appropriately. The emphasis is upon normal development as the yardstick against which to measure deficiency but, more importantly, as the goal of a holistic approach to human functioning. However, there is also reference to the kinds of outcomes that might be expected if things go wrong, particularly areas in which intervention, instruction, or informed social policy might make a difference. The effects of malnutrition, alcohol, smoking, and drugs on the prenatal organism is an example. Another instance occurs in the case of battered wives or children, a situation in which the health service professional's sensitivity to the issues might point the road toward life or death.

The developmental point of view discerns the broad outlines of problems, highlights, and rhythms of existence at different ages. Understanding of "ages and stages" assists in placing much behavior into perspective (so that we need not fear that the fiercely rebellious 2-year old is going to remain thorny for the rest of his life or so that we can listen and abide as grandfather launches into an oft-told reminiscence).

A developmental point of view, however, is balanced with a clear sense of the importance of environment in supporting or even determining some outcomes, especially with regard to certain capabilities and competencies. Further, each age has its own health hazards; my co-author, Joan Hassol, has attended to these in a series of "companion" chapters that detail the considerations for health care accompanying each stage.

My teachers, my students (often the best teachers), and many writers walk through these pages, sometimes anonymously. It is frequently impossible to identify the original sources of ideas that have become so much a part of my own thinking. Responsibility for liberties taken with the interpretation of these ideas, however, must be claimed as my own.

A number of individuals need to be acknowledged specifically. Frances Goodwin once again, as for my previous text (*Psychology of Human Behavior for Nurses*), edited with persuasion and insistence when prose failed to live up to the goal of comfortable understandability. My colleague, Grayson Murphy, read and commented on Chapter 2, and Wendell Pols, Reference Librarian at Roger Williams College, cheerfully tracked down the most obscure references, having only minimum information. Our indefatigable editor, Ilze Rader, sustained us through many long nights. My family contributed confidence and optimism that the project would, indeed, one day be finished. To each and all, a hearty "thank you!" It could not have been completed without you.

LORRAINE BRADT DENNIS

PREFACE

Few professions allow as intimate, consistent, and influential contact with as wide a spectrum of people as the health professions. Health professionals are advocates, educators and caregivers.

This text is designed to introduce students to a variety of health-related topics in which these various roles play themselves out in the daily functioning of professional life. The rapid development of the biological sciences has radically changed our concepts and definitions of health and health maintenance. We can no longer think of health as a static state. Rather, we now know that at each stage of life there are different yet appropriate ways of defining health, i.e, the health issues confronting adolescents are different than those confronting the elderly. Health issues are discussed for each stage of human development, with a particular focus on normal development and prevention.

My involvement with the creation of this volume is due in no small part to the persistent encouragement of several people who provided the human contact that made the long hours in the library and the isolating vigil before a demanding typewriter possible, and sometimes even exhilarating.

To Dr. Ann Burgess, my grateful thanks for insisting that I could do it; to Dr. Lorraine Dennis, my heartfelt appreciation for your patience, enthusiasm, and confidence; and to Ilze Rader and Carol Robins Wolf, my thanks for quietly and kindly reminding me of deadlines and for letting me say what needed to be said.

To my family: Sometimes, if one is particularly lucky, the opportunity to realize a fantasy arises. Thank you all for helping make that fantasy a reality.

JOAN HASSOL

CONTENTS

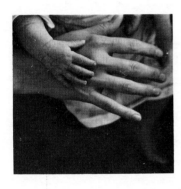
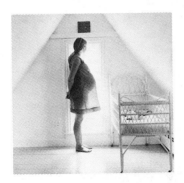

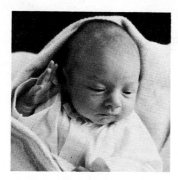

CHAPTER **3**

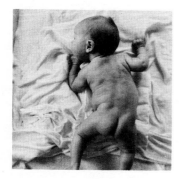

CHAPTER **4**

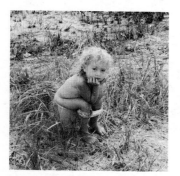

CHAPTER **5**

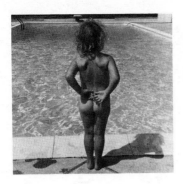

CHAPTER **6**

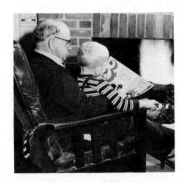

CHAPTER **7**

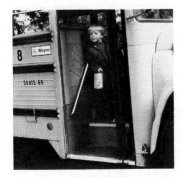

CHAPTER **8**

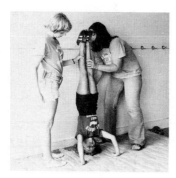

CHAPTER 9

HEALTH CONCERNS IN SCHOOL-AGE CHILDREN   152

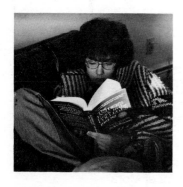

CHAPTER 10

THE ADOLESCENT: IDENTITY   168

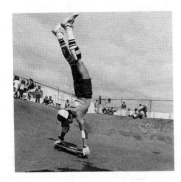

CHAPTER 11

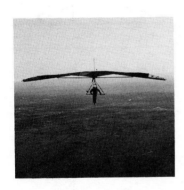

CHAPTER 12

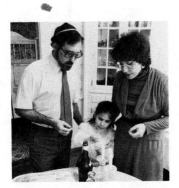

CHAPTER 13

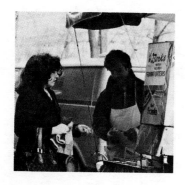

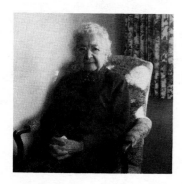

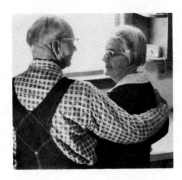

CHAPTER **16**

HEALTH CONCERNS IN THE OLDER ADULT 284

Introduction to
HUMAN DEVELOPMENT
and HEALTH ISSUES

CONSIDERING DEVELOPMENT

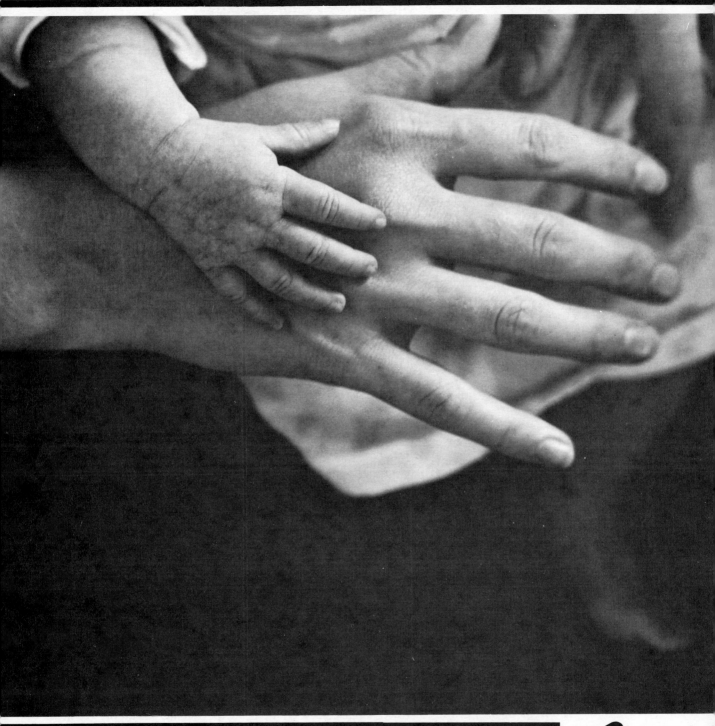

CHAPTER 1

THE STUDY OF DEVELOPMENT

First, a vantage point—a kind of road map to point out where we are going, together with something of the why and how. Let's begin with a look at the term *development*. What does it mean?

Development refers to the series of changes that occur with passing time in an orderly and predictable sequence, taking place by means of an integration of biological and environmental factors. Development includes, but is not synonymous with, *growth*, which refers to the increase in size, height, circumference of head, limbs, and waist, or length of fingernails that is brought about by proliferation of cells.

The distinction between the two terms is not always clear because they are sometimes used as if they were interchangeable. However, it is important to understand that there is a difference. For example: the growing infant lengthens arms, legs, and torso, gains body and organ weight, and acquires teeth and more hair. The development of the infant's nervous system makes possible a brand new capability, translating distance into eye-hand coordination and conveying the message to appropriate neurons for activating certain muscles. The result is a deft finger-thumb opposition that literally transforms the baby's hand into a marvelous tool for manipulation and construction. Just days before, baby was still attempting to pick Cheerios off the highchair tray with a whole-hand closing. Now baby is gleefully managing the smallest particles. Development is the process, often coupled with growth but providing the complex articulation of structure and function, that makes finger-thumb opposition and other capabilities possible.

THE SCIENTIFIC METHOD

The previous section has used a couple of terms—*orderly* and *predictable*—that come from the language of scientific inquiry and need to be examined more closely. Understanding these terms is important because the "facts" of psychology (including developmental psychology) are sought and tested according to a generally agreed-upon set of procedures often called the *scientific method*. Students should know something of these procedures in order to evaluate the information that pours forth in the name of "science."

The fact of the matter is that we live in a scientific age, use the products of scientific technology every day, and, as students, dutifully memorize the steps that are said to make up the scientific method, all with only the foggiest notion of what science is. In the case of most of the readers of this text, careers are enmeshed in scientific endeavor. Could you define "science"? Try to explain what makes science different from another human activity, such as writing sonnets or decorating the Sistine Chapel. What distinguishes the lifework of Watson and Crick, 1953 Nobel Prize winners for analysis of the DNA molecule, from that of William Shakespeare? What differentiates the scientist studying psychology or biology from the philosopher studying ethics?

If you are a typical student answering these questions, you are likely to be thinking along lines of "experimental versus creative" or "objective versus subjective." "Experimental" and "objective" are certainly adjectives often applied to science, so you are on the right track, but the response is not complete. If, by "experiment" you imply trying something out, testing it, isn't that what an artist does also? Doesn't the novelist or artist or musician try different words, plots, color and line combinations, or chord progressions until the result is acceptable? And though you may counter that such a process is subjective whereas science is objective, it can be argued that scientists view data through their own eyes, have already decided upon a question relating to their own experiences, and will report the results with their own words and interpretations. Pretty subjective!

Science is distinct from other kinds of endeavors such as art or theater in terms of its subject matter and goals. Science is the attempt to understand natural phenomena. Its subject matter is nature—the universe and all natural events.

"To understand" means to know enough about a natural happening so that one can report what is going to happen with a good degree of accuracy. Scientists search for regularities, for events that recur. Once the conditions for recurrence can be specified, prediction becomes possible. And, of course, predicted information is potentially useful. So it can be said that "understanding" leads to "prediction and control." To be able to predict the path of a hurricane from the weather signs permits some control over this natural event by warning people to take in their lawn furniture and store a supply of fresh water. To be able to predict the life cycles of various insect pests makes control of their numbers possible. To be able to predict the course of many diseases provides the basis of medical intervention and practice.

Present-day science should be considered an extension of humankind's perennial search for understanding of the universe in order to better human existence. Even prehistoric groups were scientists of sorts. Like all who have followed, they sought knowledge about the world so that more of it could be brought under control. From cave drawings we know that the dwellers had accurate concepts of animal morphology and habitat—the better to stalk them and secure some supper! Stone Age skeletons of at least 50,000 years ago show restored fractures and some remarkable surgical procedures that necessitated some understanding of regularities of human anatomy and physiology. Some 3000 to 4000 years before the birth of Jesus, knowledge of the properties of certain minerals permitted melting and casting of pure copper, copper-arsenic, and copper-tin alloys. Domestication of plants and animals was built upon accumulated observations of plant and animal life cycles.

To recount the groping steps toward understanding natural phenomena taken by the peoples of the past is as exciting as telling any adventure story. Because we live in an "age of science," it is easy to dismiss the attainments of earlier observers as being of little consequence, if indeed these are accorded any respect as science at all. However, the basic assumption upon which primitive peoples fixed their practices and upon which modern science proceeds is still essentially the same. Science assumes orderly and dependable cosmic laws that govern natural events. And the aim of science is still unchanged. Science, today as yesterday, represents the attempt to discern these laws so that the events may be better predicted and thus yield more opportunities for useful application of the knowledge.

The search is for regularities of occurrences, for *patterns* and *order* (concepts from the opening section of this chapter). Whether the finding is a pattern of stars that assists navigation, or certain rock outcroppings that signal what lies beneath, or the measurement of two angles of a triangle that permits specification of the measurements of the third, discovery is still based on observation. Modern science has refined and systematized the approach. There are sophisticated statistical techniques that aid precision and a vast variety of instruments to support and enhance the human powers of observation. The findings are more easily communicated and preserved so that new generations of scientists can build upon what has been established before.

Sometimes it becomes possible to find out a great deal about an event and, especially, those circumstances necessary and sufficient to cause the event to occur. *Necessary* in this context means that the event will not occur unless the specific circumstances are present, and *sufficient* means that, if present, the circumstances will inevitably produce the event. When it is possible to discern "causation" so explicitly, one has the best possible potential for control of the event.

Three Scientific Approaches

Description (Normative Approach)

Science begins with the description of natural phenomena. In order to proceed at all, we must first ascertain "what is there," or "what is typical." The descriptive approach seeks to answer questions of observable "facts." When does the average baby begin to sit alone or to walk? Is the neonate (newborn) capable of seeing more than just light or shadow? Are male infants typically more active than female infants? Are there other early-appearing sex differences? What is the course of puberty for boys and for girls? What kinds of problems are confronted by middle-aged and elderly widows? These are the kinds of questions about human development that might be answered by a descriptive investigation.

A great deal of important information has come to us through the centuries by way of descriptive studies. The ancient Egyptian priests were using descriptive methods when they kept careful records of the various levels of the river Nile, discovering the pattern that would warn of disastrous floods. Thucydides was engaged in descriptive research when he systematically listed all known symptoms of the plague of Athens in his account of the Peloponnesian War. His aim was that the plague be recognized if it should ever break out again. Van Leeuwenhoek, assisted by the lenses with which he was forever tinkering, contributed substantially with his descriptions of the "little beasties" in a drop of rainwater and with his documentation of the motility of spermatozoa.

Good description still furnishes the basic building blocks of all science. Many examples can be listed: an accumulation of case histories informs with regard to the course of a disease. Marine biologists descend into the ocean depths to see "what is there" and gather specimens for further examination. Sophisticated spacecraft like Voyager I relay information about the rings and moons of Saturn for earthbound space scientists to study and analyze. Over many years, repeated observations of dozens of families in Yellow Springs, Ohio, gave us the first indications of persistent character traits that can be observed in typical preschool children and seem to be stable into adulthood (Kagan and Moss, 1960).

It must be apparent that accurate description will depend upon accurate observation and accurate reporting. The very presence of the investigator may distort the situation if data are being gathered from human or infrahuman subjects (such as chimpanzees). In other words, people who know they are being watched or who simply recognize a stranger in their midst may change their usual behavior. This is termed the *observer effect* and plagues all of the social sciences. Scientists go to elaborate lengths in the attempt to be as unobtrusive as possible, hiding behind one-way vision screens, pretending to be attending to something else, and sometimes living with the group under study until the presence of the "outsider" is no longer noticed.

It is also possible that an investigator, even when trying to be as careful as possible, might nevertheless be in error in what is thought to be observed. A second observer helps to guard against this. Sometimes, too, it is possible to record the events with movie or television cameras so that they can be replayed as often as necessary to obtain agreed-upon accuracy.

Furthermore, every observer is limited in the number of instances to which it is possible to attend. Scientists are exceedingly cautious about suggesting that the findings apply to a larger group of events. Because the ultimate aim is to be able to predict, isolated events are not usually valuable or important except to spark interest in the possibility of a pattern of recurrence. Scientists are trained to make decisions with regard to what confidence can be placed in the proposition that findings are representative of a larger whole.

All of this should be taken to indicate that even "simple" observational procedures are an "iffy" business. Modern science attempts to provide the ultimate safeguard by insisting that any serious investigation be *publicly verifiable*. This simply means that the scientist is required to submit findings to the scrutiny of colleagues in the field; then the study can be repeated by others and the results either confirmed or questioned. This is the step that many purveyors of beauty or health-care preparations decline to follow, often insisting that their "results" speak for themselves. However, a valid replication of such results would be very difficult to accomplish. As an example let us think about a procedure to test a potion that promises to halt and reverse the changes associated with old age.

The first step must be to fashion a definition of "youth regaining" that can be observed and measured. It will not do to simply accept the subjects' reports because of the *placebo effect*, the well-known possibility that subjects feel better because they believe a medication or preparation has acted. The kind of definition of an occurrence that can be observed and measured by any number of different observers is termed an *operational definition*. To be able to specify what will be accepted as a youth-regaining phenomenon is regarded as *operationalizing* it. What might be adequate for a claim of "rejuvenation" qualities of a product? Wrinkle count before and after use of the product? Number of pushups the individual is able to do before and after? Blood pressure and heart rate under stress before and after? It is quickly evident that a commercial enterprise would not be very interested in this kind of evidence. Failure to operationalize the definitions for "results" makes many claims of "scientific tests" very suspect. To devise an operational definition that two or more qualified observers would be able to verify is often difficult but absolutely essential for accurate description.

Association (Correlative Approach)

Scientific description supplies a great deal of information about nature. A textbook on human anatomy, for example, compiles the results of countless careful descriptions of innumerable dissections. The "facts" of human anatomy are rather well established.

Frequently, however, it is desirable and important to move a step beyond description. Sometimes it seems possible that there is a link or association between diverse phenomena. Suppose a pin is placed on the map of a large city at the site of each serious crime committed over a period of several months. It would soon become evident that certain areas have many pins, whereas other areas have few. Some sections of the city have "more than their share" of crime. There would seem to be some kind of tie or association between a particular area and the excessive number of crimes committed there.

Or suppose it is possible to study a large group of adult men over a period of years. Some of these men smoke cigarettes regularly, whereas some do not smoke at all. Over the years, it is discovered that lung cancer and heart conditions develop with much greater frequency among smokers than among nonsmokers. The smokers seem to have more than their share of lung cancer and heart disease. This would suggest a link or relationship between cigarette smoking and lung cancer or heart disease.

Or suppose a study of aptitude test scores for sixth and twelfth grade pupils also inquired about the children's television-viewing habits. It would be possible to use certain statistical procedures that would make the suspected relationship between the two sets of data (test scores and hours spent watching television) explicit. The term for this kind of study is *correlation;* it provides a statistical index of relationship.

Present-day correlation techniques make possible a more precise observation of suspected associations between phenomena. However, whether the relationship is documented by modern statistical procedures or whether the relationship is compiled by the more casual observations of early scientists, an important limitation must be observed. The existence of a relationship between events or measures cannot be offered to document cause and effect. That is, although an association or correlation between phenomena may permit some prediction of the occurrence of one with the other, it does *not* warrant a conclusion that one is the cause of the other.

For example, in the time of our great-great-grandmothers, the association between incidence of malaria and exposure to the night air of malarial regions was well known. As a matter of fact, the name of the disease means "bad air." One could predict with a degree of success that sleeping with shutters flung open to the night would increase the chances of acquiring malaria. We now know, of course, that night air does not *cause* malaria—that the cause is a parasite transmitted through the bite of an infected mosquito. Sleeping with one's unscreened windows open invited attack by the insect. So, even though a relationship seems highly suggestive, it must be appraised with caution. There is always the possibility of another factor, an "X" as yet unknown (a mosquito, so to speak!) that relates to the associated events and operates as the true cause.

This important rule is often forgotten. The newspaper report about the link between hours of television viewing and aptitude test scores is headlined "Tuning in to TV's Effect on Studies." The clear implication is that television adversely affects children's academic skills. Although this might sound reasonable, the study itself does not provide such evidence. It is a correlative study that indicates a relationship between higher number of hours of television viewing and lower aptitude test scores. However, turning off the television set will not automatically reverse such a trend. It would be necessary to inquire about other factors in the student's life that promoted excessive television watching and probably also operated to decrease language and math facility. The newspaper headline displays a common error in attributing a cause-and-effect sequence in this regard. Scientists are usually much more careful and would have reported only the documented relationship.

Experimental Approach

Descriptive research furnishes answers to questions for basic information. What is the average IQ of Harvard freshmen? What is the typical age for onset of menstruation in the Western hemisphere? What is the usual age of weaning for rhesus monkeys? What is the sequence in development of spoken language in young children?

Associative or correlative research seeks answers to a different kind of question. It attempts to determine whether two or more natural phenomena might be related. Is there an association between taking thalidomide during the prenatal period and deformities of offspring of the pregnancy? Is there a correlation between the IQ's of parents and those of their children? Is there an association between socioeconomic level and the incidence of premature births? Although the method of arriving at an association may point up a clear link, it cannot be offered as evidence that one factor is the cause of the other.

In order to provide a rigorous demonstration of cause, it is necessary to employ the third approach of science, the *experiment*. An experiment is a situation that has been carefully and deliberately arranged by an investigator in an attempt to answer a question of cause.

The investigator proposes to demonstrate that a specific factor is "necessary and sufficient" to produce a particular result. Natural factors or circumstances or phenomena under study in psychology are called *variables* because these occur in differing amounts or may be absent altogether. The variable of an experiment that is thought to be caused by (or to depend upon) another variable has a special designation. It is called the *dependent variable*.

The variable that is to be tested to see if it causes the effect (the dependent variable) must somehow be isolated from all other possible variables that might also affect the dependent variable. Because this variable is operating alone or independently under ideal arrangements, it is distinguished as the *independent variable*.

An independent variable, then, is the presumed cause of the dependent variable, which is the presumed effect. Note the caution with which that statement is worded. The scientist is not likely to report that the investigations "proved" something. Rather, the conclusions will be reported very tentatively. The scientist is forever aware that even the most careful of arrangements might have overlooked variables that interfere with or *confound* the results. Only after experiments have been verified a number of times can the findings be cited with a high level of confidence.

Let a simplified description of an experiment serve as an illustration. A farmer wishes to test the effect of a certain type of fertilizer upon a field of corn. Will the fertilizer, the independent variable, cause an increased yield of corn? In this case, the size of the resulting crop will be the dependent variable. If the farmer plants corn, fertilizes it, and obtains a bumper crop, is he justified in crediting the fertilizer? Not at all! Many other factors (variables) influence the growth of corn: amount of sun, amount of rain, type of soil, kind of seed, and method of cultivation. How can the farmer be sure that he is witnessing the effect of the fertilizer rather than the possibility that it has simply been a particularly good growing year for corn? The solution is to *control* the extraneous variables in some way so that their effects can be accounted for and "held constant," therefore not affecting the final reckoning. One way to accomplish this might be to plant two similar fields of corn at the same time, making sure that the soil and seed are the same type and that fields are situated in such a way that they receive the same amount of sun and rain. Then, by fertilizing one field and not the other, the farmer can compare the resulting yield from both fields and note any difference. If our farmer is a good scientist, he will repeat the experiment several times before giving credit to the independent variable. He will know the difficulty of making absolutely certain that the influence of all possible confounding variables has been controlled.

An experiment, then, is a deliberately arranged test for cause and effect. Its validity will hinge upon how well the investigator has succeeded in controlling the variables involved so that the operation of the independent variable will be isolated. To "hold constant" the confounding variables often involves arranging identical conditions for two groups, an *experimental group* and a *control group*, with the experimental group receiving the independent-variable treatment while the control group does not. Such a procedure is easier to describe than to accomplish. Furthermore, it is much easier when fields of corn are being considered, rather than human beings. We will elaborate on this point shortly.

It must begin to seem that scientists are the "doubting Thomases" of the world. In a sense, perhaps they are. But the orientation of the scientist is better characterized as a kind of prudence by which it is well understood that to accept knowledge as final is to close the door to further inquiry.

Actually, the general outlook is one that recommends itself to each of us. It implies a lively curiosity, a willingness to relinquish pet fancies as these are discovered to be based on false assumptions, an acceptance of change, and, most of all, a ceaseless quest for new knowledge.

DEVELOPMENTAL PSYCHOLOGY: A BRANCH OF PSYCHOLOGY

We have looked at science and have seen it to be the search for understanding of natural phenomena, a search that began even before humans kept records. Although the aim (understanding, prediction, and control) has remained the same, experience has taught scientists that the inquiry proceeds more accurately if certain rules are followed in the attempt to find answers to scientific questions. The flourishing of what we know as modern science began when the careful observations known as the "scientific method" became tied to the keen awareness of the possibility of error and to the emphasis upon verifiability.

However, it has been barely a century since the proposal that it might be possible to make scientific sense out of human behavior . . . that perhaps the method of inquiry that had already proved so fruitful for other sciences could be used to study human beings. Physiologists had long since demonstrated the circulation of blood through the capillaries, had described the structure of the ear and eye, and knew much about the nervous system. Physicists were learning the properties of gases, the laws of motion, and the principles of light waves. Physicians had begun to use anesthesia and antisepsis and were becoming acquainted with the notion of pathogenic organisms as agents of disease when the new science, psychology, was born in the laboratory of Wilhelm Wundt in Leipzig in 1879.

At first the studies concentrated upon attempting to discover the laws or regularities of perception, with emphasis upon the inner experiences of "noticing" or detecting whatever is to be perceived. The process of observing and reporting upon one's own sensations is called *introspection,* and participants were carefully trained both in what to look for and what to report, for example, in discerning the subtle difference in tones coming from two tuning forks.

From this small beginning sprang the discipline we know today as psychology, with formal instruction being offered in almost every college and university across the land. Hundreds of thousands have been trained in psychology and are engaged in a vast variety of psychology-related endeavors, including advertising, personnel administration, counseling and testing, teaching, and many different kinds of social services and research.

Developmental psychology is a branch of general psychology. Although it seems to be something of a latecomer to the field, it can be suggested that developmental regularities were among the earliest discoveries of the young science and have proved to be among the enduring blocks of information about human beings and their behavior. The physician-psychologist who was the first to describe human psychological development systematically, in detail, was Sigmund Freud.

Freudian Theory

Freud proposed not only a regular and predictable sequence of personality development, but also the dynamics that made it all "work" and solutions to help if something went wrong. His death took place in 1939 after an extraordinarily productive career, which was an important feature of the first half of the 20th century and continues to exert influence to this day.

Because his ideas ran directly counter to the mores and customs of the society, Freud became a highly controversial figure. Strong emotion is still engendered when those who feel he made an immense contribution argue with those who feel that he was utterly wrong. Nevertheless, because of Dr. Freud, the Western concept of human psychology was wholly changed. There really are "pre-Freudian" and "post-Freudian" eras. Because of Freud, such terms as *unconscious motivation, ego, defense mechanism,* and *psychotherapy* are not only ordinary aspects of vocabulary but are taken for granted in any consideration of human behavior. To Freud is also owed the emphasis upon childhood as important to later outcomes in adulthood. This was not original with Freud, but his description of the step-by-step development gave it ready currency as a workable model. Though the theory still must withstand all of the tests that the scientific community can muster, the fact of the matter is that much of what has come later owes a debt to Freud's thinking, writing, and teaching. Because it serves as a backdrop against which more contemporary theories evolved, we will take a look at some of the main features of the Freudian view of human development.

Sigmund Freud: Psychosexual Development

Eros and Thanatos

Human existence is powered, according to Freud, by two great basic instincts (Freud, 1965). In this, he allied himself almost, but not quite, with other instinct theorists.

Freud's writings have come to us through translation from the original German in which he wrote. As any language student knows, the search for a word in one language that precisely defines the "feel" of the word in another language is very difficult and frequently the actual sense of the translated word suffers. The German word used by Freud to describe the basis of human life and behavior is *trieb*. With a lack of an exact counterpart in English, this has been translated as "instinct." But the German meaning of trieb entails much more sense of driving force; it is really more akin to our word "urge."

More telling, however, in distinguishing Freud's theory on instinct from the others, is his consistent emphasis upon the goal-directedness of human behavior and upon the source of the "instincts" in the biological structure of the organism. To Freud, instincts do not float, as it were, without beginning or end in a kind of vacuum that must be envisioned for the concept of an "acquisitive instinct," "competitive instinct," or "maternal instinct." Rather, the instincts originate in the tension systems of the body on the one hand and are anchored in the object or activity that reduces this tension (the goal) on the other.

Freud thought of his two "instincts" as the fundamental sources of dynamic energy— the generator that fuels all activity and behavior. Basic to all life, he suggested, is one major aim—that of self-preservation. Allied to this is a subsidiary aim—perpetuation (preservation) of the race. In other words, for Freud, when stripped of all its trimmings, life boils down to the business of staying alive and producing others to carry on the species. This basic instinct was called *Eros*—named after the Greek god of love. All of the inner urges that impel us to build, to construct, and to take care of ourselves and our young might be thought of as expressions of this life force. It would include, of course, the sexual tensions that lead (ordinarily) to reproduction. From this basic power system come the motivations that enable building shelter, creating clothing, shielding against the elements, securing nourishment, pursuing a vocation, and fostering children. For Freud, Eros was the underlying source of all creative activity.

The second "basic instinct" was postulated later in Freud's formulations. He observed that human beings are not only constructive and preserving, but that they hate as well as love, and death is as much a fact as life. He reasoned that there must also exist, within the organism, a biologically derived force that tends to break down organic matter, to counteract creation. This is *Thanatos*—named for the Greek god of death, considered by Freud to be the source of aggressive and hostile behavior.

It is difficult for most of us to accept the notion of a "death instinct." Indeed, Ernest Jones, one of Freud's foremost students and interpreters, calls it "disturbing" (Jones, 1961, p. 158). It seems to represent a bleakly pessimistic view of humankind. If humans are born with a fundamental tendency to destroy and injure, there seems to be little recourse except to build our prisons larger, hire more police officers, and resign ourselves to ever-recurring war.

However, an inexorable logic dictated the concept of Thanatos and, to Freud's credit, he never shrank from proposing an unpopular idea. In postulating Eros as striving for the most comfortable life possible, one is forced to admit that the state of least striving (most comfort) would be sleep, or death. Thus, as Jones puts it (p. 163):

. . . death is not an unfortunate accident. Life itself inherently leads to death, is actually aiming at bringing about death, even if by a circuitous and complicated path. The aim of life is peace, in the final resort the peace that disintegration of the organic into the inorganic provides. Katabolism has the last word over anabolism.

It might be pointed out here, however, that a number of modern scholars who accept many of Freud's ideas still reject the notion of an inborn aggressive instinct. They suggest that the facts of hostility and aggression can be just as well explained as arising out of frustration of the constructive energies. Thus, if one is starving and blocked from obtaining food, the reaction would likely be one of fury. It has also been reasoned that aggressiveness has a certain life-preserving function—that the ability to be fired with rage made it possible for primitive people to protect their families from marauding tribes and ferocious beasts with the necessary strength and energy.

Expression of the Instincts: Personality

The instinctual energy is transformed into human expression by action and feeling. The ways in which the energy is expressed is learned during the process of growing from infant to adolescent. Freud, as we shall see, did not extend his thinking about developmental change beyond adolescence. For him, human beings enter adulthood as products of what has gone on before and any changes thereafter would probably have to come about by means of lengthy and intensive psychotherapy, called *psychoanalysis* in the Freudian system.

The individualized "self" through which the energy is transformed is called the *personality*. We think of personality as being unique and individual, but Freud was the first to attempt to offer a picture of the regularities pertaining, he claimed, to all human beings and to relate these regularities to both normal and pathological behavior (Munroe, 1955).

According to Freud, the personality is made up of not one, but *three*, selves. This is not a wholly alien idea. It is common to sense "being at war" with one's self when faced with a conflict. We say "one part of me wants to do this and the other part of me wants to do that." Robert Louis Stevenson constructed a classic story around this idea in *The Strange Case of Dr. Jekyll and Mr. Hyde*, and recent movies and television productions have dramatized the "split personality" in *The Three Faces of Eve* and *Sybil*. Freud called the three components of personality the *id*, the *ego*, and the *superego*.

The Id. The *id*, for Freud, was the basic energy source, untransformed by any outside influence. It was considered to be the driving force behind any kind of human activity and to have only one aim: to gratify its impulses and to avoid pain. The term comes from the Latin and means "it." This neutral designation seems to have intended the sense of existence quite apart from the real world, wholly unrestricted by concepts of time, place, propriety, or consideration of others.

The best illustration of the id in action is seen in newborn babies. When they are hungry, infants howl; when satisfied, they sleep. Newborns have absolutely no concern that the parents may be sleepy, that their crying may disturb the apartment dwellers next door, or that their excretory habits leave much to be desired. Babies are solely concerned with their own bodily needs for comfort. The id, therefore, is described as adhering to the *pleasure principle*.

Only the slightest stretch of imagination is necessary to depict what kind of world this would be if such id domination of behavior continued. Think of the chaos if each individual persistently sought only self-gratification. We would live in terror of our lives every minute, in mortal danger even at the hands of our own family. Fortunately, for us and for civilization, the id impulses are brought under control during the process of growing up.

The Ego. The aspect of the personality that begins control of id impulses is the *ego*. For a little while, because of dependence and helplessness, the infant's id-directed desires are gratified. The infant is fed when hungry, even though this may mean a delayed dinner for the rest of the family. We are tolerant of the self-centered, unsocial behavior "because he doesn't know any better." We assume, of course, that there will come a time when the child will "know better," and that is exactly what happens.

Babies begin to grow up, slowly gaining comprehension that they are not master of all they survey. There is a certain inexorable length of time to wait, for example, while mother takes a bottle of formula from the refrigerator and heats it. A rattle dropped over

The newborn is totally concerned with herself. When she is unhappy, she cries, with no concern for sleepy parents or neighbors in the next apartment.

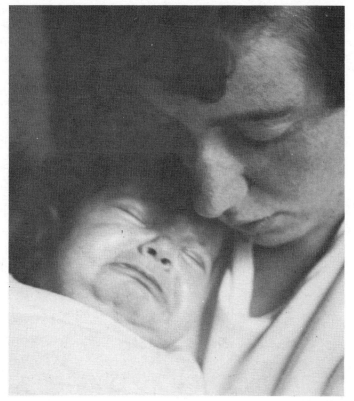

L. Hassol

the side of the highchair is gone unless someone else chooses to pick it up. Babies may attempt to pull themselves up by means of the radiator and receive a painful burn. The baby explores the contents of an ashtray and someone slaps a hand. Day in and day out, the toddler bumps into the realities of life, the realities that have no place in the id world.

Slowly, out of the id energy, then, evolves the ego—the "I" of the personality. It is the ego that provides the id impulses with a check, according to Freud. Baby begins to learn the consequences of behavior. It is the ego that now supplies the "information" that the radiator surface will be hurtful, that sampling the interesting wastebasket brings adult displeasure, that certain procedures are necessary at the top of a staircase in order to avoid a nasty fall, and that no matter how much you scream, you cannot play with the moon.

The ego, it should be noted, is not concerned with right and wrong—with morality. Its task is to limit, redirect, govern, or *repress* those id impulses that are likely to have unpleasant consequences because of the way the world is. The emphasis upon "the way it is" leads to the description of the ego as conforming to the *reality principle.*

The ego, as described by Freud, might be thought of as the gradually developing intelligence that slowly gathers comprehension of the world. The ego can be said to learn the behaviors that make baby "fit to live with." Thus, a child who is seriously mentally retarded is unable to form a properly functioning ego and must be guarded by others lest the id impulses lead him or her into danger.

The ego, then, is essential to the human being who must live and work and accommodate to the world. Freud believed ego development to be pretty well completed by the age of 5 or thereabout and that the years of infancy and childhood are thus crucial in determining its ultimate strength or weakness.

The Superego and the Ego Ideal.   Even a highly developed ego, however, would enable the individual to make only self-centered decisions. The human ability to make value judgments, to decide about right and wrong, to put the self in someone else's shoes (which makes *empathy* and *sympathy* possible), and to become civilized demands a further refinement of motivating energy. This occurs during an important stage in the child's life when a portion of the ego evolves into the *superego*, which can also be thought of as *conscience*.

The superego does not form until the child is several years old and, in Freud's theory, is the specific result of developmental events termed the *Oedipal conflict* (which will be described in the next section). The normal outcome finds the child incorporating parental views and attitudes and attempting to be as much like the same-sex parent as possible. The process is termed *identification*. The voice of conscience, according to Freud, is the internalized voice of the important controlling adults in the child's life. If the superego is well developed, the values and taboos eventually become an integral part of the self and parental control becomes self-control. The superego punishes transgressions with feelings of guilt and remorse that are exceedingly painful. The admonitions of the superego are heeded in order to avoid these feelings. The superego also rewards "good" behavior. Operating as a subsystem, the *ego ideal* provides a picture of the self as one would like to be—the goal to shoot at, so to speak. Feelings of pride and satisfaction come about when one lives up to aspects of this inner picture.

Freud did not imply that the id, ego, and superego have actual form and substance, existing like three little gnomes in the head. Rather, he intended the representations to depict the forces that he felt operate in every personality. A major problem confronting every individual, according to Freud, is that of maintaining a good working balance among these forces. The demands of the id, since these are the true source of all motivating energy, must be given some outlet. It becomes the task of the ego and superego to see that the expressions are consistent with both reality and values held by society.

An imbalance in the functioning of these forces, he suggested, results in some degree of incapacity for "normal" behavior. Id dominance, unrestrained by ego or superego, is exemplified by the behavior of the schizophrenic or manic patient in the psychiatric division of an institution. Without the curbs provided by ego and superego, the patient might shout obscenities, smear excreta, or indulge in infantile fantasies of absolute power. In a less extreme form, the result of id domination is seen in people described as "childish" or "spoiled" because they insist on their own way regardless of the rights, welfare, or desires of others. There are occasions when the id gains control in the lives of any of us, particularly under conditions of great stress. The shout of "fire!" in a theater may cause the crowd to rush pell-mell for exits, each individual intent only upon self and survival. Illness is sometimes such a threat, weakening ego and superego controls.

There are others whose ego formation seems strong but for whom the superego did not develop properly, presumably for lack of or rejection of a primary model. Many criminals and delinquents fall into this category. Their asocial behavior is directed only in terms of reality, the possibility of being caught.

Still others may be described as laboring under a heavy-handed superego. These individuals rigidly deny themselves any mite of pleasure, are constantly harassed by a sense of sinfulness, and often seek to impose their inflexible restrictions upon others. They lead cheerless, bleak, and sterile lives, preoccupied with the impossible task of keeping every impulse seeking gratification submerged.

Psychosexual Stages

In the preceding description of how life energy is expressed—used, tempered, channeled, pushed down, or permitted an outpouring in the course of daily activities—through the functions of three parts of the personality, the term "evolved" appeared several times. We could just as well have used "developed" because Freud's is a *developmental theory*.

Freud suggested that from infancy through childhood and into adolescence the energy-tensions are manifested and seek gratification in a succession of body areas. Each area is, in some sense, representative of that period of the child's life, serving as the main seat of pleasurable sensation and lending the potential of either too much or too little fulfillment. The specific sensual areas shift and change because of growth processes and because of changes in the impact of society's demands (at first, from parents and later from school and peers). The growing competence and comprehension of ego and superego take place, then, within a five-stage sequential system, each stage of which builds upon and elaborates what has gone on before.

Oral Stage.   In the beginning the baby is "all mouth." The first source of comfort and good feeling comes from the mother's breast (or from a nippled bottle) by means of sucking. The delights of the mouth for an infant are readily apparent. For Freud, this pleasure is a precursor of ultimate erotic pleasure. It is sensual (of the senses) and brings about a decrease in tension and a replete satisfaction. (You can imagine the outrage with which Victorian society received the idea that the infant is obtaining a kind of sexual joy from the feeding situation!)

The crisis of this period comes with weaning. In Freud's day, breast feeding took place for most of the infant's first year. Typically, the child was next given a cup and more solid food as mother became pregnant again or when the first teeth erupted and nursing became painful. Weaning was seen as a traumatic time for the child, and mothers received copious advice regarding how to manage the situation.

Anal Stage.   By this time, the infant has become a toddler and the zone of sensual pleasure has shifted from the mouth and stomach to the organs of excretion and most specifically to the sphincter muscles, which regulate retention and expulsion. Reared, as we all are, to view the products of excretion with disgust, the description of this period usually seems impossibly outlandish to students. It is necessary to suspend revulsion in order to note that a typical infant does not mind wet or soiled pants and that infants will play with excreta unless prevented, and to acknowledge that there really is a very sensual kind of relief afforded by emptying a full bladder or bowel.

The crisis of this period revolves around training. Again, times have changed, so that modern parents usually accomplish teaching the baby to gain sphincter control without stress or turmoil; however, in the first quarter of this century, toilet training was considered a contest of will between parent and child and was, literally, called "breaking" the child. Freud's idea was that successful progression through any stage might be hindered if the needs were inadequately gratified, leaving the individual forever yearning; or, if the needs were too well satisfied, there would be no incentive to give up the pleasure for another, more mature stage. The term for retaining an inappropriate tie to a past stage is *fixation*. One fixation of the anal stage, carried on into later life, was thought to be *miserliness*, a preoccupation with possessions and suspicion that the world is out to snatch one's precious belongings away—a grown-up repetition of the toilet-training situation.

Phallic Stage.   From the sphincters, the zone of body pleasure and interest was thought to shift to the genitals during ages 4, 5, and 6. For Freud, the sexes diverge in their development during this stage, though he is much more definitive in the description of what happens to little boys than with regard to what happens to little girls.

The small boy at this time is supposed to develop powerful wishes to have mother all to himself. Freud insisted that the intention was phallic (sexual). (By daring to make such a statement, Freud promptly lost all hope of an appointment to the University of Vienna because he became such a controversial figure.) Whether the child can actually experience sexual strivings or whether the desire for mother's undivided attention is broad rather than specific has not been settled. But in any case, the youngster perceives a powerful rival in the father and wishes he were out of the way. The enormity of daring to pit his small self against such a wrathful giant is quickly overwhelming, especially as he contemplates what would be father's revenge—castration. The only way out of the dilemma is to do an about-face. The longing for mother is renounced and repressed (therefore Freud maintained that normal men do not remember these childish impulses), and the little boy lines himself up with father, saying, in effect, "See? I couldn't have ever wished you dead. Here I am trying so hard to be exactly like you."

The entire conflict and its outcome were called the *Oedipus complex* after the Greek mythical hero who unknowingly slew his father and married his mother in fulfillment of an ancient prophecy. The normal outcome was to be identification with the father, taking on male attributes and values and developing a strong superego.

The route for little girls, as seen by Freud, partakes of the male-centered view of his era. He suggested that the little girl suddenly notices she does not have a penis and presumes that she was mutilated in some ghastly manner by her mother. She is so devastated that she will spend the rest of her life attempting to make up for the loss in one way or another. Ideally, in Freudian terms, she will settle for passive reception of a husband's penis during intercourse and obtain some satisfaction upon bearing a male child. Pathologically, she will reject the feminine role and exhibit *penis envy* by adopting masculine characteristics of striving, competitiveness, and aggressiveness.

Of all the Freudian ideas, this one is probably the most vigorously challenged. It is not necessary to identify oneself as a feminist to be irritated with the presentation of the girl as inferior, an "anatomical tragedy" (Freud, 1927) (he really did say it!), and more tellingly, the acceptance of the idea of her inferiority as a feature of normal development. Furthermore, the characteristics that Freud assigned to the normal female outcome of the Oedipus complex*—masochistic, passive, narcissistic, less fully identified with the mother, who is perceived as the culprit in the misfortune, and therefore possessing a less fully developed superego—may have been considered desirable and feminine in a Victorian-age woman but are accepted as neurotic for the active, independent, and competent woman of today.

The phallic period, for both boys and girls, closes with the coming of school days. The turmoil, anxieties, and fears are repressed and will surface during adulthood when the mature young man or woman re-enacts the old Oedipal attachments with the newly secured mate.

Latency. This is the school-age period when, according to Freud, the conflicts of earlier years go into hiding. It is supposed to be a relatively tranquil period during which the young person becomes socialized with age-mates and learns the school skills preparatory to entering adulthood.

Genital Stage. With the onset of puberty, the various unresolved psychosexual conflicts break out again, this time to be incorporated in the general lifestyle. By this time, functioning is taking place on three levels of awareness: the conscious, which is present awareness; the preconscious, which is memory; and the unconscious, which is the storehouse of the id strivings and includes all the repressed impulses of life and all the experiences that threaten a tolerable self-concept.

By means of *defense mechanisms*, the ego can permit a reasonable amount of id energy to be expressed, even though a conscious recognition would be unacceptable. For example, the insecure teenager who is really terrified of growing up and assuming responsibilities may drink too much alcohol, unconsciously returning to an earlier time when comfort came from something taken in by mouth. The genital stage normally should bring about mature sexuality, with relationships that eventually produce a new family to carry on the species.

---

*The term attached to Freud's explanation of the female experience is *Electra complex*, although it is not used much today. It refers to the desire of the female child for the male parent.

Evaluation of Freudian Theory

What do we make of Sigmund Freud and his theory? His place in history has already been suggested. With regard to the validity of the theory, much of it now seems rather dated. The Victorian era, with its rigid suppression of sexuality and its strict adherence to what are usually thought of as stereotyped sex roles, brought about its own developmental problems. With stern, forbidding fathers and swooning mothers, a fine-boned, expressive male or an active, assertive female was likely to have a hard time. Further, the theory is much better for explaining pathology and emotional troubles than it is for the good cheer, steady courage, gentle love, reasoned decision making, and rollicking humor that are characteristic of the behavior of most of the human beings whom we know.

On the other hand, the insights of the theory spark in everyday life like little flashes of light. The blissful . . . yes, orgasmic . . . look on the face of a nursing baby, the triumph with which young Master Three-Year-Old wedges himself in between mama and daddy, and the glimpses of many a defense mechanism in operation, even (with a grimace of recognition) in one's self, remind us of Freud's genius.

Freud's theory is presented here, *not because it is the final word, but because it has served and serves today as a base for scientific investigation of human development.* As we proceed through the "ages and stages" presentation of this text, we will discuss the developmental theory of Erik Erikson, which is a direct offshoot of the Freudian, and the cognitive-development theory of Jean Piaget. Psychologists are not typically fashioning grand theories that account for all human behavior anymore, but are rather content with testing much less extensive hypotheses derived from much less comprehensive theory.

WHY STUDY DEVELOPMENT?

We have just looked at the method of scientific inquiry by means of which the search for patterns of human development is conducted. We also reviewed one of the "grand old theories" of human development that succeeded in focusing attention on a hitherto taken-for-granted childhood and in making parents much more aware of the far-reaching consequences of their child-rearing practices. With this introduction, we now intend to follow the developmental processes through the life span, from beginning to end, and to link the development of each age with the implications for building and maintaining good health.

Ideally, the study of development ought to have a personal impact on the life of the student. Many students will have only just left adolescence behind, while others are likely to be still undergoing the disengagement and detachment process. They may acquire some perspective in terms of how far they have come and what lies ahead. Some students may be mature adults who will recognize their own children in these pages. They, too, may gain a clearer picture of where they are by having seen where they have been.

Every student will be confronted with decisions throughout life that have important developmental involvements. The premise of all education is that informed decisions usually have advantages over uninformed ones. The message from this branch of psychology is that there is information that has been gathered systematically and that many developmental decisions can proceed from an authoritative base. Should the pregnant woman be advised to give up smoking? What is the effect of day care or nursery school on children? What do teen-agers want to know about sex? Does divorce affect children? Are there advantages or drawbacks to living together "without benefit of marriage?" Is there a male menopause? Do most elderly suffer from loss of memory? There are empirical findings on each of these questions.

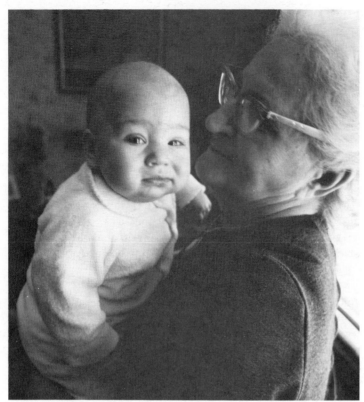

Development is a lifelong process; we change every day of our lives. Studying the life span from beginning to end prompts us to reflect on our own lives, who we are, where we have been, and what is yet to come.

Judith Kruger Michalik

The study of development also provides a framework for expectations. The "norms" for childhood offer a range of ages for the developmental mileposts. It is not that the child must be lopped off or stretched out to fit, as for a Procrustean bed, but rather that the norms are convenient checks. If an ability or characteristic is "late," the parents can be alerted to watch so that something potentially serious would not be ignored. Understanding of the developmental sequences can also prevent impossible demands that end in total frustration for both child and parents.

Furthermore, the "new look" in development extends the concept to adulthood, assisting adults of all ages to anticipate and accommodate changes in themselves and in others. To understand that adolescence is not the end of development, but rather that there is promise and potential for every adult age, offers an exciting and hopeful view. There is a song that contains the poignant question about being an adult, "Is that all there is?" We can confidently, now, answer no! There is much, much more! Development is a lifelong process with something new to look forward to at every age.

The Content of the Study of Development

Developmental studies are sometimes descriptive, sometimes correlational, and sometimes experimental. There is little doubt that research with human beings as subjects offers perplexing problems to the scientist, who must be sure that the investigation lends itself to replication by another scientist so that the findings can be checked.

Because development involves both those processes that are "built in," biologically, and those that are put into effect by the environment, the individual is literally undergoing continuous change. Some of these changes provide the new basis for the next set of changes and, important for our investigator, certain changes must come about by virtue of being subjects for an investigation (Neugarten and Datan, 1973). Think about the difficulty of attempting to duplicate any condition as precisely as would be wished for a true replication.

Nevertheless, patterns do exist and can be discerned and described, as we shall see, though we are careful about becoming too excited about findings that ought, always, to be regarded as the best-we-have-at-the-moment. Developmental patterns can be categorized in the main as follows.

Physical Changes.   This is the area for which there is a large body of information, in part because of the extensive work by other professions, including scientists with specialties in anatomy, physiology, biology, and medicine. This is also the information that has the broadest currency, and we have not included detailed accounts in this discussion.

Cognitive Changes.   Mental development has been studied for years by means of intelligence tests. More recently, a Swiss psychologist named Jean Piaget proposed a sequential-stage theory for cognitive development, much of which has been studied and verified by numerous investigators. Piaget died in 1980 at the age of 83, and although it would be exaggerating to say that he has had as great an impact as Freud, there is little doubt that we think differently today about cognitive development because of him. We will be describing some of his ideas in the course of future chapters.

Psychosocial Development.   Recall that Freud called it *psychosexual* development. The newer designation pays more heed to the social environment and the multitude of transactions in which the individual engages, with sexuality important but not of sole importance among them. The theoretician to whom we will attend in this area is Erik Erikson, a student of Freud's who succeeded in adapting Freudian concepts into a construction for contemporary times. We will be following his "eight psychological ages of man" as the framework for this presentation.

GLOSSARY

ANAL STAGE   The second stage of psychosexual development, according to Freud. The seat of libidinal pleasure is the excretory orifices, and the conflict is toilet training.

ASSOCIATIVE SCIENTIFIC APPROACH   Attempts to ascertain a possible relationship between variables.

CONTROL GROUP   The group that receives all the variable influences except that of the independent variable in an experiment.

CORRELATION   A statistical procedure that measures the extent of a relationship between variables.

CORRELATIVE SCIENTIFIC APPROACH   Attempts to assess a possible relationship between variables.

DEPENDENT VARIABLE   The presumed effect in an experiment.

DESCRIPTIVE SCIENTIFIC APPROACH   Procedures that are used to assess what is typical or what is normative.

DEVELOPMENT   The series of changes that occur with passing time in an orderly and predictable sequence, taking place by means of an integration of biological and environmental factors.

EGO The "I" of the personality that develops from contact with reality and controls the id.

EGO IDEAL A kind of goal for the self. A picture of the self as one would like to be.

EXPERIMENTAL GROUP The group receiving the treatment of the independent variable in an experiment.

EXPERIMENTAL SCIENTIFIC APPROACH Method by which an independent variable is manipulated in the effort to determine its effect.

FIXATION Freudian term for failure to pass through a psychosexual stage completely so that some tag-ends of the conflicts linger in present life.

GENITAL STAGE The last stage of psychosexual development, according to Freud. The adolescent should move to true heterosexuality and, at the proper time, choose a mate.

GROWTH Increase in size, height, circumference, or length, which is brought about by a proliferation of cells.

ID The portion of the personality that, according to Freud, expresses energy in its most fundamental aspect, not bounded by reality and guided only by the pleasure principle.

IDENTIFICATION The child incorporates parental views, attitudes, values, and behavior.

INDEPENDENT VARIABLE The presumed cause in an experiment.

LATENCY The fourth stage of psychosexual development, according to Freud. The previous conflicts are laid to rest as the school-age child joins peer activities and concentrates on school tasks.

OBSERVER EFFECT The presence of the investigator may distort the situation that is being observed.

OEDIPAL CONFLICT For Freud, this ultimately results in the acquisition of masculinity. It begins when the small boy desires his mother but fears father's revenge and resolves the conflict by repressing his desire and attempting to become as much like father as possible (identification).

OPERATIONAL DEFINITION Definition of a variable in terms of the measures used to assess it.

ORAL STAGE The first stage of psychosexual development, according to Freud. The seat of libidinal pleasure is the mouth, and the conflict is weaning.

PHALLIC STAGE The third psychosexual stage of development, according to Freud. During this stage, the paths of boys and girls diverge, with resolution of the Oedipal conflict and the Electra conflict setting each on different routes to masculinity and femininity.

PLACEBO EFFECT Subjects are affected by their expectation that a substance will act.

SUPEREGO The conscience. It develops from the internalized prohibitions and values of parents.

VARIABLE In psychology, a factor, characteristic, trait, or influence that is present in varying amounts or degrees.

REFERENCES

Freud, S.: Some psychological consequences of the anatomical distinction between the sexes. International Journal of Psychoanalysis, 8:133–142, 1927.

Freud, S.: *New Introductory Lectures in Psychoanalysis*. Edited and translated by J. Strachey. New York: W. W. Norton & Company, 1965 (originally published, 1933).

Jones, E.: *Papers on Psychoanalysis*. Boston: Beacon, 1961.

Kagan, J., and Moss, H. A.: The stability of passive and dependent behavior from childhood through adulthood. *Child Development*, 31:557–591, 1960.

Munroe, R.: *School of Psychoanalytic Thought*. New York: Holt Dryden, 1955.

Neugarten, B., and Datan, N.: Sociological perspectives on the life cycle. In Baltes, P. B., and Schaie, K. W. (eds.): *Life Span Developmental Psychology: Personality and Socialization*. New York: Academic Press, 1973.

IN THE BEGINNING

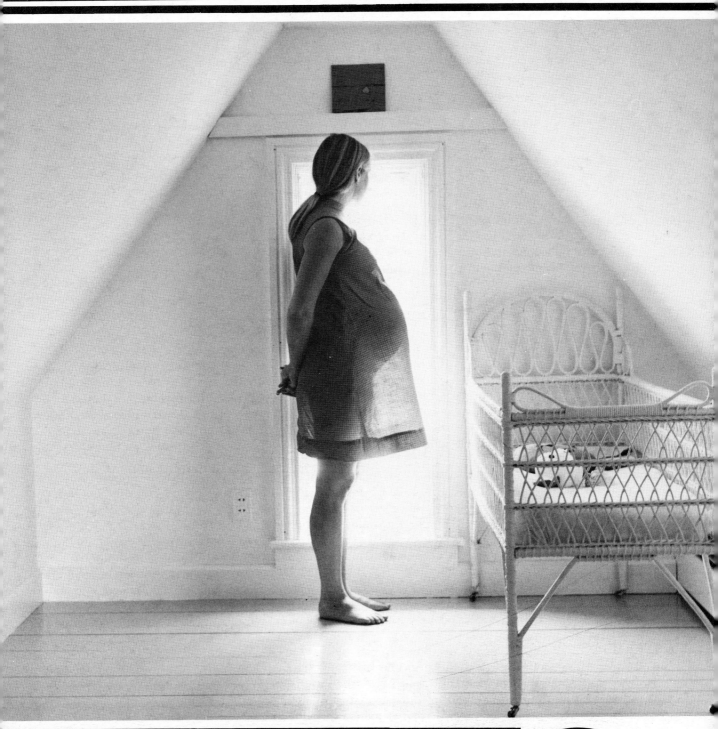

CHAPTER 2

A baby is born! Over all the world, in every society, this is an event of tremendous significance. The high, thin wail announces not only the miracle of a new life, now launched, but also the promise of what the baby may become. Parents pay heed to this potential as they weave dreams about the baby's future. Right now, the baby is small and helpless, but later . . . perhaps a ballerina, an Olympic contender, chief of the tribe, healer, builder of bridges, or a tiller of the soil? All things are possible in the minds of fond parents who cradle the tiny bundle.

But not quite all . . . because parents themselves dream and aspire for the child in terms of the society in which they live. Parents in the United States will not ordinarily list "chief of tribe" as a likely possibility for a small son. Nor is the Watusi mother likely to consider the chances of becoming an Arctic explorer for hers. So the circumstances of birth, by opening up certain possibilities and closing off others, provide an augury of the baby's future.

However, we are ahead of the story. In order to understand the future, it is necessary to begin at the beginning. How much of the future is irrevocably determined at birth? What are the biological "givens," the built-in characteristics with which the baby starts the life journey?

CHARACTERISTICS OF ALL ORGANISMS

The baby is, first of all, a human organism. To identify an *organism* is to say at once a great deal about possibilities. All organisms, from the simplest one-celled to the most complex multicelled, share certain fundamental attributes. For every organism, simple or complex, these characteristics are basic to each particular mode of life. The characteristics are interdependent, constituting a system, which means that consideration of a single characteristic must take all the others into account. The following enumeration, then, should be recognized as an arbitrary delineation of what is, in reality, an integrated, functioning whole.

1. All living systems are composed of cells, each of which is a discrete entity consisting of a substance called *cytoplasm*. Each cell is limited by its surrounding *cell membrane* and contains the director or "brain" of the cell, the *nucleus*. Cytoplasm is known to contain a number of chemical compounds, but it is much more than a mere aggregate of these elements. The still mysterious secret of life seems to lie in the organization of these compounds into an extremely complex colloidal system that is capable of maintaining itself in a steady state, despite continuous introduction of new material and elimination of some of its own substance. The limiting membrane separates internal from external, keeping out—within limits—much that is noxious and yet permitting a continuous exchange of substances between the internal and external environments.

2. All organisms tend to maintain a constancy of internal conditions. This is sometimes called the principle of *homeostasis*, described by biologists as a "steady state." Many internal balances are necessary to sustain life. The chemical events known as *metabolism* result in nutrition, growth and repair of the system, and elimination of waste. In the process, fluids, minerals, salts, and other vital tissue components are regulated. Some organisms, including humans, need a constant internal temperature so that when outside conditions present a possibility of overheating, the organism's cooling mechanism swings into operation, causing perspiration, which, upon evaporating, cools one off. If the temperature becomes too cold, shivering occurs, stepping up consumption of body fuel and generating more heat. Many animals can fluff their fur, creating a dead-air space next to the skin and thus insulating against heat loss. Some organisms can protect themselves against an unfavorable external environment that threatens their internal equilibrium by changing the character of the limiting membrane, thus forming a spore or cyst. Some organisms can accomplish an internal metabolic rearrangement or

can produce an adaptive enzyme that renders an unfavorable substance harmless. In humans, the various inflammatory processes, allergic reactions, and mechanisms for coping with pathogenic invaders fall into this category. All organisms, in other words, are equipped with a means for attempting to preserve and regulate a degree of inner constancy.

3. All organisms carry out basic physiological processes. Organisms obtain nourishment from the external environment, digest it, circulate the nutritive elements, and eliminate waste products. This is a homeostatic arrangement, already described, that can be thought of as maintaining a kind of *dynamic equilibrium*, an equilibrium that is constantly in the process of change. This also implies an open system rather than a closed system, with an intricate series of chemical reactions furnishing energy for sustaining the equilibrium.

4. Organisms have the ability to sense their environment and to react to that sensing. This is sometimes called the principle of *irritability*. Cytoplasm registers changes in the environment and tends to respond adaptively. In simple organisms, the sensing apparatus is crude and the possibilities for reacting are limited. Thus, the single-celled ameba will move away if a drop of acid is introduced into the water near it, adapting by means of the irritability and motility of its one lone cell. In higher organisms, the sensory apparatus is marvelously elaborate and the range of possible responses is relatively vast.

5. Every organism has a life cycle that includes growth, development, reproduction of its kind, and decline. This book will be reviewing the basic features of human life cycle development.

THE UNITY OF ALL LIVING THINGS

Human babies, therefore, have certain "built-in" capacities by virtue of sharing in the properties of all organisms. Human babies can be expected to partake in the ceaseless interchange between the internal and external, between the self and the environment. Each normal human baby will, of course, be equipped to perform the basic physiological functions associated with nourishment, utilization of nutrients, and the elimination of waste products. Each small being will also maintain other important internal constancies. Large portions of the external environment are available to the baby's sense organs and response capabilities. We can expect the baby to grow, develop (through a long period of dependency upon others), perhaps eventually to reproduce, become aged, and certainly to die.

This biological base links the human baby with an ameba and creates the essential unity among all living things. The basic organismic capacities are, in simple forms of life, biological predecessors of much that becomes psychological in higher organisms. For each organism, the modes by which it exercises these capacities—maintaining constancy of internal conditions, performing physiological functions, sensing, and responding—as well as the details of its particular life cycle and its special cytoplasmic morphology, entail great differences.

The individual qualities of each organism are passed on from one generation to another. One ameba is much like another, one eagle has characteristics in common with other eagles, and human share their attributes with all humankind. To understand the means by which human beings fulfill and recreate their own organismic potential, it is necessary to take a look at human heredity.

HUMAN HEREDITY

The previous section described the kinship of human beings with all living organisms. Now let's examine the similarity of human beings one to another and, in addition, the individual's special similarity to familial ancestors.

Human life begins with the union of two germ cells, the spermatozoon from the father and the ovum from the mother. The new cell that is formed is called a *zygote*. At the moment of conception, the heredity of the individual who will develop from the zygote is set for all time. Thereafter, every cell in the individual's body will carry the particular unique (except in the case of identical twins) inheritance in the form of 23 pairs of chromosomes located in the cell nucleus. The way this comes about will be reviewed briefly.

Reduction-Division

Ordinarily, the cells of the body are replaced when worn or damaged, and they are increased in number by a process of cell division termed *mitosis* (Fig. 2–1A). This

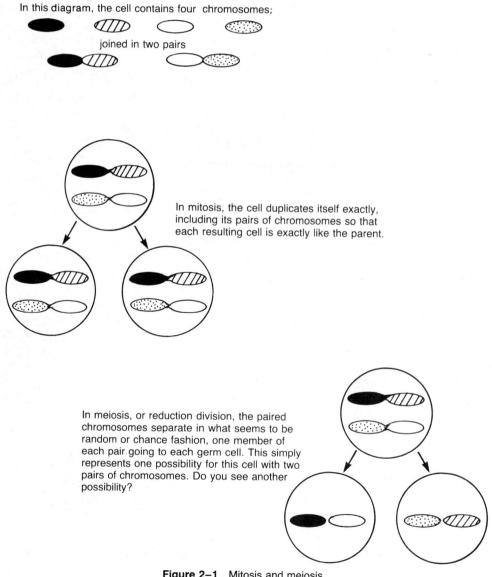

In this diagram, the cell contains four chromosomes;

joined in two pairs

In mitosis, the cell duplicates itself exactly, including its pairs of chromosomes so that each resulting cell is exactly like the parent.

In meiosis, or reduction division, the paired chromosomes separate in what seems to be random or chance fashion, one member of each pair going to each germ cell. This simply represents one possibility for this cell with two pairs of chromosomes. Do you see another possibility?

Figure 2–1 Mitosis and meiosis.

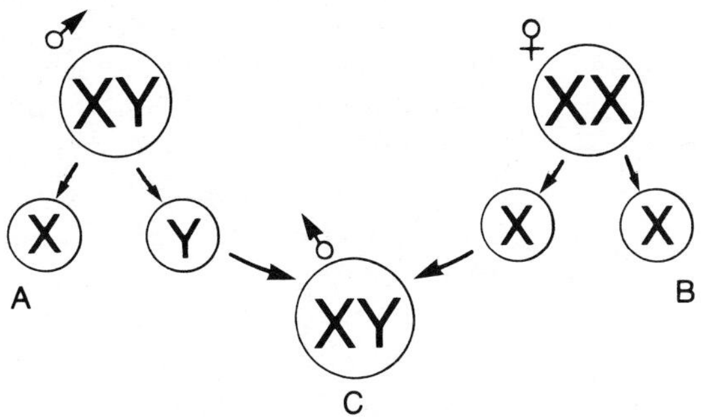

Figure 2–2   (A) In the male, reduction-division results in germ cells, half of which carry an X chromosome and half of which carry the Y chromosome. (B) In the female, reduction-division results in germ cells, each of which carries an X chromosome. (C) The sex of the child depends upon whether one of the father's X or Y chromosome gametes chances to fertilize the ovum. In this case, the child will be male.

involves an exact reproduction of the parent cell, including its chromosomes, so that each resulting cell is precisely like the one that divided to produce it, carrying the same 23 pairs of chromosomes.

The germ cells (spermatozoa for the male and ova for the female), technically known as *gametes*, undergo a special process of cell division known as *meiosis* or *reduction-division* (Fig. 2–1B). Germ cells begin, like every other cell in the body, with a full complement of 23 pairs of chromosomes. As germ cells mature, however, during meiosis, the pairs of chromosomes separate in what seems to be random fashion with one member of each pair going to each new cell. Thus, the new mature cells receive only half of the original chromosomes. Instead of 23 pairs of chromosomes, each germ cell carries 23 single members of what were once chromosome pairs. Reduction-division, then, refers to the process by which the original chromosome pairs are divided and the total number of chromosomes is reduced for each new mature germ cell.

Fertilization, the union of two gametes, results in a brand new assortment of chromosomes, 23 from the male germ cell pairing with 23 from the female cell, to create the new zygote. When the zygote divides and redivides into the cells of the developing organism, it does so by the process of mitosis, with each cell becoming a duplicate of the original zygote. Thus, an individual's heredity depends upon the particular combination of 23 chromosomes from the germ cell of the father and 23 chromosomes from the germ cell of the mother.

In view of the fact that during reduction-division, the chromosomes were sorted randomly, it is possible to suggest that there are 2^{23} or more than 8 million different assortments of chromosomes that could occur for each spermatozoon and each ovum. This means that each father and each mother has more than 8 million different possible combinations of characteristics that might be passed on to their children. An individual's heredity is drawn from a pool of some 150 trillion possible chromosome combinations, resulting first from the chance assortment of chromosomes for each germ cell and the subsequent chance of union of those two particular cells. The sorting of the chromosomes, occurring for every germ cell during its maturation, helps to explain why children who have the same parents and are reared in similar surroundings may differ so widely in appearance and other characteristics.

Chromosomes and Genes

The emphasis upon the individuality of each newborn baby is thus not misplaced. The baby's heredity is a unique combination of factors, one half from the father and one half from the mother. However, it should be noted that the particular chromosomes of the mother and father constitute the "pool" from which all the chromosomes of their offspring are derived; therefore, brothers and sisters are likely to resemble each other, having drawn their chromosomes from the same "pool" by virtue of having the same mother and father.

Human chromosomes are tiny paired structures, so small that counting them had been very difficult until a technique was invented for spreading the cellular material thin enough so that the chromosomes would not lie on top of each other. Then, with advanced methods of lighting and photomicrography, it was possible to ascertain the count of 46 chromosomes (23 pairs) for human beings. The exact structure and number are different and distinct for each species, ranging from as few as two to as many as 127 pairs (Sinnot et al., 1958).

Chromosomes are carriers of the actual hereditary factors called *genes*. As a result of the 1953 Nobel Prize–winning efforts of Watson and Crick, the gene is known to be made up of a complex substance called deoxyribonucleic acid (DNA). The molecular pattern of this compound appears to have the form of a double spiral staircase, with the two spirals linked by a particular arrangement of specific biochemicals like the steps of a staircase. The exact order of these "steps" along the spiral, as well as the varying proportions, seems to constitute a coded message of hereditary information. The spiral staircase, or double helix, can "unzip"—divide and reproduce in mirror-image fashion—providing identical sets of hereditary instructions for every duplicating cell.

Sex Determination

Expectant parents are always curious about the sex of a prospective child. Boy or girl? So much hinges upon the outcome. Many a queen was put aside in ancient times for failing to produce the male heir necessary to continue the dynasty. This practice really did the poor woman a gross injustice because it is the father who determines the child's sex.

The chromosomes that determine sex are of special interest not only because of their effect on whether the child will be male or female, but because of their association with certain traits that are *sex linked*.

The pair of sex-determining chromosomes of the normal female are identical and are given the designation of X and X. The male carries one X chromosome and one of a different type, termed the Y chromosome. Thus, two X chromosomes will result in a female, and an X and a Y will produce a male. Because of the process of reduction-division, the gametes of the female will each carry one X chromosome. However, half of the gametes of a male will carry the X and the other half will carry the Y (Fig. 2–2). If a spermatozoon with a Y chromosome chances to fertilize the ovum, the child will be a boy. If, on the other hand, the spermatozoon carries the father's X chromosome, the child will be a girl. Thus, the father who is disappointed at having fathered a daughter has no cause for blaming his wife!

Theoretically, there should be an equal chance of the zygote's being male or female, since half the spermatozoa carry an X and the other half carry a Y. In fact, however, more males are conceived than females, at a rate of approximately 120 to 170 males for every 100 females. Since males have a higher mortality during uterine development, the ratio of male to female births is 105:100 (Rugh et al., 1971).

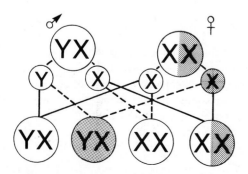

Figure 2–3 In color blindness, a normal male and a female with genes for color blindness on one X chromosome have one chance in four of having a color-blind son and one chance in four of having a daughter who carries the color-blind gene as a recessive trait.

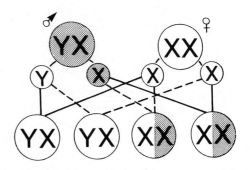

Figure 2–4 A color-blind male and a normal female would have normal sons, but the father would pass on his color blindness to all his daughters, who would carry the gene as a recessive trait.

This greater vulnerability of the male has been attributed to the possibility that the Y chromosome may be somewhat defective. It is only about one third as large as the X chromosome and contains a proportionately smaller share of DNA. Furthermore, the Y chromosome does not seem capable of countermanding the expression of traits carried by the X chromosome, such as color blindness or hemophilia. Such characteristics will be manifested in a son, if he has inherited an X chromosome that is a carrier from his mother, because his Y chromosome cannot counteract the effect. However, a daughter would manifest the characteristic only if she were to have received two defective X chromosomes, one from the father and one from the mother. The patterns of inheritance are traced in Figure 2–3 through 2–5. Sex-linked characteristics, then, are those that follow the distribution of the X chromosome in both sexes, finding expression in the male because of the incapacity of the Y chromosome to cover or repress their effects, but expressed in the female only if both X chromosomes carry the trait.

Dominance and Recessiveness

An important attribute of the gene is *dominance* or *recessiveness*. Genes, like the chromosomes of which they form a part, are paired, one member of each pair coming from the father and the other from the mother. If the parental genes for blue eyes, for example, are the same (each parent contributing a gene for blue eyes), the child's eyes will be blue. But what if one parent's gene was for brown eyes while the other contributed a gene for blue? When the genes are different, the effects of one may prevail, covering up the effects of the other. Such a gene is said to be *dominant*, and the ineffective gene is termed *recessive*. A dominant gene will produce the trait no matter what kind of a gene it is paired with, whereas a recessive gene must always be united with one like itself in order to take effect.

In the case of brown eyes versus blue, brown eyes are known to be dominant. Therefore, a child receiving two different genes, one for brown eyes and one for blue, will have brown eyes.

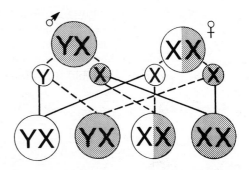

Figure 2–5 A female can show color blindness in her phenotype only if she inherits the trait from both mother and father.

The appearance of a trait, so that it can be observed, is termed the *phenotype*. The term *genotype* refers to the actual genetic endowment, including qualities that may or may not be manifested in the phenotype. When the organism has two different genes for a particular trait, the genotype for that trait is said to be *heterozygous;* when the two genes controlling a trait are the same, the genotype is termed *homozygous.* With a phenotype of blue eyes, the individual would be known to be homozygous; since the gene for blue eyes is recessive, it would take two of the same kind to produce such a phenotype.

Much of what is known about dominance and recessiveness has been worked out with plants, animals, and insects such as the fruit fly. For human beings, our information is much less complete. Some traits thought to be dominant in human beings include drooping eyelids, white forelock (known as "blaze"), baldness in men, certain forms of glaucoma and polydactylism (extra fingers or toes), and the Rh-positive blood factors. Conditions known to be caused by recessive genes include albinism (complete lack of pigment in the skin, hair, eyes, and nails), sickle cell anemia, the metabolic disorder called phenylketonuria (PKU) and the Rh-negative blood factor.

What Do We Inherit?

What do we inherit? When this question is asked, ordinarily the inquirer is interested in specific characteristics: Did Victoria get her grandmother's red hair? Did George inherit his father's bad temper and ability in math? Did Susan's migraine headaches come from Aunt Mary? Although some characteristics known to be inherited have already been described in this chapter, it must be confessed that we are far from having all the final answers.

Physical Features?

There is little doubt that many physical features are transmitted genetically. The color of one's eyes, hair, and skin, the structure and distribution of hair, facial contours, blood type, and some kinds of malocclusion of the teeth—these can be attributed to heredity. Yes, Victoria, red hair is inherited, but from both sides of the family. It is a recessive characteristic that could be manifested only if one had acquired the appropriate hereditary components from father and mother.

The list can be extended, but it is necessary to introduce a new factor that plays a part in determining the outcome of gene action. The factor is environment—the external circumstances in which a gene must operate. For example, the tendency to be tall or short or to be stocky and muscular or lean and lanky is known to be inherited. However, the socioeconomic circumstances of one's life, especially dietary and nutritional factors, also influence height, body type, and weight. Impoverished environments are associated with impoverished growth. Children of unemployed parents have a slower growth rate in general than children with one or both parents employed. Japanese who migrated to California before World War II had children who were taller than those who stayed in the home country. Young boys, ages 1 to 3, from very poor areas of the United States average 2.6 inches shorter than their age-mates in more affluent sections of the country (Schaefer and Johnson, 1969). Although there is probably a genetic limit to how tall the child of short parents might become, environmental factors contribute to determining whether the child will achieve this ultimate possibility.

Special Abilities?

A similar observation must be made with regard to special abilities such as those that characterize a William Shakespeare, a Wolfgang Mozart, or an Isaac Newton. In such

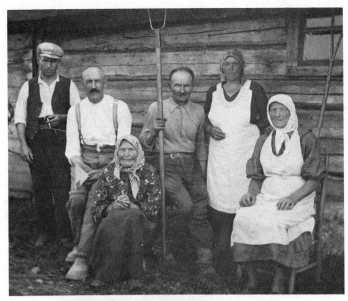

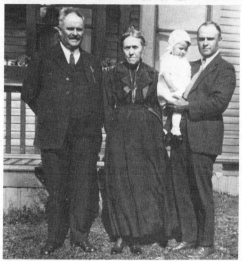

Family photographs have a fascination for all of us. We look into the faces of other generations and know that they are a part of us and that we are a part of the generations to come.

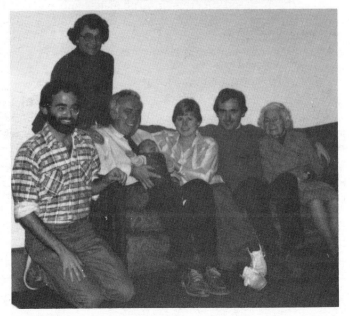

instances, some kind of extraordinary endowment must be assumed. Even with years of the best training and most devoted effort, probably very few of us could become an Olympic contender or a concert pianist. On the other hand, fulfillment of the hereditary potential is impossible without appropriate environmental opportunities. Can George inherit his father's ability in mathematics? The answer would be a qualified "yes": Genetic factors seem to be involved, but there also must be the environmental supports.

Intelligence?

A regularly occurring question concerns the influence of heredity upon intelligence. It has ignited a rather explosive controversy in recent years, sparked mainly by the hypothesis of Arthur R. Jensen (1969), which suggested that the average difference of 15 points between the IQ scores of blacks and whites (favoring the whites) is due to genetic differences rather than to environment. Jensen based much of his argument on analysis of resemblances between IQ test scores for twins, for siblings, and for parents and their offspring. To understand Jensen's contention, it is necessary to describe the rationale for this procedure.

Identical twins are developed when one zygote, in the course of dividing and subdividing, splits into two parts, with each part proceeding to form a separate individual. Because the chromosomes of the zygote are replicated with each division, the two individuals will be genetically identical. They will be of the same sex and will resemble each other closely. *Fraternal twins*, on the other hand, are formed when the mother chances to produce two ova that are fertilized by two different spermatozoa. Though sharing a prebirth environment, fraternal twins are no more alike than ordinary *siblings* (children born to the same parents) in terms of genetic endowment.

If intelligence is inherited, identical twins with their identical heredity should be very similar in intelligence. And, as a matter of fact, this is pretty much what has been found. Identical twins, when tested with standard intelligence tests, do resemble each other more than fraternal twins or ordinary siblings are likely to resemble each other.

It can be suggested, of course, that identical twins are usually dressed alike and perhaps are treated more alike than fraternal twins or ordinary brothers and sisters are. A study of identical twins who were separated at an early age and reared in different households helps in assessing this possibility. Cyril Burt (1966), a British psychologist, provided most of the information in this regard. He studied pairs of unrelated children who had been raised together in orphanages and pairs of identical twins who had been adopted soon after birth by different families. He found that the unrelated children reared together showed very slight resemblances in IQ scores, whereas identical twins reared apart were more similar, one to another, than fraternal twins and siblings reared together.

Jensen relied heavily on Burt's evidence in presenting his case for heredity as the major factor ("accounting for 80%") in intelligence (Jensen, 1973). Recently, serious questions have been raised regarding the validity of Burt's data. Because Burt has died and many of his records have been burned, the doubts cannot be laid to rest and must be considered a large flaw in the Jensen argument (Kamin, 1974). There is another caveat regarding the findings of the "separated twin studies": Adoptive homes ordinarily must meet certain standards, and the environmental surroundings of adopted children are not as drastically different as those typical of white children and black children in our society.

Still another formidable obstacle to obtaining clear and unequivocal answers to the relationship of intelligence to heredity is the difficulty of deciding precisely what is meant by "intelligence." Ordinarily, investigators (including Burt) have accepted the scores on standardized tests as measures of intelligence. However, the tests tend to rely heavily on the kinds of skills necessary for school success. Though school skills are important and

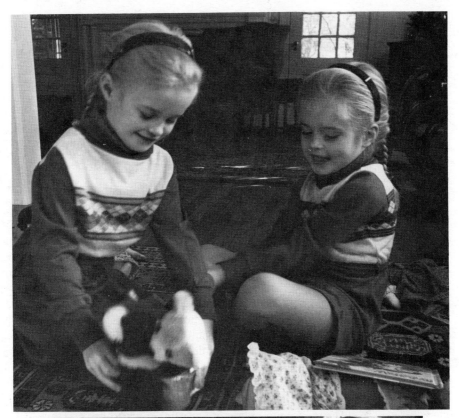

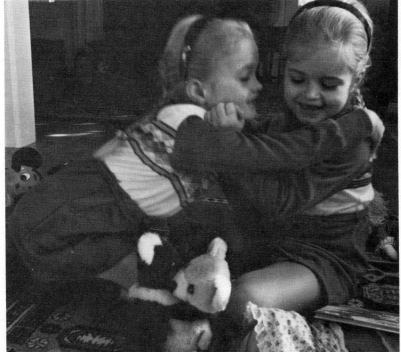

Judith Kruger Michalik

Identical twins will be of the same sex and will resemble each other closely. Identical twins who have been separated at birth and raised in different households are studied eagerly by researchers because such situations provide a way to distinguish between the effects of heredity and environment.

highly valued in our society, do such skills reliably indicate more intelligence than the sharpened senses and wit that can ensure survival in a ghetto?

These are not academic questions raised to quiet an empty controversy. Jensen's speculations about possible genetic differences between races (if, indeed, it is possible to define "race") have provided support for those who wish to reestablish racial segregation and those who begrudge the programs of compensatory education for ghetto children. The present answer to questions of heredity as a factor in intelligence is that there *is* no answer—that assertions in this regard are only speculation. One's capacity for coping with life circumstances is a product of the interaction of genetic and environmental circumstances, in proportions that are not known (Anatasi, 1958).

Temperament and Personality?

When we inquire about the inheritance of traits of temperament or personality, the answers are even more uncertain. Did George inherit his father's temper? One argument could certainly make the case for environment rather than heredity, noting the many times that George must have seen his admired father "blow his top." This would suggest that George learned to rage and shout at slight provocations, with father providing the model for such activity.

The case for genetics would have to show that George possessed a "hair-trigger" tendency to react while he was still an infant, before the environment had a chance to take effect. A study that followed 231 children from earliest infancy into adolescence described them in terms of "reactivity" by means of repeated observations and interviews with parents (Chess and Thomas, 1968; Chess et al., 1973). Included in the descriptions is "the difficult child" with slow adaptability and intense reactions and with behavior characterized by fussing, crying, temper tantrums and protests. Thus, it is possible to suggest that such a child is "born with" the kind of extra irritability that we tend to call "bad temper."

However, the possibility of the inheritance of behavior tendencies, temperament, and personality traits is still very unclear. With a simplistic description of gene action, one is led to think of each gene as having a singular task. In fact, however, most physical and behavioral characteristics are under the direction of *polygenes*—genes that work together with complex additive or complementary effect. This adds greatly to the difficulty of any attempt to separate the strands of heredity from those of the environment. Individual activity levels for newborn infants that seem to persist through at least the first few years of life have been demonstrated (Escalona and Heifer, 1959), but this does not provide conclusive evidence for the inheritability of behavior because, as we shall see, it disregards possible influences from the prenatal environment.

Illnesses?

Nor are we certain about the role of heredity in transmission of certain physical and mental illnesses. It is known that many afflictions seem to have a familial history— diabetes, tuberculosis, allergies, heart disease and high blood pressure, cancer, epilepsy, sinus trouble, and migraine headache, to mention a few. However, since the question of whether or not the condition will actually occur in a specific individual seems also to depend upon environmental circumstances, we speak of inherited tendencies.

One might suggest, then, that Susan and Aunt Mary owe their migraine headaches to a common inherited tendency. Similarly, there is some modest evidence for genetic transmission of *schizophrenia* (a blanket term for a complex of mental disorders characterized by such symptoms as thought disorders, hallucinations, and delusions).

Data on twins, assembled in 1953, indicate that if an identical twin is diagnosed as schizophrenic, the chances are 86 in 100 that the other twin will develop the same disorder. However, if one fraternal twin develops schizophrenia, the other twin runs a risk of only 14 chances in 100 of becoming so afflicted (Kallman, 1953). More recently, studies of *consanguinity* (relationship by blood) have tended to confirm belief in the possibility of an hereditary component for schizophrenia, showing that the risk rises in direct proportion to the closeness of the genetic relationship with an afflicted relative (Mittler, 1971).

Nevertheless, the conclusion that mental illness is inherited is still too hasty. Why do not all identical twins show concordance for schizophrenia? The answer may be along the lines suggested by Anatasi (1958) in a thoughtful essay that is now more than 20 years old but still has pertinence for today. She suggests that the question of how much is contributed by environment is a futile one; rather, one should be inquiring into how these two forces—heredity and environment—interact with one another to affect development. Perhaps what appears to be transmitted is not schizophrenia itself, but an entire series of dispositions, tendencies, and sensitivities. When an individual with such a combination of tendencies confronts environmental trauma and stress, the response might be in the form of schizophrenia.

The Importance of Heredity

Although the information about exactly "what" is inherited by an individual may seem less certain than might be desired, the importance of heredity to development cannot be doubted. The genetic transmission of sex, for example, determines the attitudes and expectations of parents toward the child from the very beginning. Boy or girl? The moment that important question is answered, a whole stream of forces is set in motion. One whole set of possibilities is invoked and another set discarded. Even the way one holds the baby is different if he is young "Butch" than if she is dainty "Rosemarie."

One's particular body structure and muscular coordination have a bearing on future development and behavior. The boy who is slight of build and light in weight may be a bitter disappointment to papa, who had dreamed of cheering for his son's football team. How many sad stories could be told of brothers or sisters who compared themselves unfavorably with each other because one seemed to be much better endowed? How many lesser Cyrano de Bergeracs have gone through life with a chip on the shoulder because of a prominent nose or protruding ears?

Again, it is appropriate to point out the interaction between heredity and environment. If the society into which the child is born places a premium on light skin, the inheritance of a dark skin will inevitably affect the kinds of transactions possible in that society and will have special effects on behavior.

We have noted the difficulty of disentangling the effects of heredity from those of the environment when the focus is upon specific individual characteristics. However, when the inquiry is directed toward humankind in general, the role of heredity is clear. Human heredity dictates the human exercise of the organismic capacities listed at the opening of this chapter. Humans inherit all of the morphological details that distinguish them as members of the genus *Homo*, species *Homo sapiens* ("thinking man"). Human beings inherit their remarkable cytoplasmic structure, which maintains its "steady state" by means of intricate internal mechanisms and biochemical balances, many of which are still unexplained. Much of the future of medicine will be written in terms of the biochemical processes taking place inside and outside human body cells.

Human heredity also determines growth and development that is orderly, sequential, and considerably slower than that of other organisms. This means that the human baby remains dependent for a very long time, making the human family necessary in one form or another in order to nurture the young and to make possible the learning of complex cultural patterns of behavior.

Like all other organisms, humans are sensitive to and responsive to the environment.

Lacking a natural endowment of heavy protective covering such as hide or fur, humans must shield themselves and their dependents from extremes of weather.

Because of their endowment, human beings walk upright, freeing the forelimbs for intricate manipulation. These limbs, however, do not make possible flight like that of birds, nor are they especially well suited for bare-handed combat. The human eye is somewhat less keen than that of the hawk, and the sense of smell is not well enough developed for tracking prey. The distance for human running and the speed with which it can be accomplished are unremarkable.

Indeed, it might seem that human beings are, by nature, poorly equipped for survival in a world of fang and claw and in bitter cold and jungle heat. And this would be so, were it not for the genetic gift of a brain structure and nervous system capable of marvelous operations. Human capacity for the use of symbolic processes, for example, offers the advantage of transmission of cumulative experience not possible for any other organism. Because of the human being's ability to learn and to invent, most of the limitations of physical endowment have been overcome. Human beings have not only adapted to their environment; in most instances, they have become masters of it.

Human heredity, then, has both set genetic limits and provided the possibility of triumphing over them. This is a most remarkable paradox that will be explored further as we proceed.

PRENATAL ENVIRONMENT

The discussion has emphasized the importance of heredity in establishing both limits and potentialities for each human being and has introduced the possibility of enormous variation among individuals, so that even children from the same family may differ a great deal among themselves and from their parents. Also noted was the importance of the environment, seen as interacting with heredity. The environment can provide opportunities for the expression of an hereditary trait, for example, encouraging the development of a Wolfgang Mozart. Or it can set up circumstances and barriers so insurmountable that even the best hereditary potential never has a chance.

Although the hereditary factors that one carries in every cell of the body are fixed at conception for all of one's life, the genes do not operate in a vacuum. Indeed, genes would be unable to manifest any effect at all without an interchange with the environment. Although *environment* is usually taken to denote the external world and all of its various direct or indirect impingements on the individual, there are two other influential but lesser known environments that will be discussed now. These are the intercellular environments, which provide the media for gene interaction, and the uterine environment, which is the abode of the developing baby.

Intercellular Environment

Recall that new life begins with the union of a spermatozoon and an ovum to form a zygote, which is a fertilized cell carrying 23 chromosomes from the spermatozoon that have matched up with 23 chromosomes in the ovum to make a full complement of 46 chromosomes for the human organism. An orderly process of division and redivision (mitosis) will begin, whereby chromosomes will be replicated. The zygote first becomes two identical cells; these become four and the four become eight. The process of developing the billions of cells that make up the human body is under way.

At first, each cell is precisely like the cell that divided to produce it. However, as you know from other studies, the human body is composed of many different kinds of cells. There are striated muscle cells, spindle-shaped cells of involuntary muscles, irregular cardiac muscle cells, and cells with elongated processes that make up nervous tissue, to describe but a few. Each of these is identifiably different from the others, and each has a wholly different function. How do different cells, with different forms and functions, develop from cells that are busily replicating so that each is exactly like another?

The dramatic answer, when it is finally unraveled, is likely to win its discoverer a Nobel prize. The bits and pieces of information so far uncovered promise that this still unsolved enigma is truly one of the most remarkable of the life processes.

As we have noted, the first cells of early embryological development are all alike. They are *undifferentiated*. However, at some specific period during development, according to some kind of built-in timetable and by some amazing process that is not at all understood, the parent cell gives birth to a particular kind of cell —a nerve cell or smooth muscle cell, for example. The cell has differentiated. Thereafter, the specialized cell will produce only its kind and no other.

Transplantation studies on a number of lower forms of life, such as salamanders and frogs, suggest that the intercellular environment (that is, where the cell is located on the embryo) plays a role in cell differentiation. Early in development, an undifferentiated cell can be readily transplanted from one spot to another on the embryo. For example, undifferentiated tissue from the area that will become the neural groove, forming the primitive nervous system, can be moved to another area where it will develop in a manner consistent with its new location. But it will be quite unlike what it was destined to become had it remained where it was. Thus, what was originally designed to be nervous system tissue may become skin tissue after a transplant. Apparently, what a cell is to become is influenced, to some extent, by the environment of cells surrounding it (Balinsky, 1975).

However, it is necessary to recognize the influence of heredity. The environment is not the sole determinant of the fate of undifferentiated tissue. If undifferentiated cells from the mouth region of an embryo of one species are transplanted to the embryonic mouth region of another species, the cellular environment will indeed promote formation of a mouth, but it will be a mouth characteristic of the original donor, not the host! (Balinsky, 1975). Cell differentiation and development seem to be influenced by both the intrinsic genetic properties and the cellular environment.

Critical Period

Still a third factor, in addition to heredity and environment, is crucial to the process of cell differentiation —the "timetable." Cell differentiation proceeds according to a kind of inherent schedule. First, one group of cells begins to multiply more rapidly and, thereupon, to specialize, forming the particular tissues and organs associated with the new kinds of cells; then another group of cells begins to undergo differentiation.

This orderly pattern of embryological development seems to be fixed, with a certain amount of time allotted for the emergence of each organ system. It is as if each specific type of tissue and the structures it is to form has its own "time for ascendancy" or "critical period." During its critical period, the organ system is both highly responsive to growth-stimulating influences and highly vulnerable to disruptive ones. If some unfavorable occurrence interferes at that time, it does not have a second chance; focus of growth passes to another system.

Cell differentiation is ordinarily completed by the end of the first trimester (three lunar months) of pregnancy. It is therefore possible to explain the differential effects of a deleterious agent in terms of when, during the pregnancy, it was introduced. For instance, German measles (rubella) contracted by the mother during the first trimester can result in brain damage, blindness, deafness, or cardiac deformities in the baby, depending upon the time of the infection. However, if the mother contracts German measles later in the pregnancy, after the organ systems have been established, the fetus is not likely to be harmed.

In related instances, thalidomide, taken during the early months to prevent morning sickness, produced stunted limbs, flattened noses, missing external ears, and malformations of the digestive and circulatory systems (Schardein, 1976; Taussig, 1962). Cleft palate seems to result from some interference with the "schedule" during the seventh to tenth weeks, the period during which the bones of the palate form and normally close. The eighth week brings development of the base of the skull, the wall of the heart, the nasal bones, and the fingers—all structures that are damaged in Down's syndrome (mongolism). Something, perhaps influenced by that strange extra chromosome, must occur at this time, blighting the structures and resulting in an afflicted child (Ingalls, 1957; Robinson and Robinson, 1965).

Even in embryological development, then, we can glimpse the interrelationships of the three factors that must be taken into account over and over again in attempting to understand human behavior—heredity, environment, and the timetable of development.

The timetable—the orderly pattern of development—is seen here as the essentially unyielding schedule for cell differentiation. We will see it continuing throughout fetal life as the organs and systems take shape and become functional. We will discuss it further as an enduring influence after the baby is born, operating as a kind of built-in schedule, influencing when the baby will sit, creep, and walk, setting the stage for many types of learning, regulating the onset of adolescence, and, perhaps, determining developmental changes during adulthood.

The timetable has been termed *maturation*. It was once considered to be relatively immune from any environmental effects. Mothers were urged to refrain from "pushing" babies into attempts at sitting or walking and were encouraged to think of the maturation process as a natural unfolding of appropriate skills, one by one. This "leave well enough alone" notion has been modified because of mounting evidence pointing to the necessity of environmental support for normal development. Children reared in impoverished circumstances fail to develop "normally" and are often mentally, physically, and socially behind schedule (Dennis, 1973; Hunt and Kirk, 1971).

Maturation was also viewed as important only during childhood and youth. Again, this seems to be too narrow an outlook. There is a gradual accumulation of evidence suggesting orderly changes and a continued sequential patterning of physical, mental, and emotional development throughout the adult years (Gould, 1975; Kimmel, 1974; Mass and Kuypers, 1974; Reese and Overton, 1970). Thus, in our discussion, we will regard maturation as the timetable that, within a certain range of variability and if favored by a benign environment, orders the developmental events of one period and influences the events characteristic of the next.

Intrauterine Environment

Now, having considered the beginning of human life and having noted the importance of the interaction of heredity, environment (intercellular), and the maturational timetable, it is necessary to take heed of still another environmental influence—that of the uterine surroundings wherein the tiny organism begins to live and grow.

Although it is customary to reckon an individual's age as beginning with birth, this method ignores some 10 lunar months of existence before that event. There is a tendency, too, to think of the prenatal environment as pretty much the same for all developing babies. But this neglects possible variations in intrauterine conditions that may subject one fetus to stresses quite different from those exerted upon another. We are becoming increasingly aware of threats to fetal development from maternal malnutrition, infectious diseases, drugs, radiation, psychological stress, and blood incompatibilities. Most of these will be discussed in detail in the next chapter. Here we will attempt to provide the conceptual framework within which the forthcoming details can be placed.

Malnutrition

Investigations of the effects of malnutrition are not as precise as one might wish because malnourished mothers are typically from an environment of poverty, suffering from other debilitating conditions, and often unable to obtain adequate medical care. Therefore, it is difficult to know if it is the malnutrition, some other factor, or a combination of conditions that is influencing the outcome. However, there is increasing documentation of the relationship between premature birth or "small for date" babies (unusually small for gestational age) and malnutrition (Gruenwald, 1970). The most frightening findings indicate the possibility of reduction in brain weight, abnormalities in brain wave activity, and abnormalities in the brain's cellular protein, RNA, and DNA composition resulting from nutritional deficiency during pregnancy (Chase et al., 1972).

Again, we are reminded of the "critical period" hypothesis: There is evidence that the consequences of malnutrition are most devastating when the brain of the developing organism is in its period of most rapid growth. This occurs during the period of pregnancy and for the first 2 years of postnatal life. By the end of the child's second year, the structure of the human brain is virtually complete (Dobbing, 1970). The implications of these findings are disheartening when we view the wide incidence of maternal and infant malnutrition in the form of chronic starvation and protein deficiency found around the world (Birch, 1971; Higgins et al., 1973).

Maternal Diseases

We have already seen that an infectious disease such as German measles (rubella) can be devastating during the critical period of the first trimester. A number of other diseases are also known to be potentially harmful. These include toxoplasmosis, hepatitis, cytomegalovirus (CMV), chickenpox, mumps, Asian influenza, poliomyelitis, and typhoid fever, all of which are associated with a high incidence of stillbirths, miscarriage, blindness, mental deficiency, deafness, microcephaly, and other deformities, especially when contracted during the early months of pregnancy (Prichard and MacDonald, 1976).

Wasting diseases such as tuberculosis, cancer, and malaria often seem to bring about kinds of disabilities similar to those linked with malnutrition. Diabetic mothers have more than their share of stillbirths, with defects of the circulatory and respiratory systems and early mortality of their offspring. Untreated syphilis can be transmitted to the developing fetus; a child born with congenital syphilis is likely to have impaired vision and hearing as well as deformities of bones and teeth. (Treatment with penicillin during the first half of pregnancy can prevent transmission of syphilis to the child.)

Drugs and Other Chemical Agents

A certain proportion of prenatal history can be written in terms of what the placental filter will permit to pass through to the fetal circulatory system and what it restrains. It is now known that many substances in the maternal blood stream, including a wide variety of the molecules of drugs and other chemicals, cross the placental "barrier" quite readily (Butler and Goldstein, 1973; Jones, 1973; Nora et al., 1967; Oulette et al., 1977; Sharma, 1972; Simpson and Linda, 1967).

The tragedy of the thalidomide babies showed that drugs that did not harm the mother could harm the baby. Study of another drug, diethylstilbestrol (DES), has shown that the damage caused by a substance given during pregnancy may not become evident until years later. DES was prescribed for a half million women between the 1950s and

1970s—before doctors recognized that it could cause vaginal cancer and other kinds of reproductive organ abnormalities in the daughters of women who took it.

Thousands of different types of drug products are introduced in the United States each year, and it is always possible that a particular drug may have effects on the fetus that are not known at present. Therefore, physicians now recognize that even well-known drugs should be taken during pregnancy only when absolutely necessary, and they recommend that pregnant women (or any woman who *may* be pregnant) take no medication, no matter how harmless it may seem, without consulting a doctor.

Maternal Age

A number of statistics attest to the fact that it is quite possible to become a mother at an age that is too young or too old. The mortality rate for infants is highest for mothers under the age of 15, next highest for mothers ages 15 to 19. It drops during ages 20 to 29, when it begins to increase again, rising dramatically after age 35. The maternal death rate is also considerably increased during these late years of reproductive life. This does not indicate that all babies born to mothers on either side of the decade of their twenties are foredoomed to developmental distress; however, when parents can choose, they might be wise to plan families for the most advantageous age period.

Maternal Emotion

There was a day when women were counseled to listen to beautiful music and think happy thoughts in order to provide a tranquil and favorable atmosphere for the developing baby. We now understand that there is no direct nervous system connection between mother and baby. It is also possible, therefore, to reassure mothers that a frightening experience is not likely to "mark" the baby.

However, several studies hint at a link between maternal emotional states and birth difficulties, as well as worrisome fetal and postnatal behavior. It is believed that the hormonal products of anxiety and emotional tension can cross the placenta and result in increased activity of the fetus, which carries over into irritability and hyperactivity of the neonates (Sontag, 1966).

Social Environment

It is clear that the course of development during the prenatal months can be affected by an enormous number of circumstances. Indeed, there is astonishing evidence that points, not to ongoing events in the uterus, but to events in the past—the "grandmother effect," whereby malnourished mothers gave birth to babies who, growing up in better economic conditions, were more fortunate in their own nutrition and especially the nutrition of their own pregnancies. Nevertheless, these daughters were more than twice as likely to have stillborn infants and premature deliveries as mothers without history of malnutrition for the previous generation. It may not be possible to wipe out effects of wretched prenatal conditions with just one generation of changed circumstances.

It is a fact that all the hazards cited prove to be more widespread and pervasive among the poor than among those more affluent. The United States ranks sixteenth among the world's nations with regard to infant mortality; that is, 16 nations do better than we do in saving their newborns. These are proportionate figures, and they have nothing to do with overall population. But the statistics do point to the discriminatory distribution of medical care. Poor women (most frequently, poor minority women) are two to three times as likely to have birth difficulties, premature babies, or babies who are otherwise in jeopardy at birth. Often the women have received little or no medical treatment prenatally, sometimes because the need for it is not recognized. The reduction of infant mortality and birth defects will depend, at least in part, upon improved availability of services to poor women and improved education of all pregnant women.

The preceding sections may have made pregnancy seem frought with danger. It is important to remind ourselves that the vast majority of pregnancies are uneventful and quite normal and that being informed can help to avoid the hazards.

Knowing about pregnancy and delivery and birth is especially important for psychological well-being during this period. The ordinary woman, looking forward to her labor and delivery, is likely to have at least a slight nagging recollection of horror stories about Aunt Mary's experiences. Because birth, in our culture, tends to be a carefully shielded event, a pregnant woman cannot call upon her own previous experiences as she might were she carrying a baby in a tribal village, where birth (and death) are public events with neighbors and relatives gathered around to lend support, give comfort, and join the celebration. In such a case, she would have been present at many births, observing, assisting and preparing for her turn. In contrast, our pregnant women have tended to be isolated, possibly sharing with a mate, but sometimes very much alone.

Like all of life's milestones, the event of pregnancy benefits vastly from human contact, caring, reassurance, and cheer. Pregnancy is not an illness, but a dramatic series of body transformations occupying the better part of a year. For the parents who eagerly await a child, it can be a year of incredible excitement, learning, and joy.

GLOSSARY

CONSANGUINITY   The property of being related by blood; kinship.

DIFFERENTIATED CELLS   Cells that have become specialized.

DOMINANCE   The power of a gene to exert its full phenotypic effect even if paired with another different gene.

DYNAMIC EQUILIBRIUM   An equilibrium that is constantly in the process of change.

ENVIRONMENT   The external influences, direct and indirect, that affect an individual.

FRATERNAL TWINS   Twins developed from different zygotes, therefore genetically no more or less alike than siblings.

GAMETES   Germ cells, either male or female.

GENOTYPE   The actual genetic endowment carried by the genes that may or possibly may not be manifested in the phenotype.

HETEROZYGOUS   A situation in which the organism carries differing genes for a particular trait.

HOMEOSTASIS   The tendency to maintain a "steady state" within the cell or body with respect to food, fluid, air, sleep, heat, and cold.

HOMO SAPIENS   Literally, thinking man.

HOMOZYGOUS   A situation in which the two genes controlling a trait are the same.

IDENTICAL TWINS   Twins developed from the same zygote, therefore genetically identical.

IRRITABILITY   The capacity of the organism to sense the environment and react to that sensing.

MATURATION   The process of developmental change, which is extensively controlled by genetic factors.

MEIOSIS Reduction-division. A special process of germ cell division at maturity, with each resulting cell carrying 23 single members of what were once chromosome pairs.

METABOLISM The life processes that involve ingestion and utilization of nutrients to make energy, with subsequent excretion of waste products.

MITOSIS Ordinary cell division with resulting cells that are exact reproductions of the one that divided to produce them.

ORGANISM A living creature.

PHENOTYPE The appearance of a genetic trait in the form of an observable characteristic.

POLYGENES Genes that work together with complex additive or complementary effect.

RECESSIVENESS An attribute describing a gene that, when paired with a dominant gene, is not effective in the phenotype. In order to exert its effect, it must be paired with another like itself. Two recessive genes can be manifested in the phenotype.

REDUCTION-DIVISION See **Meiosis.**

SCHIZOPHRENIA A complex mental disorder characterized by thought disturbances, hallucinations, and delusions.

SEX LINKED Traits that follow the distribution of the X chromosome in both sexes, finding expression in the male but expressed in the female only if both X chromosomes carry the trait.

SIBLINGS Children born to the same parents, thus sharing the same gene pool.

UNDIFFERENTIATED CELLS The first cells of early embryological development that are all alike.

ZYGOTE The new cell, formed by union of ovum and spermatozoon.

REFERENCES

Anatasi, A.: Heredity, environment and the question of "How?". *Psychological Review*, 65:197–208, 1958.

Balinsky, B.: *An Introduction to Embryology.* 4th ed. Philadelphia: W. B. Saunders Company, 1975.

Birch, H. G.: Functional effects of fetal malnutrition. *Hospital Practice*, March 1971, pp. 134–148.

Burt, C.: The genetic determination of differences in intelligence: A study of monozygotic twins reared together and apart. *British Journal of Psychology*, 57:137–153, 1966.

Butler, N. R., Goldstein, H.: Smoking in pregnancy and subsequential child development. *British Medical Journal*, 4:573–575, 1973.

Chase, S., Welch, N., Dabiere, C., Vasan, N., Butterfield, J.: Alterations in human brain biochemistry following intrauterine growth retardation. Pediatrics, 50:403–464, 1972.

Chess, S., Thomas, A., Birch, H. G.: Behavior problems revisited: Findings of an anterospective study. In Chess S., Thomas, A. (eds.): *Annual Progress in Child Psychiatry and Child Development.* New York: Appleton-Century-Crofts, 1973.

Dennis, W.: *Children of the Creche.* New York: Appleton-Century-Crofts, 1973.

Dobbing, J.: Undernutrition and the developing brain. In Himwich, W. (ed.): *Developmental Neurobiology.* Springfield, Ill.: Charles C Thomas, 1970.

Escalona, S., Heifer, G. M.: *Prediction and Outcome.* New York: Basic Books, 1959.

Gould, R.: Adult life stages: Growth toward self-tolerance. *Psychology Today*, 8(9):74–81, 1975.

Gruenwald, P.: Fetal malnutrition. In Waisman, H. A., Kerr, R. (eds.): *Fetal Growth and Development.* New York: McGraw-Hill, 1970.

Higgins, A. C., Crampton, E. W., Moxley, J. E.: A preliminary report of a nutrition study of public maternity patients. *Montreal Diet Dispensary*, 1973.

Hunt, J. M., Kirk, G. E.: Social aspects of intelligence, evidence and issues. In Cancro, R. (ed.): *Intelligence, Genetic and Environmental Influences.* New York: Grune and Stratton, 1971.

Ingalls, T. H.: Congenital deformities. *Scientific American*, 197:109–116, 1957.

Jensen, A. R.: How much can we boost I.Q. and

Scholastic Achievement? *Harvard Educational Review*, 39:1–123, 1969.

Jensen, A. R.: *Genetics and Education*. New York: Harper and Row, 1973.

Jones, K. L.: The deformed children of alcoholic mothers. *Science News* 104(1):6, 1973.

Kallman, F. J.: *Heredity in Health and Mental Disorder*. New York: W. W. Norton & Company, 1953.

Kamin, L.: *The Science and Politics of I.Q.* Hillsdale, N. J.: Eribaum, 1974.

Kimmel, D. C.: *Adulthood and Aging*. New York: John Wiley & Sons, 1974.

Mass, A. S., Kuypers, J. A.: *From Thirty to Seventy*. San Francisco: Jossey-Bass, 1974.

Mittler, P.: *The Study of Twins*. Baltimore: Penguin, 1971.

Nora, J. J., Nora, A. H., Sommerville, R. J., Hill, R. M., McNamara, D. G.: Maternal exposure to potential teratogens. *Journal of the American Medical Association*, 202:1065–1069, 1967.

Oulette, E. M., Rosett, H. L., Rosman, N. P., Weiner, L.: Adverse effects on offspring of maternal alcohol abuse during pregnancy. *New England Journal of Medicine*, 528–530, Sept. 8, 1977.

Pritchard, J., and MacDonald, P. C.: *Williams Obstetrics*, 15th ed. New York: Appleton-Century-Crofts, 1976.

Reese, H. W., Overton, W. F.: Models of development and theories of development. In Goulet, L. R., Baltes, P. B. (eds.): *Life Span Developmental Psychology: Research and Theory*. New York: Academic Press, 1970.

Robinson, H. B., Robinson, N. M.: *The Mentally Retarded Child: A Psychological Approach*. New York, McGraw-Hill, 1965.

Rugh, R., Shettles, L. R., Einhorn, R. N.: *From Conception to Birth: The Drama of Life's Beginnings*. New York: Harper & Row, 1971.

Schaefer, A. C., Johnson, O. C.: Are we well fed? *Nutrition Today* 4:2–11, 1969.

Schardein, J.: *Drugs As Teratogens*. Cleveland: C. P. C. Press, 1976.

Sharma, T.: Marijuana: Recent research and findings, 1972. *Texas Medicine*, 68(10):109–110, 1972.

Simpson, W. J., Linda, L. A.: A preliminary report on cigarette smoking and the incidence of prematurity. *American Journal of Obstetrics and Gynecology*, 73:808–815, 1957.

Sinnot, E. W., Dunn, L. C., Dobzhansky, T: *Principles of Genetics*. New York: McGraw-Hill, 1958.

Sontag, L. W.: Implications of fetal behavior and environment for adult personality. *Annals of the New York Academy of Science*, 134:782–786, 1966.

Taussig, H. B.: The thalidomide syndrome. *Scientific American*, 962:29–35, 1962.

THE INFANT:
Basic Trust

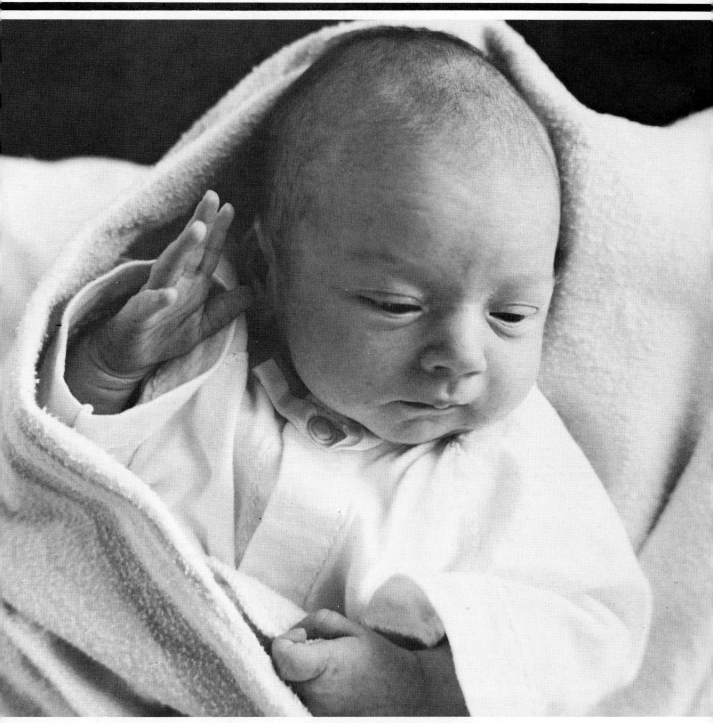

CHAPTER 3

THE FIRST MEETING

The newly born baby is placed in the mother's waiting arms. Tentatively, she touches the infant's hand with her finger tips, first with one hand and then the other. She touches her baby's toes, then holds a foot, massaging its instep with her thumb. Within a few minutes, she begins to stroke the legs, arms, and trunk with her whole hand, all the while keeping up a running "conversation" with the newcomer and maintaining eye contact for a period of time that would be wholly uncomfortable under ordinary conversational circumstances with someone who is older.

Try it! Initiate a dialogue with a partner and notice that, as the speaker, you establish eye contact for only a few seconds before looking away. Try maintaining the eye contact during the entire time of speaking and discover how uncomfortable it is. Meanwhile, the listener typically keeps eyes fixed upon the speaker's face each time the speaker returns for the few seconds' gaze. When it is the listener's turn to speak, the behavior patterns are reversed; now the listener establishes contact, averts gaze, and reestablishes it in a regular pattern.

However, it is apparent that eye-to-eye contact over a long period of time is very important to the new mother. Because touching with the finger tips, followed by whole-hand stroking, cooing sounds, and looking into baby's eyes, seems to be so universal, the suggestion has been made that this particular behavior may release maternal caretaking responses (Klaus, 1973). It has also been noted that the unsedated neonate remains in a wide-eyed awake and alert state for almost an hour after birth, able to follow movement with the eyes, and seemingly exceptionally attentive to the sights, sounds, and other sensory impressions of the world.

HOW INFANTS ARE STUDIED

Less than 25 years ago, it would have been impossible to say much about infants except to assert that they exist in a "booming, buzzing confusion," as first described by William James. He was convinced that neonatal vision consisted of light and darker shadows and that the other sensory impressions were equally deficient. For the next half-century, there was very little evidence to contradict these impressions. The reflexes of the baby could be elicited, and the developmental landmarks—such as smiling, eruption of the first tooth, and the abilities to roll over and sit alone—were mapped. But, though it was possible to induce an infant to track a slowly moving object with the eyes, there didn't seem to be any way to ascertain whether the infant actually saw the object or whether it was just a blur moving across a lighted background.

The first real breakthrough came in 1957, when R. L. Fantz invented a way to "ask an infant a question" about what the baby sees. If, reasoned Fantz, an infant is presented with visual stimuli and consistently prefers to look at one stimulus more than the other, could it not be suggested that the infant truly does distinguish the details?

Fantz designed an umbrellalike canopy, which was placed across the infant's crib. It had a "peek-hole" in the top so that an investigator could look down and time what was being mirrored in the infant's eyes—that is, what the eyes were fixated upon. The visual stimuli were large cards with various kinds of designs, including a bull's eye, horizontal stripes, and a checkerboard pattern. Each of these was presented in random position, paired with a standard unpatterned gray field. Babies ranged in age from 1 week to 15 weeks old. All preferred the patterns to the plain stimulus. But were they perhaps simply responding to the "shadows"?

Fantz accomplished another study with babies ranging from 4 days to 6 months old. This time he paired two stimuli—a stylized face and a face with scrambled features—with ovals that had solid patches of black equal to the area covered by the features (to control for shadow contrasted with brightness). All possible pairs were presented to each infant. At all age levels, infants looked longest at and "preferred" the facelike and scrambled face stimuli to the black patches; these results suggested that even very young babies are sensitive to and can differentiate between visual perceptions. Even more importantly, it became possible to obtain information about infants that had heretofore been considered impossible (Fantz, 1961).

Almost immediately, other means of "asking babies what they perceive" were discovered. It was found that infants changed their rate of sucking; they made instrumental responses (such as kicking in order to help keep a mobile turning); their skin conductance changed; and their total body movement, respiration, and heart rate changed: All these signs can be used as indicators of perception.

Can the infant tell the difference between a regular "suckable" nipple and an ordinary piece of rubber tubing? The answer is found in an investigation conducted by Lipsitt and Kaye at Brown University. Babies were presented with nipple or tube in random alteration, and the strength of the sucking was measured by counting the number of sucking responses per unit of time. The results showed that the baby clearly preferred the nipple, even though no substance was being supplied by either object. When slightly sweetened milk was offered through the tube, the sucking response increased markedly, decreasing again when the milk was no longer offered (Lipsitt and Kaye, 1965). It seems clear that the very young baby can discern and make appropriate responses to several different environmental conditions with evidence of considerable competence!

A sensitive and useful measure of what the baby can perceive is termed *habituation*. The phenomenon can be described as the instance when an infant seems to become bored with and no longer attends to a stimulus. For example, if a visual stimulus such as a checkerboard card is presented, taken away, and presented again in a regular series, the infant tends to look at each presentation for a time. But after a while, the infant no longer attends. The baby gets used to it and attention shifts. The baby becomes *habituated* to a stimulus that is presented repeatedly. However, if the stimulus is changed (the checkerboard is exchanged for a bull's eye), the baby becomes attentive again. The descriptive term for this phenomenon is *dishabituation*—a renewed interest in a changed stimulus after habituation to an original one.

Notice the exciting implications of this phenomenon. Now it becomes possible to ask an infant several "questions." How long does it take before boredom sets in? What kinds of stimuli hold attention the longest? How small a difference can be noticed? After the stimulus has caused habituation, will the baby attend again to one that is only slightly changed, such as in the difference between the sound *buh* and *puh*? (The answer to that last question is yes.)

Even more importantly, the ability to habituate and dishabituate indicates cortical processing of information and memory storage. If the baby doesn't show interest in a stimulus on the 12th trial, we can assume that what was perceived earlier is remembered, especially when there is revived interest if the stimulus is changed. It means that the new stimulus has been compared with an existing perception of the old and has been found different and therefore interesting (Sameroff, 1975).

How can the investigator accurately assess when the infant has become habituated? When this phenomenon was first investigated, observers simply watched for behavioral signs of disinterest. Baby looked away from the stimulus, became restless, or began to cry. A little later, however, it became possible to measure the psychophysical signs with suitable equipment. Galvanic skin reflex, respiration, brain-wave activity, and, most recently, cardiac rate were found to provide sensitive indicators of attention. The process of attending has come to be called the *orienting response*.

The orienting response was first described by the Russian physiologist, Ivan Pavlov. This phenomenon was studied in Russian laboratories for some time before American investigators understood what a fine tool it might become for infant study. During the past decade, habituation, dishabituation, and an associated response, *offset*, have been used to provide a virtual explosion of information about infants. (*Offset* is the response that occurs after a regular series of stimuli has become habituated so that the infant no longer attends. If the stimuli series is halted, the infants may respond as if they had missed the expected occurrence of a stimulus, even though they are no longer attending.)

These responses have been used to make a number of determinations, for example:

1. How long the baby remains affected by maternal medication during childbirth.

2. What kinds of differences the young baby is capable of discriminating in regard to auditory or visual stimuli.

3. Whether premature babies of various postnatal ages show evidence of being able to habituate.

4. The effects of malnutrition on cortical activity.

5. The attempt to map the developmental course of central nervous system maturation.

6. The possibility of central nervous system dysfunction.

COGNITIVE DEVELOPMENT

In large measure, because of the burgeoning investigations of the past two decades, the time of infancy is no longer dismissed as relatively unimportant in terms of psychological development. It has, of course, always been possible to observe and assess a baby's physical growth and rapidly changing motor capabilities. But the response repertoire of the infant seemed so limited, at least for the first few months, that it was difficult to recognize any kind of major cognitive or intellectual development taking place. However, the new methods of investigating infant capacities have produced such remarkable findings that we are forced to regard the newborn baby as an extraordinarily competent being with proficiencies that exceed any prior assumptions.

For example, T. G. R. Bower, in a series of fascinating studies (1976), has demonstrated that infants during the first week of life not only defend themselves from an approaching object by pulling the head back and raising hands and arms in front of the face, but can also distinguish between an object on a hit-path that appears to be coming directly toward the face and one on a miss-path that will move harmlessly past the head. These looming objects were actually visual images presented on a screen so that there was no air rush associated with passing that might have caused the defensive movement.

In a ramification of this procedure, Bower and a colleague rigged a rotating, shadow-casting device that presented the infant with a series of shape changes and culminated with a forward rotation, which appeared about to strike the baby on the nose. Babies less than 2 weeks old moved their heads as far away as they could when the forward rotating edge approached. Bower's discussion of this defense behavior acknowledges that it is probably inappropriate to describe the infant as "knowing" that the approaching object was harmful.

However, there is another mind-boggling demonstration of infant perception. Dunkeld observed that a baby less than a week old will imitate an adult in sticking out the tongue, fluttering eyelashes, and opening and closing the mouth (Dunkeld, cited in Bower, 1977). It is necessary, somehow, to account for these infants "knowing" they have a tongue, eyelashes, and mouth and that these correspond to what they are seeing, to say nothing of the social interaction that the game entails.

One of the most important contributors to ideas on the cognitive development of infants was Jean Piaget (1952), a Swiss psychologist who died in 1980. According to Piaget, cognitive development proceeds in stages that are sequential and continuous. Each stage builds upon those that have preceded it. Therefore, no stage can be skipped, and the accomplishments of later stages depend, in some measure, upon what has gone before.

For Piaget, intelligence consists in coping with the environment. His was the global

This baby, less than two hours old, responds to her mother's game of sticking out her tongue.

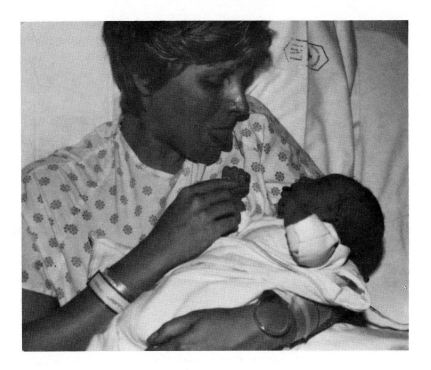

view of the biologist, also borrowing from his lifelong interest in the philosophy of knowledge. In his universe, then, it is possible to consider the "intelligent" functioning of an ameba swimming away from a drop of acid placed in its tank, as well as the intelligent functioning of the scientist applying logic and mathematics to obtain a hypothetical picture of the whole.

Furthermore, the sequence of the development of intelligence is the same for all organisms. The term used by Piaget is *invariant*, meaning "the same"; however, only a human being progresses all the way to the highest level, which includes ability to use abstractions, to think about hypothetical situations in a logical way, and to organize rules and operations into complex systems.

In Piaget's view, the development of intelligence results from the biological nature of the organism (what it is—groundhog, eagle, or human—in addition to its specific attributes) and therefore determines in considerable part the possible interactions with the environment. If the biological nature is somewhat flexible, the organism can interact in more numerous ways with the environment and become more varied or different within the species. Thus, the possibilities for differing kinds of interactions are extremely limited for an ameba, and one ameba is much like another. However, as any dog lover will attest, dogs have "personalities" and can truly be said to be different from one another, even within a particular breed.

Piaget was not as interested in the variations in cognitive functioning among us as in suggesting the general processes that hold for all of us. All of us, he stated, begin our interactions with the environment by means of reflexive, built-in responses. Many creatures do not progress further than this very beginning of the period that he described as the first step for intelligence—the *sensory-motor period*. The interactions, in the beginning and thereafter, always take one of two forms—assimilation or accommodation.

Assimilation is the taking in, processing of, and incorporation of information obtained by way of the senses. An analogy is the taking in, processing of, and dispersal of food elements. Similar to the way in which nutritive molecules are transformed into energy and tissue, environmental information flows into the basic cognitive unit called a *schema* (plural: *schemata*), a complex mental structure incorporating actions and ideas that are associated.

For example, one of the infant's first interactions with the environment is likely to be feeding, by means of either bottle or breast. The nipple in the mouth will elicit the reflexive behavior of sucking and swallowing. During repeated feedings, baby will be taking in many associated aspects of the feeding situation—odor, the feeling of the caretaker's arms, the sound of the voice, being rocked, and the internal sensation of warmth and comfort. All of these elements will form the schema, including the baby's own responses of kicking and waving of arms in anticipation of being fed when the now familiar elements are present.

Assimilation, then, accounts for the construction of most schemata. A schema should be thought of as a composite; especially, it must be considered to include the organism's active coping with, managing, and controlling the environment. Piaget has said that "thought is internalized action," and the sensory-motor period includes the motor aspects as coequal with the sensory. If schemata were involved only with assimilation, however, it would be difficult, if not impossible, to deal with a changing environment and even a changing (maturing, for example) organism. Therefore, a second process, *accommodation*, is present.

Accommodation describes the ability to adjust an existing schema to fit a changed circumstance. For example, an infant with a schema for creeping toward sofas and chairs and using them to achieve a standing position may try the same behavior using a hot radiator. Now the schema must be changed, *accommodated*, to take into account the reality of hot radiators as unsuitable for pulling oneself to a standing position.

The twin processes, assimilation and accommodation, are conceived of as functioning together to bring about a kind of cognitive balance (termed *equilibrium*) that enables us to form a mental picture of the world that fits our perceptions and capabilities of the moment, but that promotes growth, extension, and change as the balance is threatened by new information, new capabilities, and different environments. Early in life, the food-getting schema is limited to mother and breast. Later, as baby grows and develops teeth and eye-hand motor coordination, the schema—expanded by the twin processes of assimilation and accommodation—will include spooning food from a dish on the highchair tray, and much later perhaps buying a fancy restaurant meal for a best girl friend.

During infancy, the sensory-motor period progresses through a series of stages that come about because the baby's maturing systems promote increasingly complex relations with the world; these, in turn, encourage new perceptions and modes of reaction. One of the dramatic developments is the comprehension of *object permanence*. This is the gradually dawning realization that objects have a stable identity—that things stay the same, even if they are out of sight.

Such a notion typically strikes students as so elementary as to be hardly worth mentioning. However, imagine for the minute how it would be if you didn't know that your car will remain where you park it, that the contents of your dresser will not disappear when the drawers are closed, or that the man going around the corner will continue on his way, though out of sight. Without the concept of object permanence, there would be no possibility of predicting or expecting; life would be chaotic.

We are not sure how the realization comes about. It is possible to observe its appearance when baby looks for a toy that was laid down a few moments before or watches the doorway expectantly for mother to appear. The fascination that peek-a-boo has for the 7- and 8-month-old child is probably an early "testing" of the concept. Also, there is the impish delight with which toys are hurled over the side of highchair and crib as fast as and as long as some kind soul can be persuaded to retrieve them.

Underlined by Piaget's work is the recent recognition of the importance of infancy for later development. We have paid heed to the importance of childhood for personality and emotional development ever since the works of Sigmund Freud, but infancy was not seen as an especially significant time period for enhancing cognition. Indications are beginning to accumulate that the path that leads to competence in classrooms and in school work and the path that leads to later school-related learning difficulties diverge and separate at about age 10 months. One source of this proposition is the Harvard Preschool Project (White, 1975). The group associated with this project noted that differences could be perceived before the age of 6 years between the child who would have success in school and the child who would likely fall behind in school tasks. The decision was made to attempt to track the development of such a difference back through early childhood to see how it originates. First, however, it was necessary to define the nature of the difference between the "competent" 6-year-old and the one who was much less competent.

After extensive observations of young children in preschool, kindergarten, and first grade, it seemed apparent that a competent child ranks high in several kinds of abilities:

1. Knows how to ask for help from an adult.

2. Has a good measure of independence, that is, engages in planning and carrying out of projects, seeking help only when necessary.

3. Is able to anticipate consequences of behavior.

4. Possesses superior language ability.

5. Is a zestful, self-confident problem solver.

Furthermore, these differences between competent and less competent children were observable. The child who did not rank high on these abilities was much more dependent (either retiring or disruptive) and often given to impulsive behavior with unplanned-for consequences. The child tended to use language minimally and functionally ("gimme dat," "git out") and with almost no ability to pretend or use the imagination.

The surprise came when it was discovered that the differences among 3-year-olds were as vivid as those among 6-year-olds. It then became necessary to look into the earlier life of children. The investigators went into homes with tape recorders to watch every aspect of a child's infancy and toddlerhood with questions about toys, the kinds of interaction taking place and with whom, the language being used by the caretakers, and the details of the child's daily life.

Results showed that children seem to be very much alike until about the age of 10 months or the time at which they begin to move about actively—creeping, pulling themselves up on furniture, and walking with its aid. At this stage, the arrangements and routines of child care (which tend to be similar up to this point) become quite different. It probably has much to do with the mother's view of the change from a passive to an active child. If this stage is seen as a nuisance for the mother, then confinement will be the rule—playpen, plastic chair, or crib. If it is seen as a time of great danger, restraint will also be the rule, probably with considerable hovering and intervention from mother. If this period is seen as a time of enhanced and interesting capabilities, however, the child's curiosity will be encouraged, the household will be "arranged for wandering baby," as Dr. Spock (1976) put it in an early version of his famous book, and exploration will be both induced and relished. The last practice seemed to be characteristic of households that produced competent children.

In these households, language usage was extensively directed at the child. The most interesting difference, however, was that the mothers of competent children did not spend a great deal of time with the child or engage in a lot of deliberate teaching. Rather, they seemed to interact with the child in extremely effective "small takes," often for not more than 20 seconds, but in such a manner that the child looked upon adults as resource people who could supply help and information as necessary (White and Watts, 1973).

Awareness of the importance of infancy in laying down the basic building blocks of intelligence has some wide implications for our society. The latest statistics indicate that in the 1980's almost 45 per cent of the nation's children will live a portion of their lives in a one-parent family. Some of those children will undoubtedly be of preschool age, and most single parents will have to work. It seems important that the society begin to look to the quality of care that will be offered for those children, whether it is at grandma's, at a day-care center, or in the home of a friendly neighbor. Tired, worried mothers are not likely to provide a steady, enriching background, nor is a tired, worried day-care worker, who is paid less than grocery store clerks. The friendly neighbor may be plopped in front of the television set with the baby on the sofa beside her, safe from harm, but hardly engaged in exciting infant adventures. For all parents, it is vital to get the message out: The time of infancy is important! It will never come again. Do not be misled by what seem to be the infant's limitations. We now know that children begin to learn from the very first day and, it seems apparent, the more they learn, the more they want to learn.

BASIC TRUST

It is important for the reader to understand that though we are going to be talking about cognitive development and emotional development, as if these were two separate and distinct entities, it is only an artifice of language that permits us to do so. Keeping in mind, then, the fact that the infant actually develops "all of one piece," we will turn the focus to emotional development.

Although the proposition that our most enduring emotional attributes have their beginning in childhood is almost taken for granted these days, it is good to remind ourselves that the idea is not so very old. The author of that notion, Sigmund Freud, died just as World War II was getting under way, and he himself was a refugee from the Nazis. As of 1982, his daughter Anna was still practicing psychiatry in England. The fact that we are so comfortable with the idea that loves and hates of childhood extend their influence into the later years attests to the power of Freud's theory.

However, Freudian theory has some serious limitations for today's thinking, including the fact that it did not extend the notion of development beyond adolescence. Most contemporary psychologists feel that this is too narrow a view, failing to credit the impressive capacity of human beings to learn not only from successes and mistakes in dealing with the environment, but also from the sorrows and joys of changing interpersonal relationships during the course of a lifetime.

Erik Erikson (1963) has provided a model for considering emotional development. This model borrows extensively from Freud, but also attends to the newer insights regarding the different circumstances of learning as well as what is learned. The process he describes is not as inexorable as Freud's, and in Erikson's view, the adult years are recognized as being as important for character formation as the period of childhood and youth.

Erikson's "ages and stages" theory suggests that the central core of one's emotional character (including attitudes toward the world and others, self and sex, work, mate, offspring, and, finally, death) is evolved gradually through the qualities of interaction with the significant people in the environment. To this interaction, each individual brings a unique set of potentialities for relating. One infant is *not* exactly like another. Some babies like being held close and caressed; some seem to be, from the beginning, "non-cuddlers" (Schaffer and Emerson, 1965).

Erikson sees the conditions of each "age" (the helplessness of the tiny baby, the burgeoning capability of the 2-year-old, the increased awareness of the 4-year-old, and so on, through all the stages of life) and the particular circumstances of the people and events in the surroundings combining to produce an especially profound personality characteristic. This, in turn, will tend to direct and color future transactions. Each stage, so to speak, is constructed upon those that have been previously passed. If one stage has been faulty, the rest build on a shaky foundation. But Erikson is quick to insist that all is not lost, that later circumstances can "shore up" and strengthen the wobbly base; it is only that it is more difficult to accomplish after the stage has gone by.

Though we are going to be describing Erikson's *"eight psychological ages of man"* (beginning with the age of infancy) as if these belonged to discrete age periods, it should be pointed out that these must not be regarded as beginning at one specific age and ending at another. Rather, the ages are approximate, varying from one individual to another. Also, it should not be thought that successful passage through one stage means that the battle is won once and for all. The hazards of life require continual confrontation, and each crisis will pose a challenge that may be surmounted or, possibly, may necessitate a retreat. However, according to Erikson, if the particular psychological attribute was secured during its "proper" period, recovery may be attained more easily during a period of serious threat.

Erikson envisioned a kind of ground plan for the human life cycle, whereby the life of the individual can be divided into fairly distinct periods, each one critical, both in the particular contribution to basic personality and in furnishing the underpinning of further development. For infancy, the developmental task is that of acquiring the primary orientation toward the world and its people, which he terms *basic trust*. This first and most lasting outlook seems to be engendered by the quality of caring that the infant receives at the hands of the caretakers.

In the beginning, the internal sensations regularly signal hunger, with feelings that must be painful and that the baby registers by crying. Happily for most babies, mothers usually respond promptly, doing what they can to alleviate the distress. When this happens over and over again, the baby can begin to associate mother with relief, with comforting, and with the pleasurable sensations of being picked up, rocked, fed, and caressed. Little by little, babies learn that when they are cold or wet or hungry, there will be someone to care and redress their misfortune. The baby can begin to develop a kind of faith or trust that these needs will be satisfied. At about 4 months, babies are likely to stop this "hungry crying" when someone approaches, anticipating or trusting that they will be fed.

Basic trust, Erikson suggests, describes the baby's gradually growing sense of the world as a dependable place and of the people in it as well intentioned. The ability to trust seems to serve as the cornerstone of a healthy personality. In simple words, it means that the baby comes to feel, as a deeply ingrained, "pre-language" attribute of being, that the world is a pretty nice place, and that people tend to be helpful.

Whatever the problem, when the cry of distress is answered promptly, the infant develops a basic trust in the world.

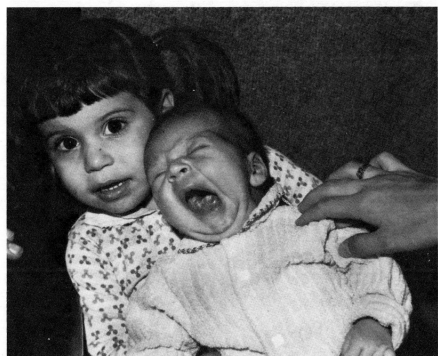

Contrast, for a moment, this trusting baby with one who is not as fortunate, who is rarely picked up, whose distress signals bring delayed and grudging attention, and who is treated harshly or with rejection. It can be suggested that this infant's first impressions of the world will be filled with apprehension—a pervading sense that life is difficult and painful and that people are no help at all.

Such a child is thought to develop a diffuse anxiety and insecurity—a mistrust of a cruel world. These children may become preoccupied with their own needs because of the constant uncertainty that these needs will be fulfilled. Having been given so little opportunity for responding positively to others, their relationships are likely to be demanding, hostile, or simply cold and withdrawn.

When we consider these first generalized impressions that the infant receives of the world and the people in it, it is possible to understand why a sense of basic trust (or

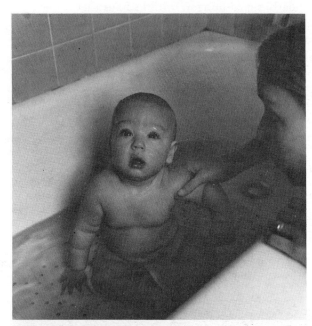

The well-loved baby's outlook tends to be one of cheerful confidence. Who can resist a happy child who reaches out to us? When the world responds, the infant's perceptions are strengthened and she learns to reach out again.

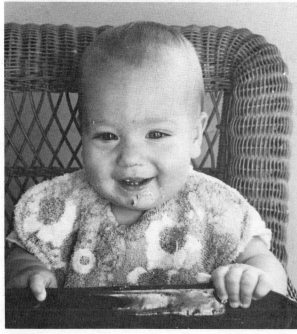

Judith Kruger Michalik

failure to develop it) has such a far-reaching effect. A well-loved baby's approach to others tends to be one of cheerful confidence. A view of the world as a happy place colors a child's attitudes toward all future events. Who can resist a joyful, chortling cherub? Even the most dour among us beams and responds in kind, thereby reinforcing the infant's perceptions. On the other hand, a child who expects little but pain and neglect in the world tends to approach others sullenly, convinced of their malevolent intentions. And people tend to turn away from such an unpleasant child, unwittingly perpetuating this view of the world.

The earliest experiences in the heart of the family, then, become prototypes for future relationships with others. From the significant adults in their lives, infants acquire expectations that are extended to people in general. The happy or painful circumstances of infancy cast long shadows over the life to come.

Basic trust, then, is intended to convey the flavor of these early satisfying experiences with the world, together with a growing sense of confidence in the infant's own powers. Gradually, the body responds with some precision to its bidding. The child can finally pick up bits of food from the highchair tray with a deft pincers movement of finger and thumb; this begins to extend the circle of confidence. The unsubdued frolicking of older brothers and sisters may startle baby at first, but the infant will soon attempt to join the good-natured roughhouse with squeals of delight. Grandparents, visitors to the household, the paper deliverer, the mailman—the circle of cordiality becomes wider and wider, building and fortifying the basic trust.

Therapists for the mentally ill find a remarkable sameness in case histories of their most disturbed patients. Again and again, it becomes apparent that emotional deprivation lies in the background of the severest disorders. So unloved were these infants that they could not develop the basic trust that enables the fashioning of binding ties with one another (Erikson, 1968). And because human beings cannot exist in such emotional isolation, they may suffer the psychological breakdown we call mental illness.

ATTACHMENT

Erikson's concept of the development of basic trust clearly seems to place a first responsibility on the mother for establishing the kind of relationship that will enable the

The rewards of close early and continuing contact with the infant can be shared by both mother and father.

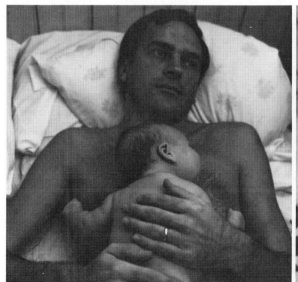
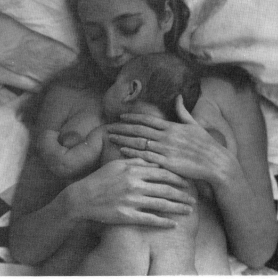

Judith Kruger Michalik

infant to build the sense of dependability. Freud's formulations, too, place heavy emphasis on the mother-infant relationship. Father does not enter the Freudian picture until the child is about 4 years old. In this book, we have also bowed to convention and described the early events of infancy as if these were ideally managed by the mother.

It seems important, however, to pause and inquire seriously about the origins and implications of ideas about the mother-infant relationship that have taken on a strange kind of intensity in our time. Every student reading this book has likely taken sides in some aspect of the controversy, the matter can be summed up with the assertion that "mother's place is in the home." The statement is often elaborated by some reference to "normal" families, implying a money-earning father and home-making mother, with any other arrangement thereby considered "abnormal" or deviant. Frequently, the notion of a "maternal instinct" is invoked, together with reference to the fact that animal mothers, care for the young in animal groups. From all this, the conclusion is derived that the mother as the principal child-rearing agent is "biological," therefore "natural" and therefore "right."

There can be little doubt that a number of factors arising during the late 19th and early 20th centuries contributed to an emphasis upon "mothering" that has only recently been questioned. An early influence was, of course, Freud's description of the importance of the first 5 years of childhood in determining, literally, the psychological course of the remainder of one's life. Feeding, weaning, and toilet training were seen as critical periods that form the base for later neuroses, with mother as the dominant figure steering the course through these stages. Another factor was that advances in medical care ensured that more infants would live to adulthood so that parents could literally afford a larger emotional investment in children without the ever-present possibility of childhood death from one of the prevalent infections. This, coupled with the Freudian injunctions, has made parents feel more responsible for outcomes in regard to their children. These factors meshed with complex industrial society arrangements. Men began to work at some considerable distance away from the home. Homes became organized into small, rather mobile units, that could be uprooted at the employer's convenience, and middle-class ideals came to include a home in suburban areas of cities. So, the predominant middle class pattern became one of father commuting miles to work while mother—taking care of the home and children—came to be seen as the major influence on the child. The social scientists underlined the pattern with their studies of, first, "maternal deprivation" and later, "attachment."

The early studies of infants in institutions focused attention on lack of normal developmental progress, which was interpreted to result from the absence of the mother. Infants failed to thrive even though physical care and nutrition were adequate. Spitz (1945), Goldfarb (1945), and Bowlby (1952) concluded that children who lacked mothering could languish and even die, but that if they survived they would exhibit a curious inability to relate to others—a flattened emotional capability. (It is interesting to note that none of these studies attended to the absence of fathers!)

It was Bowlby who translated the concern for lack of mothering into the theory of attachment. He described emotional bonds developing between mother and child that have, as a psychobiological function, the maintenance of proximity with each other. Infant behaviors such as crying, sucking, rooting, and smiling are thought to be proximity-promoting behaviors that will later become more active, directed toward a specific person, and include following and clinging.

Attachment theory, in the beginning, simply presumed that the "specific" person would be the mother. Bowlby believed it to be "essential for mental health" that the infant and young child should experience a "warm, intimate and continuous relationship with his mother (or permanent mother-substitute) in which both find satisfaction and enjoyment" (Bowlby, 1969). Many of the studies that followed sought to explore different aspects of attachment, including the patterns of attachment at different age levels. There were a number of attempts to find increasingly sensitive measures of attachment (i.e., behavior in a fear situation, kinds of protest when mother leaves, and reunion behavior) and the differing practices that might produce different strengths of attachment (Ainsworth, 1967, 1969, 1972, 1974).

Margaret Mead, a well-known anthropologist, was one of the first to question the prevailing view that care by a single, continuous mother figure was a necessary condition for the development of healthy interpersonal relations. She criticized the provincialism of Western psychologists in their presumption that, because our society places a heavy value on an exclusive mother-child bond, this is necessarily natural and right (Mead, 1962).

Mead pointed to other kinds of arrangements that seemed to be successful in other cultures, suggesting that perhaps children who grow up "mothered" by many women in the tribe are more secure than those who have had an exclusive and intense relationship with only one woman. Loss of an individual mother would be more catastrophic than the instance in which the child could easily and comfortably turn to someone else.

Now, some years after Mead's cautions, there is a growing feeling that study of attachment ought to be changed to study of *attachments*. Milton Kotelchuck (1976) asks what hard evidence exists to support the notion that children relate uniquely to their mothers. The answer is that there is no evidence whatsoever; it has always just been assumed. Kotelchuck's studies confirm the proposition that children relate to both parents similarly, both in a laboratory situation and in the home.

More than 70 per cent of the children studied were responsive to the presence of their fathers, protesting their departure and welcoming them back. There is some evidence that paternal caretaking practices make a difference. There seems to be a minimum level of paternal caretaking necessary for a relationship to exist. In a study in Guatemala, where men had almost nothing to do with their young infants, young children responded less to the departure of their fathers than did children in the United States (Lester, 1974). More telling, and in line with Mead's suggestion that multiple caretakers may cushion children's distress at separation, is the finding that children from families in which fathers share considerable caretaking responsibilities do not display the voluble dismay when left alone that is evidenced by those whose mothers have cared for them almost single-handedly.

An overemphasis on the biological mother as the most important source of attachment has served politicians as the excuse to refrain from attending seriously to extrafamilial care needs for children in the United States. "The mother's place is in the home" as a stated value simply fails to recognize that ours is the first society that has insisted that mothers rear children alone. Other societies have always made use of a multitude of support systems—nannies, unmarried or widowed relatives including the ubiquitous grandmother, apprenticeships at an early age, and reliance on the extended family system of the peasant village or tribe. The insistence that children be raised by the mother fails to attend to the fact that there is no evidence for the superiority of mother-reared children (Schaffer and Emerson, 1964).

Nor does this stated value note the effects of parenting when the mother or father is care-worn, anxious, irritable, or otherwise affected by poverty and troubles. With the divorce rate edging closer to one in two, many parents are not going to be able to abide by the idealized pattern. It seems unconscionable to add guilt to their burden that they are somehow damaging the child's future ability for attached and loving relationships.

None of the foregoing is intended to suggest that the family as provider of comfort and the dependability that engenders basic trust ought to be supplanted. It is, however, a plea for a new and broader look at the "folk wisdom" that often comes to be built into research and the pronouncements of social scientists. (Note, for example, how many of the manuals instructing women about how to be good mothers are written by men and the almost nonexistent availability of manuals aimed at fathers.)

The time has come, one might hope, to look at the possibilities for enlarging early environments and, coincidentally, for instituting good support services for harried parents.

Studies of child-care centers, when these places are well planned and staffed, have not turned up the widespread adverse effects predicted by opponents (Caldwell, 1970). On the contrary, not only did the day-care infants, assessed at 30 months, equal home-reared infants in strength of attachment to the mother; they also showed an increased developmental level not seen in the home-reared group.

Environmental stimulation and encouragement for motor exploration, opportunity to build basic trust and affectional ties—these, together with physical care and good nutrition, are the requisites of infancy. Healthy, humane, resourceful parents and caretakers are necessary to join the interaction, play the infant games, and provide the steady base for infant venturing. If those with whom the infant has contact can all share the baby's joys and sorrows, so much the better!

A prescription for the well-being of future families ought to include the notion of loving, enriching child-care centers where mothers and fathers can bring children for portions of the day, not only because they may be going off to work, but also because the child can benefit from a new set of circumstances that provide cooperative social experience with other trusting, dependable, interesting children and adults. The prescription would also call for more flexible work schedules that allow more parent-time with children for fathers as well as mothers. The existence of new modes such as these would begin to pay serious attention to the charge that the United States, contrary to its rhetoric, actually puts families and children last on the list of priorities for helpful programs (Bronfenbrenner, 1971). Health care, wholesome nurturing, and proper nutrition are vital for well-being in infancy; when these are readily available for all infant citizens, we can begin calling ourselves a caring society.

GLOSSARY

ACCOMMODATION   Piaget's term for the process by which a schema is adjusted to fit changing information and circumstances.

ASSIMILATION   Piaget's term for taking in, processing, and incorporating information.

ATTACHMENT   The affectionate reciprocal bond, typically between infant and caretaker, that produces desire for contact and distress upon separation.

BASIC TRUST   The term used by Erikson to describe the quality of a happy infant's orientation toward the world and its people.

DISHABITUATION   A revival of attention with a new stimulus after a previous stimulus has caused habituation.

EQUILIBRIUM   Physiological or psychological "balance."

HABITUATION   The process of becoming familiar with and no longer remaining attentive to a stimulus.

INVARIANT   The "same" function for all species.

OBJECT PERMANENCE   The infant's realization (concept) that objects continue to exist even if they are out of sight.

OFFSET   If a regular series of stimuli is presented until habituation occurs and the series is then halted, one responds as if missing the expected occurrence of the stimulus.

ORIENTING RESPONSE   Attending to a response by focusing the appropriate sensory organs upon it.

SCHEMA   For Piaget, the cognitive unit that comprises the comprehension of environmental events.

REFERENCES

Ainsworth, M. D.: *Infancy in Uganda*. Baltimore: Johns Hopkins University Press, 1967.

Ainsworth, M. D.: Object relations, dependency and attachment. *Child Development*, 40:969–1026, 1969.

Ainsworth, M. D.: Individual differences in the development of attachment behavior. *Merrill-Palmer Quarterly*, 18:123–143, 1972.

Ainsworth, M. D.: Infant-mother attachment and social development. In Richards, M. P. M. (ed.): *The Integration of the Child into the Social World*. Cambridge, England: Cambridge University Press, 1974.

Bower, T. G. R.: Infant responses to approaching objects: An indicator of response to distal variables. *Perception and Psychophysics*, 9:193–196, 1976.

Bower, T. G. R.: *A Primer of Infant Development*. San Francisco: W. H. Freeman, 1977.

Bowlby, J.: Maternal Care and Child Health. Geneva: World Health Organization. Monograph No. 2, 1952.

Bowlby, J.: *Attachment and Loss: Attachment*, vol. 1. New York: Basic Books, 1969.

Bronfenbrenner, U.: Who cares for America's children? *Young Children*, 26(3):157–163, 1971.

Caldwell, B.: Infant day care and attachment. *American Journal of Orthopsychiatry*, 30:397–410, 1970.

Erikson, E.: *Childhood and Society*, 2nd ed. New York: W. W. Norton & Company, 1963.

Erikson, E.: *Identity, Youth and Crisis*. New York: W. W. Norton & Company, 1968.

Fantz, R. L.: The origin of form perception. *Scientific American*, 204(5)66–72, 1961.

Goldfarb, W.: Psychological privation in infancy and subsequent adjustment. *American Journal of Orthopsychiatry*, 15:247–255, 1945.

Klaus, M., Kennel, J.: Care of the Mother. In Klaus, M., Fanaroff, A. (eds.): *Care of the High-Risk Neonate*. Philadelphia: W. B. Saunders Company, 1973.

Kotelchuck, M.: The infant's relationship to the father: Experimental evidence. In Lamb, M. (ed.): *The Role of the Father in Child Development*. New York: John Wiley & Sons, 1976.

Lester, B., Kotelchuck, M., Spelke, E., Sellers, J., Klein, R.: Separation protest in Guatemalan infants: Cross-cultural and cognitive findings. *Developmental Psychology*, 10:79–85, 1974.

Lipsitt, L. P., Kaye, H.: Change in neonatal response to optimizing and nonoptimizing sucking stimulation. *Psychonomic Science*, 2:221–222, 1965.

Mead, M.: A cultural anthropologist's approach to maternal deprivation. In *Deprivation of Maternal Care: A Reassessment of Its Effects*. Public Health Papers No. 14. Geneva: World Health Organization, 1962.

Piaget, J.: *The Origins of Intelligence in Children*. New York: International Universities Press, 1952.

Sameroff, A. J.: Early influences on development: Fact or fancy? *Merrill-Palmer Quarterly*, 21:267–294, 1975.

Schaffer, H. R., Emerson, P.: The development of social attachments in infants. *Monographs of the Society for Research in Child Development*, 29(3), 1964.

Spitz, R.: Hospitalism: An inquiry into the genesis of psychiatric conditions in early childhood. Part I. *Psychoanalytic Studies of Childhood*, 1:53–74, 1945.

Spock, B.: *Baby and Child Care*. New York: Pocket Books, 1976.

White, B. L.: *The First Three Years of Life*. Englewood Cliffs, N.J.: Prentice-Hall, 1975.

White, B. L., Watts, J. C.: Important characteristics of primary caretakers. In White, B. L., Watts, J. C. (eds.): *Experience and Environment: Major Influences on the Development of the Young Child*. Englewood Cliffs, N.J.: Prentice-Hall, 1973.

HEALTH CONCERNS IN PREGNANCY, CHILDBIRTH, AND INFANCY

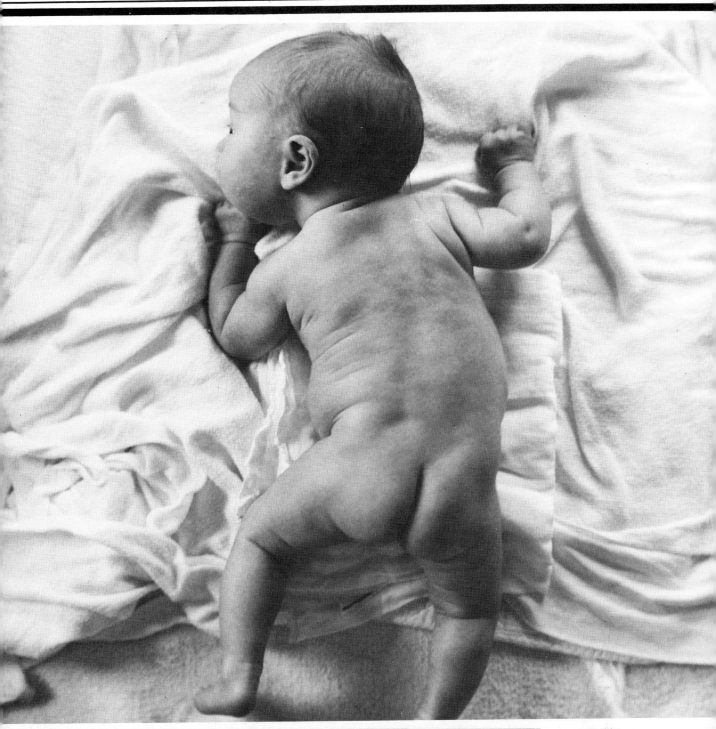

CHAPTER 4

Before 1900, nearly all births in the United States took place in the home. Only 2 or 3 per cent of deliveries took place in hospitals. Today the statistics are just the opposite. Almost all births take place in hospitals; only a small percentage occurs at home. The change to hospital deliveries was accompanied by an emphasis on cleanliness, prevention of infection, and medical technology to ease labor and delivery and to save lives of both mothers and infants. The changes in medical practice have dramatically reduced infant mortality rates. In 1910, about 100 of every 1000 infants born in the United States died before reaching 1 year of age. By 1977, the infant death rate had been reduced to 14 per every 1000 babies born alive (Fig. 4–1). The causes of infant deaths are shown in Figure 4–2.

Hospital routines became established because they were believed to promote the health of the mother and baby. By the late 1940s it had become generally accepted that the woman expecting a baby would be hospitalized for a week or more; the baby and mother would be separated immediately after birth, the mother staying in bed to rest, the baby being whisked away to a nursery to be with all the other newborns. There, the baby would be taken care of by trained nurses, possibly for many hours, before being

Figure 4–1 Infant mortality rates in the United States, 1915–1977. (From Healthy People: The Surgeon General's Report on Health Promotion and Disease Prevention. DHEW (PHS) Publication 79–55071, 1979.)

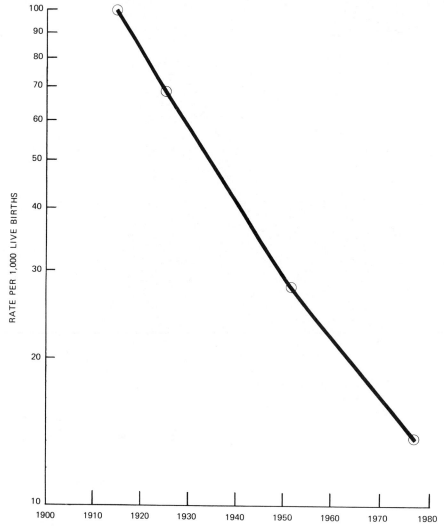

NOTE: 1977 data are provisional; data for all other years are final. Selected years are 1900, 1925, 1950, 1977.

Source: National Center for Health Statistics, Division of Vital Statistics.

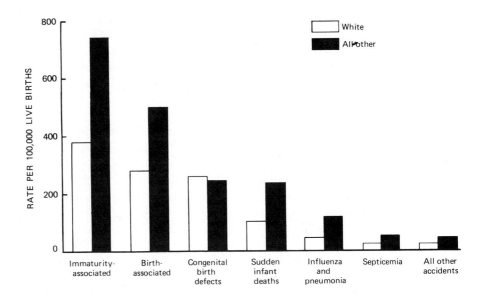

Source: Based on data from the National Center for Health Statistics, Division of Vital Statistics.

Figure 4–2   Major causes of infant mortality in the United States, 1976. (From Healthy People: The Surgeon General's Report on Health Promotion and Disease Prevention. DHEW (PHS) Publication 79–55071, 1979.)

returned to the mother. The father, expected to pace nervously in the waiting room until the physician or nurse emerged from the delivery room, would be limited to seeing the mother and baby during rigidly controlled visiting hours.

In the hospital, the mother would likely be taught how to prepare infant formulas, how to sterilize bottles, and how to feed the baby by bottle on a strict 4-hour schedule. Most of these practices began for good reasons. For example, separation of mother and baby and limited visits by the father began as safeguards against the spread of disease. However, sometimes hospital routine and convenience became more important than the concerns of the families whom the routines were meant to protect. The mother, after entering the institutional setting, was separated from her family, treated as a dependent "patient," and had very little to say about the circumstances of one of the most important events of her life—the birth of her baby.

Listening to the conversation of a healthy pregnant woman today, you might hear the terms "Lamaze instruction," "rooming-in," or "birthing center." You might hear a woman talking about her husband being present during labor and delivery or about plans for leaving the hospital the day after delivery. These trends represent a shift in emphasis from a childbirth experience in which the mother had almost no control of events to one in which more and more women are evaluating options, making decisions, and participating in the delivery process. But you might also hear talk of fetal monitoring, amniocentesis, or ultrasonography, the sophisticated technology that is also part of childbirth today. In few areas of health care practice is change more evident than in the care of women during pregnancy and childbirth. These changes are not without controversy.

In this chapter we will examine the physiological changes in pregnancy, the major causes of infant mortality, the technological developments that affect pregnancy and childbirth, and the progress of the newborn baby.

PREGNANCY

Who is the maternity patient? According to Webster's Third New International Dictionary, one definition for a *patient* is someone undergoing medical treatment; a sufferer.

But we know that pregnancy is not a disease. Indeed, many women state that at no other time do they feel more fulfilled or healthy, especially if a new baby is acceptable or anticipated with enthusiasm. If the pregnancy is normal, and the "patient" is not ill, then it is clear that the role of those caring for the mother-to-be is not to cure or treat but to support and assist the woman and her family during an essentially normal experience.

Assessment of Health Status

Many women receive their maternity care at prenatal clinics. For some, this might be the first time in many years that they have been involved with any health system. How they feel about this experience may be related to how they have interacted with the medical system in the past.

A pregnancy does not occur in a vacuum, it occurs in the context of the woman's whole family. How is it affecting the family? Are the baby's father or other family members available for support? Are there other children in the family? How old are they? Will help be available when the mother goes home or will she be going home alone to manage by herself?

Age and Pregnancy

The stresses placed on all family members anticipating a new member are great. If the mother-to-be is an unmarried teen-ager, the stress will be even greater. There is ample evidence to indicate that the increased pressure placed on a teen-ager might have some effect on the baby. Ferreira (1960) points out that increased stress produces an increase in uterine activity, constricts the blood vessels, and increases uterine contractions, which causes an increase in fetal heart rate. All this can produce tension and irritability in the mother. MacFarlane (1977) states that she can predict which babies will be irritable after birth by talking to the mother beforehand. There is also some indication that anxiety and stress during pregnancy may be one cause of prematurity and later postnatal distress.

Pregnancy After 35

Approximately 10 per cent of all babies born in the United States annually are born to women over 35. For the mother-to-be who is over 35, there are special issues. There has been a great change in our society in recent years. More and more women are marrying later, working longer, and postponing childbearing for a variety of reasons. Some want to continue their careers. Others are concerned with economics. Having waited a long time to have children and having had an independent lifestyle, some women may find it difficult to accept or anticipate the dependency needs of a new baby. The pregnant woman may be concerned about the amount of energy needed to deal with a toddler or a teen-ager. Underlying these expressed fears may be the fear of a difficult labor or a defective child. Perhaps this is one of the reasons many older women having a first baby are likely to seek medical care early in the pregnancy and to take good care of themselves.

Risks of Late Maternal Age

The risks associated with late maternal age increase as the age of the mother increases, with the major concern focusing on women over 35 years of age. Of 4500 women over the age of 40 having children in New York City in 1973, two thirds had normal pregnancies and deliveries (McCauley, 1976). Complications were encountered in more than 20 per cent of these pregnancies and were termed "coincidental," meaning that although the pregnancy did not cause the troubles, it probably aggravated them. Hypertension, diabetes, and kidney diseases were cited among the most common complications.

Cesarean sections were performed on 13.6 per cent of the women—twice the rate for younger women—probably because of the fact that as pelvic structures age, they become fibrous and less elastic, making a normal delivery more difficult. The mortality rate among the infants born was 9 per cent, much higher than the usual rate of 1.8 to 2.6 per cent for hospital-born infants. Twice the national average—6.8 per cent of the infants—had some congenital abnormalities, most often heart disease and Down's syndrome, the latter being the most common abnormality among all children born to older mothers.

Confirmation of Pregnancy

Although most pregnancies are first confirmed by a urine test, a pelvic examination is necessary to reconfirm the pregnancy. Many women do not know what their internal organs look like, and in fact may not know how conception occurs. An anatomical model can be very helpful in enabling a woman to understand the position of the uterus, ovaries, cervix, and vagina. During the first visit, a complete physical examination will be done. Blood pressure, urine, a hemoglobin count to determine the presence of anemia, weight and height, and Rh type will all be evaluated. A complete history will be taken, with attention given to past pregnancies and deliveries and any other relevant medical issues.

Physical Changes in Pregnancy

Pregnant women notice their breasts changing. Small-breasted women are frequently delighted that their breasts are now larger, and large-breasted women will notice how much heavier their breasts are and how often they have to buy larger bras as the pregnancy continues. It is important for all pregnant women to wear bras in order to prevent strain on the tissues of the breast and to maintain support.

By the fifth month of pregnancy, the breasts are functionally prepared to produce milk, and many women may notice a yellow leakage if their nipples are pressed. Women do not actively lactate during pregnancy, probably because of the higher levels of the hormones estrogen and progesterone in the placenta (Pryor, 1974). During this time, the placenta is also producing another hormone called *human placental lactogen*. Once the baby is born and the placenta is delivered, the estrogen and progesterone levels drop, the pituitary gland starts producing the hormone *prolactin*, and lactation can begin.

During the 9 months of pregnancy, additional changes take place. Table 4–1 lists some of these common signs.

Health Issues During Pregnancy
Nutrition

Every expectant mother needs to understand the importance of good nutrition during pregnancy. Her nutritional status will be influenced by her age, pre-pregnancy weight, current food habits, and dietary problems, if any, during past pregnancies. Her feelings about a changing body image may also influence her dietary choices if she tries not to gain weight.

Weight Gain. During the 1950s, 1960s, and even part of the 1970s, it was commonplace for physicians to admonish their pregnant patients not to gain weight. Indeed, many

TABLE 4–1 PHYSICAL CHANGES DURING PREGNANCY

Period of Occurrence	Signs and Symptoms
First month	Fatigue Frequent urination Breast swelling Possible nausea Darkened area around nipples Missed period
Second month	Fatigue Darkened area around the nipples Possible nausea Breast swelling
Third to 4th months	Expanding waist Increased appetite Breast enlargement Detection of fetal movement Possible low back discomfort
Fifth to 9th months	Braxton Hicks contractions Possible constipation Low back pain Frequent urination (9th month) Increased fetal movement Increased weight gain

women were told to lose weight. It is now known that there is a correlation between maternal weight gain and the birth weight of the baby. Brewer (1977) states that "maternal malnutrition during pregnancy is responsible for the annual death of 30,000 infants and birth defects in 200,000 children in this country. The condition called metabolic toxemia of late pregnancy is directly caused by malnutrition."

A weight gain of 25 to 30 pounds is normal for most pregnant women. Although obese women have to be more closely monitored for other risk factors, they should not be put on an overly restricted diet. According to Brewer, 2600 calories are needed daily. If calories are eliminated, maternal protein will be metabolized for energy, cutting down on the protein available for the baby. Since 90 grams of protein are needed daily, this depletion can lead to low birth weight, neonatal death or congenital defects. During pregnancy the important aspect is the rate of weight gain, rather than the amount gained. A gradual gain is normal; a sudden gain of 10 to 12 pounds in a 2-week period can indicate potential trouble.

Use of Salt. Another aspect of nutritional information concerns the use of salt in the diet. Although many physicians caution patients on the use of added salt (a warning to be heeded by all people), Brewer also suggests that when salt is restricted to prevent hypertension during pregnancy, the kidneys react by releasing the enzyme renin. Renin in the blood stream causes the arterioles to constrict; this, in turn, causes the blood pressure to rise. Pregnant women should eat a well-balanced diet that includes foods from the four basic food groups, while limiting salt and "empty calories." Each day's intake should include the foods listed in Table 4–2.

Menu Planning. Although most complete proteins are found in animal sources, a vegetarian diet can also supply the needs of a pregnant woman. Good sources of vegetable protein are found in soybeans, tofu (bean curd), cottage cheese, milk, eggs, and a variety of nuts and grains. A recent addition to this group has been the introduction of sunflower butter, with the same consistency as peanut butter, the slightly nutty flavor of sunflower

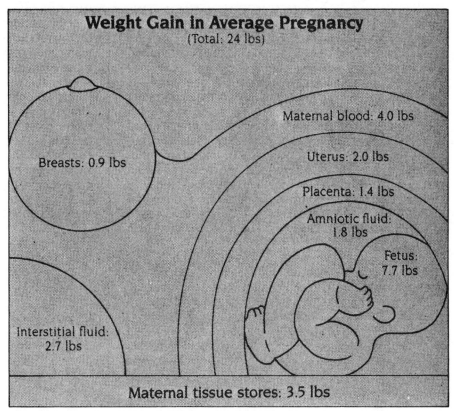

Figure 4–3 Weight gain in pregnancy. (From Whelan, E.: Fashions in feeding, Part 1: Maternal nutrition. *Childbirth Educator*, Vol. 1, No. 1, Fall 1981, p. 18.)

seeds, and the added bonus of increased vitamin B. These will all provide good protein. There are many excellent vegetarian cook books available. A vegetarian diet can be both interesting and nutritous.

With a little ingenuity and the use of herbs and spices, most women will be able to eat well and without extra expense throughout the 9 months. In fact, these menu plans could be used by any family trying to eat economical and nutritionally sound meals, all without the use of added salt.

All pregnant women should take supplemental vitamins and minerals, since there is an increased need for these during pregnancy. Even those who eat green leafy vegetables and whole-grain products and drink lots of fluids ought to supplement the diet. Teen-agers, or any woman with poor eating habits in the past, will find it more difficult to readily change well-entrenched patterns, and for these women, supplements become even more important.

Drugs and the Developing Fetus

In recent years, attention has focused on the effects of drugs on the fetus. The problems associated with the ingestion of a variety of drugs became evident during the thalidomide episode in the 1950s and 1960s. It is now known that there are times in fetal development when the fetus is particularly sensitive to drugs. The list of dangerous substances becomes longer each year. As a result, expectant mothers today are warned to take *no unprescribed medication* during pregnancy. Responsible physicians have also become extremely cautious in prescribing drugs for the pregnant woman.

Many drugs affect the fetus during the early stages of development, when the fetus is most vulnerable. However, because the last 3 months of pregnancy bring about the most rapid growth of the fetal brain, it should be apparent that drug ingestion at this

TABLE 4–2 DIETARY RECOMMENDATIONS DURING PREGNANCY

Food Groups	Quantities
Milk	Four glasses—skim, buttermilk, or whole; may substitute yogurt or cottage cheese
Eggs, cheese, or meat	Two eggs; one serving of fish, chicken, lamb, pork, or lean meat; may substitute soybeans or other beans, peanut butter, or peas and rice
Green vegetables	Two servings of green leafy vegetables—e.g., lettuce; collard, beet, or turnip greens; or cabbage
Yellow vegetables	One serving daily of squash, carrots, or other yellow vegetable
Bread	Whole wheat bread is best; two to three slices a day; may also include whole wheat cereals, oatmeal, or other whole grain cooked cereal
Fruit	One citrus fruit such as orange or grapefruit daily; may substitute glass of juice (not a sweetened juice drink)
Carbohydrates	May substitute rice and potatoes for bread; avoid pastry and cake, potato chips, and "empty calories"

time is equally dangerous. The new fetal brain cells produced late in pregnancy are involved in the formulation of interconnecting nerve cells in several regions of the brain. Also, most of the nerve cells of the cortex that have to do with coordination develop between 6 months prenatally and 18 months of age (Lewis, 1978). Some drugs destroy the stores of chemicals that act as messengers, conveying signals from one nerve cell to another. Hormones controlling cell division may also be affected. Some drugs, although they do not produce gross deformities, nevertheless produce dangerous symptoms in the newborn. Babies of mothers addicted to heroin, morphine, or methadone are often born suffering from withdrawal symptoms severe enough to cause profound respiratory distress, convulsions, and even death. These babies require special care in the attempt to control the reactions.

Alcohol

One of the most toxic substances affecting fetal development is alcohol. Early Greeks recognized its potential for damage and prohibited drinking on the wedding night for fear of producing a damaged child. Aristotle observed that drunken women brought forth languid, morose children.

Today, alcohol consumption during pregnancy is recognized as a major health problem. It is estimated that 4000 to 5000 infants are born each year in the United States with *fetal alcohol syndrome* a characteristic set of abnormalities, including facial deformities and mental retardation.

Jones and co-workers (1973), replicating a 1971 study, reported on 11 unrelated babies born to alcoholic mothers. Patterns of retarded growth, as well as facial, limb, and cardiovascular defects, were noted. Basing the investigation on a study done in Seattle, Washington, they found that maternal alcohol consumption was the third leading cause of mental retardation in that city.

Fielding (1978b) listed facial defects in these children as being as definitive in appearance as those that mark Down's syndrome. These include a shortened jaw, an unusually thin upper lip, and the absence of the epicanthal folds in the eyelids. In addition, there may be a deficiency in weight, length, and brain weight. The newborn may be irritable and shaky, and may have a weak sucking reflex.

Both Fielding (1978b) and Streissguth (1978) note that a much lower level of alcohol than previously thought to be damaging produces symptoms. As little as 1 ounce of alcohol consumed daily before pregnancy results in as much as a 90-gram loss in birth weight. When the same amount of alcohol was consumed during pregnancy, there was a 160-gram decrement in weight. Although there is an urgent need to determine whether there is *any safe level* of alcohol consumption, it is now recognized that it is the amount consumed in a brief period of time that does the damage. Pregnant women should be alerted not to have more than two drinks a day, even if this occurs only on rare occasions. There is evidence that even low concentrations of alcohol in the fetus could result in permanent functional disturbances (Rossett et al., 1976).

The reasons for the defects are still under investigation. The question is whether alcohol itself is the direct toxin or whether alcohol's metabolite (acetaldehyde) and other factors must be present to produce abnormalities. One idea is that the concentration of alcohol in the fetus quickly rises to the level present in the mother's circulation. The unborn baby's ability to eliminate the alcohol occurs only after the development of its liver enzymes during the last part of pregnancy. In addition, pregnant women tend to retain alcohol for longer periods of time and their alcohol consumption thus affects the fetus for longer periods (Hinkers, 1978).

Smoking

Smoking has also been linked to a variety of birth defects. Nicotine, which is the most active alkaloid constituent of tobacco, exerts its action on the peripheral vascular system, causing constriction of the blood vessels. The heart rate and output then increase. This vasoconstriction causes a rise in blood pressure (Piran, 1978). Carbon monoxide, the other component of tobacco smoke, combines with hemoglobin to produce a pigment called carboxyhemoglobin. This pigment reduces tissue oxygenation and thus reduces the oxygen-carrying capacity of the mother (DiMasico et al., 1978). The effect of this lack of oxygen is to significantly lower the birth weight of the baby. The number of cigarettes smoked daily seems to be directly related to lowered birth weight. Women who smoke 10 to 12 cigarettes daily produce smaller babies. Because the fetus gains approximately $1/2$ pound a week during the last 4 weeks, women who smoke heavily during this time run a higher risk of producing a "small-for-date" baby. The risks of spontaneous abortion, early separation of the placenta, or precipitous delivery of the placenta also rise in mothers who continue to smoke heavily during the last 3 months of pregnancy (Zabriskie, 1963).

Sexual Activity

Many women are concerned about sexual activity during pregnancy but are not comfortable discussing sexual issues with their mates or with health professionals. Sexuality does not cease during pregnancy. Activity may slow and change, but many people remain sexually active throughout the 9 months.

Our understanding of sexual response has been greatly enhanced by the studies of Masters and Johnson (1966). By observing and interviewing 111 women and 79 of their husbands during the course of their pregnancies, they determined that certain physiological responses are more pronounced in the pregnant female. Uterine contractions, generally felt during orgasm, become longer and more sustained.

In a study of 260 pregnant women, Solberg and colleagues (1973) noted that 47 per cent of them felt physically unattractive, particularly during the last trimester. Masters and Johnson (1966) found a higher proportion of the women in their sample reporting that this was a major factor in their declining sexual activity. In studies done by Solberg and associates (1973) and Falicov (1973), all their samples reported an increase in coital activity during the first trimester. Masters and Johnson (1966) reported an increase in desire and frequency during the second trimester, owing to the lack of risk of getting pregnant, the presence of genital engorgement, and an increase in vaginal lubrication. Other investigators report mixed responses. During the last trimester, there was diminished interest on the part of all women involved. Most couples ceased intercourse by the 8th month, although only a small proportion were advised to do this.

This last point is of some interest. For many years, physicians had advised expectant women to cease sexual activity 6 to 8 weeks before the expected due date. It is now accepted that this is necessary only under limited circumstances. If the mother has a history of premature births, if there is spotting or bleeding, or if the presenting part (that part of the baby that comes through the birth canal first) is nearly in or in the birth canal, then intercourse is not advised. Once the membranes have ruptured, there is an increased risk of infection and intercourse should cease. Although some women near term have gone into labor after intercourse, there is no indication that sexual activity during the last trimester will cause a premature birth.

Genetic Counseling

About 25 per cent of birth defects are due primarily to genetic factors, and hereditary defects are the second leading cause of death in infants and children through the age of 4. Genetic counseling today is the only readily available strategy for prevention of such disorders.

Genetic counseling is not routine but is appropriate when there is a history of familial defects or a past history of a child born with a hereditary disease or chromosomal abnormality, or when the mother is a carrier of a disorder that affects only male children.

Chromosomal Disorders

A chromosomal disorder is one in which there is a defect in the chromosomes, resulting in a condition that may have life-long implications. One such condition is *Down's syndrome*, which may produce a profoundly retarded child. Down's syndrome, which affects about 5000 newborns a year in the United States, is more common among babies born to women who are in their 40s when they give birth. There are other diseases that are attributable to a trait of a gene that causes some abnormality. Some genetic abnormalities are dwarfism, congenital cataracts, extra fingers or toes, webbed fingers or toes, and the condition called Huntington's chorea. There are other chromosomal afflictions as well, particularly those that produce an irregularity in the sex chromosomes, causing incomplete sexual development, feminizing characteristics in male children, and masculinization in female children.

Genetic Screening

There are now screening programs available for couples who are concerned about genetic disorders. The couple can be evaluated before deciding to become parents to determine whether they are carriers of genetic characteristics that might produce a defective child. Such a screening program is available for Jewish people of eastern European background, who may be carriers of Tay-Sachs disease. A degenerative neurological condition that eventually results in death for the child, it is genetic in origin. If these genes are identified in the prospective parents, the couple can have the opportunity to decide if they will risk having children.

Another fairly common genetic trait that can cause trouble is the "sickle cell," a defect in red blood cells that can produce sickle cell anemia in offspring if both parents have the trait. Sickle cell anemia causes poor development, weakness, lowered resistance to infections, and pain and swelling in joints and muscles. The sickle cell trait is most often found in black people or people of Mediterranean descent. A simple blood test is available to determine the presence of this trait, and the results can be known in 30 minutes.

Amniocentesis

In some cases, a simple blood test is not sufficient to determine fetal abnormalities, but other diagnostic tests can be done to determine the condition of the developing fetus. One such test is *amniocentesis*.

By examining cultured cells from a sample of the amniotic fluid in which the fetus is suspended in the uterus, a physician can determine whether the baby will be born with any one of a number of hereditary defects. The procedure must be timed carefully. If done too early, there is the chance of obtaining false results. The woman must have an examination using ultrasonography (described in the next section) to determine the exact position of the fetus. For prenatal diagnosis, the procedure, which must be done by qualified physicians only, should take place between the 14th and 16th weeks of pregnancy. With the use of local anesthesia, a long needle is precisely inserted through the abdomen into the amniotic sac and a small amount of fluid is withdrawn, generally about two tablespoonfuls. This fluid is then cultured. The results take 2 weeks to be available.

Although there may be anxiety surrounding the procedure on the part of the couple, they will have the opportunity to decide on a course of action if there is evidence that the baby will be born with a serious defect. Many health professionals recommend that amniocentesis be performed only if the parents have decided beforehand that an abortion would be a possibility. If the couple decide to terminate the pregnancy, more extensive counseling will be necessary to prepare the woman for a second-trimester termination.

Ultrasonography

Another tool used to determine the development of a fetus *in utero* is the ultrasound examination. Sound waves are beamed into the mother's body and bounce off different tissues in predictable patterns. These sound wave patterns can be displayed on a television screen and then printed on Polaroid film. Because ultrasonography does not involve the use of potentially harmful x-rays, this technique is considered safer than x-ray examinations to determine the maturity of the fetus, to diagnose prenatal abnormalities, and to confirm fetal life when there has been a history of repeated spontaneous abortion.

Preparation for Childbirth

Today many women want to be awake and to participate actively in giving birth. In answer to those needs, there has been a resurgence of interest in the various childbirth options available.

The Lamaze Method

One of the most popular and widespread methods of preparation for childbirth is the Lamaze method. Perfected by a French physician, Fernand Lamaze, it is based on Russian Pavlovian psychology. A series of exercises have been designed to condition the mother's reflexes in response to pain. Since pain is the first stimulus recorded by the brain, the exercises focus on sending stronger, non-pain signals to the brain, rendering the pain signals secondary (Miller and Brooten, 1977).

When Grantly Dick-Read began his "natural childbirth" work in 1932, he devised a series of exercises and breathing techniques that helped mothers deliver their babies with less need for painkillers and anesthesia (Dick-Read, 1968). The Lamaze method incorporates many of Dick-Read's principles and includes the husband or other coach as a supportive member of the childbirth team. Families involved in the Lamaze method are encouraged to participate in childbirth education classes in which partners practice breathing techniques and exercises, as well as "rehearse" the forthcoming delivery. The husband or other coach is present in the labor and delivery room to encourage, support, and coach the woman. This sharing of the birth experience often helps strengthen relationships between all the members of the family.

In some hospitals, "birthing rooms," set up more like a bedroom at home, are used. When a woman is admitted to a birthing room, she stays there throughout her labor and delivery and is not moved to the delivery room. These rooms provide a warm, homelike atmosphere and tend to reduce tension and fear for women in labor.

The Leboyer Method

Some hospitals are experimenting with relatively new procedures. In 1975, the French obstetrician Frederick Leboyer aroused the interest of both professional and lay people with the publication of his book, *Childbirth Without Violence*. Instead of the cold noisy atmosphere of most delivery rooms, he advocates a quiet, warm room, with dimmed lights. Upon birth, the umbilical cord is not cut immediately but is left attached until the last bit of maternal blood has pumped through. The baby is washed in warm water and given immediately to the mother. At no time is the baby handled vigorously, nor does suctioning occur unless resuscitation is necessary. Although the book is controversial, the emphasis placed on a nontraumatic entrance into the world is worth considering.

Childbirth Education Classes

It is common for couples to participate in childbirth education classes, many of which are sponsored or supported by hospitals. Although there is no mandatory licensing program for childbirth educators, many of them are registered nurses and are members of the two major childbirth education organizations—the American Society for Psycho-prophylaxis in Obstetrics (ASPO) and the International Childbirth Education Association (ICEA).

Childbirth education classes tend to attract well-educated, middle-class couples; in general, these classes have not yet reached minority groups and lower socioeconomic couples. In many areas, these classes offer more than information about the physical process of childbirth. They can also become informal support groups, offering the expectant parents a chance to talk with other couples and share information and concerns

---

TABLE 4–3 CHILDBIRTH EDUCATION CLASSES CONTENT*

1. Signs and symptoms of labor
2. Stages and phases of labor and delivery
3. Procedures in the labor and delivery area of the hospital; medications
4. Breathing exercises
5. Exercises to improve muscle tone and posture to make birth easier
6. Relaxation exercises
7. Basic anatomy and changes in anatomy during pregnancy
8. Nutrition in pregnancy and during breastfeeding
9. Consequences of alcohol consumption
10. Consequence of smoking
11. Avoiding nonprescription drugs
12. Growth and development of the fetus and infant

*Adapted from Sasmor, J. L., Grossman, E.: Childbirth education in 1980. *Journal of Obstetric and Gynecologic Nursing*, May–June 1981.

about childbirth and raising children. Topics commonly covered in childbirth classes are listed in Table 4–3.

Blood Typing

The pregnant woman will have her blood type checked to determine whether she carries the Rh-positive or Rh-negative factor. The Rh factor is a substance found in the red blood cells of most women (85 per cent). Such women are identified as Rh positive. Blood typing is important only for a small number of women (15 per cent) who have been identified as Rh negative.

If an Rh-negative woman has an Rh-positive mate, there is the possibility that the mother will develop antibodies in her own body to counteract what is essentially a foreign substance (an Rh-positive baby). These antibodies can destroy the baby's red blood cells. There is little risk in first pregnancies, since the baby may already be born before the mother produces the antibodies. Smith and co-workers (1978) suggested that the most likely time for the mother to begin producing these antibodies is at the time of delivery.

As the placenta separates, a small amount of fetal blood may enter the mother's circulation. If this happens, these fetal red blood cells can stimulate permanent maternal antibodies. During subsequent pregnancies, these antibodies, passing from the mother to the baby through her placenta, could harm the baby. It is for this reason that mothers who are Rh negative and have an Rh-positive mate must have their antibody level checked several times during the pregnancy. Most of the time, particularly in first pregnancies, the antibody level remains safe. After the birth of the child, the mother is given an injection of a substance called Rhogam, which prevents the antibodies from building up in subsequent pregnancies.

There is no complication if the mother is Rh positive and has an Rh-negative mate. Similarly, a baby who is Rh negative does not cause the mother to build up her antibodies.

LABOR AND DELIVERY

Signs of Labor

Gaskin (1978) describes the signs of impending labor as follows:

1. The baby drops lower down into the pelvic cavity about 2 to 3 weeks before delivery. The mother feels increasing pressure on her lower abdomen and might have to urinate more frequently. At the same time, she feels less full in the upper abdomen and is able to eat and breathe more easily than before. This stage is called "lightening."

2. The head of the baby settles into the lower pelvis and becomes "engaged." In women who have had a baby before (multiparas), this may happen only hours before labor begins. In a first-time mother (primigravida), it can occur days before.

3. There is an increase in vaginal secretions.

4. The mucous plug, which has been firmly in place in the cervix, comes out, generally accompanied by a "bloody show"—blood-tinged mucus.

5. On vaginal examination, the cervix will be much softer to the touch. Generally, the cervix feels hard, like the tip of the nose, but gets softer as it starts to get thinner.

Stages of Labor

The actual birth process occurs in four stages. There is no complete answer as to why and when labor starts, but there appears to be a relationship between the onset of labor and placental aging, which is implicated in the fall in the production of progesterone (Moore, 1978).

TABLE 4–4 STAGES OF LABOR

Stage	Signs and Symptoms
First stage (Several hours; 8 to 10 hours in a first pregnancy)	
Early	"Bloody show" Possible ruptured membranes Increasing contractions lasting 45 seconds to 1 minute, occurring up to 5 minutes apart Dilation of the cervix to about 5 cm
Late	Contractions increase in intensity, and time between contractions decreases Cervix dilates to about 8 cm
Transition	Cervix dilates to about 10 cm Intense contractions
Second stage (From a few minutes to several hours)	Cervix completely dilated Baby's head (or presenting part) moves into birth canal Irresistible urge to push Birth
Third stage (Up to 20 minutes)	Delivery of the placenta
Fourth stage (One to 24 hours after birth)	Uterus starts to contract to its normal size Restoration of physiological stability

Many investigators believe that labor actually begins as long as 6 to 8 weeks before the actual birth, when the mother experiences *Braxton Hicks contractions.* These are mild sensations of tightening in the upper part of the uterus. The effect of these contractions is to pull the lower or passive part of the uterus up, and in the process, the cervix begins to thin out and dilate, or "efface." The stages of labor are summarized in Table 4–4.

Anesthesia and Drugs During Childbirth

One of the main reasons for prepared childbirth is to lessen or eliminate the need for painkillers and anesthesia during labor and childbirth. There are two main categories of drugs used in childbirth. *Analgesics* are drugs that lessen pain. *Anesthetics* eliminate the feeling of pain, either by putting the patient to sleep or by creating a temporary loss of feeling in the area affected by the pain (Boston Women's Health Book Collective, 1979).

All medications cross the placental barrier and reach the fetus. Some have the effect of depressing functions in the newborn, such as respiration and the sucking reflex. If tranquilizers are given to relax the mother, she may become so relaxed that her labor slows down. According to Scanlon (1974), Demerol, a drug often used to lessen pain, has the effect not only of repressing vital functions in the newborn, but, in addition, of inhibiting the newborn's responsiveness to stimuli such as cuddling, consoling, and startling.

General Anesthesia

A painkiller that compels the mother to be completely asleep is potentially dangerous. A general anesthetic has a severely depressant effect on the fetus. It is most often used in the last few moments of labor or in a cesarean section.

Local anesthesia

A local anesthetic is used in a specific region. The vulva, the whole lower spine, or just the lower pelvic area might be anesthetized. Although it does not affect the mother's entire body, there is still risk to the baby.

Hypnosis

An alternative to chemical anesthesia is hypnosis. In some large medical centers, there are physicians who will coach expectant mothers by practicing hypnotic suggestion. Some physicians use hypnosis to perform cesarean sections. Flowers and associates (1960) indicate that many first-time mothers have found that hypnosis lessened the first stage by as much as 3 hours and the transition stage by an equally proportional amount.

Routine Hospital Procedures

Shaving

Other procedures are routine in hospitals, but they might be considered alien to many women. It is often routine to shave the whole pelvic area to reduce the risk of infection. There is some evidence that the risk is only slightly greater for those who are not shaved, but often the woman is not given a choice. Today, in many hospitals, only the area around the vagina is shaved, so that the itching that accompanies hair regrowth is reduced.

Enemas

Another procedure is the cleansing enema, frequently given when the woman enters the hospital. The theory is that if there is less material in the intestine, the labor will be easier. There is also less risk of contamination to the whole pelvic area during delivery. An enema given during active labor can be uncomfortable and anxiety provoking. Again, there are options that the mother can choose, including the use of a small self-contained enema that she could give to herself at home at the onset of labor. Since many women develop diarrhea normally during the last few days before labor starts, there may not be much in the lower intestine to evacuate.

Consumer pressure has prompted many hospitals to reevaluate their routine procedures to eliminate those that do not truly contribute to the well-being of mother, child, and family (Boston Women's Health Book Collective, 1979). Thus, some procedures, although helpful on occasion, are being eliminated or reduced in frequency.

Cesarean Section

In all births, there are events that are unpredictable. Sometimes, unforeseen complications may lead to the necessity of performing a cesarean section. Originally performed only in emergencies (for instance, when the baby's condition radically changed, when the head was too large for the birth canal, or when there was excessive bleeding in the mother), cesarean sections are now being performed at an increasing rate. Some estimates are as high as 10 per cent of all births and rising. With the fear of malpractice suits, many physicians do not want to take chances; at the slightest indication of fetal distress (as shown by fetal monitoring), a section might be done. If unprepared for such an event, the mother is likely to be upset. She will require anesthesia, be taken to an operating room, in most instances be separated from her husband, and will have a more prolonged recovery period. In some hospitals, spinal anesthesia is used, so that the mother is totally awake, and the father is permitted in the operating room, but this varies.

Midwifery and Home Births

In recent years, there has been an increase in the presence of midwives to assist in and actually perform deliveries in the United States. The history of midwifery is as old as civilization. By tradition and custom, women have always assisted other women during labor and delivery. During the 14th century, barber-surgeons took up the practice of obstetrics, but it was not until the middle of the 18th century that male midwives were accepted in England.

Hippocrates instituted the training of midwives in the 5th century B.C., but there was no consistent training or use of midwives throughout the world for many centuries. In 1630, the first midwives arrived in the American colonies. They had only haphazard training and supervision, and midwifery had not become an accepted part of the American medical scene (Spert, 1968).

In 1925, the first American midwives, trained in England or Scotland, began to practice in Kentucky with the Frontier Nursing Service, under the direction of Mary Breckinridge. These midwives originally went on horseback from home to home, delivering babies in an area of the country that was remote, with few hospitals easily accessible to families. Still in existence, the Frontier Nursing Service midwives now travel in jeeps and cars, still rendering prenatal, postnatal, and delivery services to a population that has grown to respect and depend on them. Since 1931, when the first school of midwifery in the United States opened under the auspices of the Maternity Center in New York, many other programs have been established, and midwives are gaining acceptance as part of the obstetrical team in many institutional settings. Midwives today are nurses who have had extensive additional education, who can deliver babies, and who are responsible for the prepartum and postpartum care of the mother. The advantage often cited for the use of a midwife is the time taken for supportive education of the mother. It represents another step away from regarding childbirth as a disease. Some studies have shown that women who received care from a nurse midwife are more satisfied with their childbirth experience than women who received care from a physician.

The scope of midwifery practice and its legal status vary from state to state. In some states, physicians have attempted to limit the practice of midwives to settings in which they are closely supervised by a physician, asserting that this is necessary for the safety of the mother and child. Organizations of nurse-midwives, on the other hand, assert that they are qualified to take total responsibility for prenatal care and delivery and that physicians have vested economic interests in limiting midwifery practice, since midwives charge far less than most obstetricians do for the services provided.

Along with the increasing awareness of midwifery as an existing force, the home birth movement, which developed momentum during the 1960s, has become another alternative that some women have considered. The controversy surrounding home births is heated. On one hand, some feel that home births are potentially dangerous, even for low-risk mothers. Unforeseen complications, such as a prolapsed umbilical cord, premature delivery of the placenta, and too-small pelvic dimensions, can all be cited. Those who advocate home births feel that the birth of a baby is a natural event that should take place within the context of the family. In home births, the father is usually more actively involved; the mother can be more comfortable in a semisitting position to deliver; there is no separation from other children; and the risk of contracting a hospital-borne (nosocomial) infection is eliminated.

The most accepted home delivery teams have a physician and midwife in attendance, with a back-up ambulance crew outside the home in case of an emergency. It is unlikely that the home birth movement will ever become typical in the United States. However, it seems possible that the changes in thinking about pregnancy could encourage more women to consider selecting a home birth as their choice for delivery. Although changes in childbirth have been slow to become institutionalized, there is an increased awareness of the many options available with emphasis on natural processes, while retaining the most useful tools of modern technology. The end result should be a decrease in maternal and neonatal disease and death.

A BABY IS BORN

Excitement pervades the delivery or birthing room every time another human being enters the world. Whether a baby is born in a large, modern medical center or a small community hospital the care that the baby receives immediately after birth and during the next few days will be of the utmost importance. During these initial days, the changes that the newborn undergoes are more profound, physically, sensorially, and even perhaps emotionally, than at any other time in life.

Neonates

Without warning, the newborn, known at this stage as a *neonate*, is thrust from a warm, fluid-filled environment where respiratory and circulatory needs have been met, into an environment with no closed boundaries. Washed by chilly air and assaulted by unfamiliar sounds, the baby must breathe spontaneously and make the necessary changes within the circulatory system for an independent life. Within 24 hours, all other systems should read "go," with adequate functioning of gastrointestinal, neurological, renal, and endo- crine systems. How well a baby accomplishes these tasks depends on many factors— genetic makeup, absence of abnormalities, prenatal care of the mother, the circumstances of birth, maternal temperament, and the care and surveillance of the caregivers. The newborn will have to be watched carefully, observations noted accurately, and an ongoing health assessment instituted.

Caring for the newborn starts during the mother's pregnancy. A woman's nutrition, physical condition, length of labor, ease of delivery, and emotional state all have an important bearing on the well-being of the baby.

All new babies are different. Like thumb prints they each have distinctive charac- teristics that set them apart. Looking at a nursery filled with newborns, one is immediately struck by the varieties present. Some will appear "wiry" and athletic, others peaceful, some pudgy, others lean. Some will seem calm and remain so; others will respond tensely to handling, somehow sensitive to the cautiousness of a first-time, inexperienced mother.

Infant Assessment—the Apgar Scale

In order to secure a standard, or base line, of an infant's condition, several assessment scales have been developed. Such scales provide a quick, accurate indication of the baby's present condition as well as potential warning signs. The most widely used is the Apgar Scale (1953). Table 4–5 lists the signs that are examined and scored.

Heart rate, respiratory effort, muscle tone, reflexes, and color are assessed on a scale of 0 to 2. A final rating is then calculated, with 10 being the highest score possible. A baby whose score is under 4 is seriously at risk and needs resuscitation. A score of 4 to 6 implies that some concern is warranted; generally, the baby's condition is guarded, and possibly clearing of the airway and supplemental oxygen will be needed. A score of 7 to 10 is considered a good Apgar rating, indicating that the infant scored as high as 70 to 90 per cent of all infants. The scale is used at 1 and 5 minutes after birth (Pillitteri, 1977).

Physical Appearance

In appearance, the baby may have a molded, elongated, asymmetrical head. This molding is due to pressure on the head as the baby moves through the birth canal. These signs

TABLE 4–5 APGAR SCALE

Sign	Score		
	0	1	2
Heart rate	Absent	Slow, below 100	Above 100
Respiratory effort	Absent	Slow; irregular weak cry	Good strong cry
Muscle tone	Flaccid	Some flexion of extremities	Well flexed
Reflex irritability			
Response to catheter in nostril	No response	Grimace	Cough or sneeze
Slap on sole of foot	No response	Grimace	Cry and withdrawal of foot
Color	Blue, pale	Body pink, extremities blue	Completely pink

may disappear within a few days or they may take as long as several weeks to disappear. Babies' backs are short and their chests round. If full term, they will be covered with a white, cheesy-like substance, the *vernix caseosa*, which is a skin lubricant. Although this is a protective device against amniotic fluid while the fetus is in the uterus, it is generally cleaned off, particularly from skin folds, as it could become the breeding ground for bacteria (Pillitteri, 1977).

Some newborns may be covered with fine, downy hair, *lanugo*. This rubs away within 2 weeks.

Another characteristic that may be disconcerting to new parents is the appearance of what look like little white pimples (milia) on the baby's nose and chin. These are immature sebaceous glands. As the glands begin to function, the "pimples" are no longer seen.

Babies' eyes are, without exception, either slate gray or blue and do not change to their permanent color until around 3 months of age. Sometimes the eyes will appear red and swollen within 24 hours of birth. This can be due to silver nitrate, which is dropped into the newborn's eyes at birth to prevent a gonorrheal infection from organisms that could have been present in the vaginal tract and entered the baby's eyes during delivery. The use of drops is required in some states. Other states have mandated the use of an antibiotic ointment; still others do not require any preventive measures.

Newborns may also look as if they have very big noses. As their faces grow, their noses assume normal proportions.

First Physical Examination

The first physical examination of a newborn will include inspection of the genitals, anal area, back, and extremities to make sure that all the excretory openings are open, that there are no obvious skeletal defects, and that the external sexual organs are present.

The infant's *state of arousal* is noted at birth, as this will have a bearing on the baby's ability to respond to the environment. The state of arousal tends to have an important reciprocal effect, since mothers tend to be more responsive to alert babies. Initial possibilities for response can be classified into several kinds of reflexes (Table 4–6).

Other reflexes have an unknown purpose. These include those elicited by touch

TABLE 4–6 REFLEXES PRESENT IN THE NEWBORN

Reflex	Purpose	Response
Rooting	Survival	Searching for a nipple
Startle	Adaptation	Jumping or withdrawal movement
Swimming	Adaptation, survival	Swimming motions when placed on firm surface
Creeping	Competency	Creeping when placed on hard surface when very young
Flexion	Competency	Same as above
Grasping	Competency	Firm holding on fingers; ability to "hang on"

stimuli. According to Newman and Newman (1978), "Reflexes provide the starting point for making contact with the environment."

Breastfeeding and Bottle Feeding

Milk Production.   As soon as the baby is born, the mother's breasts start producing milk (contrary to the myth that milk "comes in" 3 days after birth). The practice of not letting the baby nurse for the first 12 to 16 hours after birth, the limiting of nursing to 5 minutes on a side to prevent sore nipples, and the adherence to a rigid feeding schedule all combine to produce overflowing, hard breasts with nipples that are difficult for the baby to grasp. When the newborn cannot grasp the whole areola around the nipple, the baby will suck and chew only on the nipple, causing it to become painful and cracked.

Babies can start to nurse immediately at birth, provided they are not groggy from absorbing too much medication during labor and delivery. This is another reason to use as little medication as possible during delivery. Babies who have other physical problems and are in special care nurseries might not be able to nurse immediately. However, because breast milk is easier for most babies to digest, even mothers whose premature babies have to stay in the hospital for prolonged periods of time are urged to come into the hospital to nurse them at regular intervals. Mothers are also encouraged to pump their breasts and bring the milk into the hospital, if they are unable to come in themselves. When the baby is ready to go home, the mother's milk supply has been well established and the baby can start nursing.

The nursing process requires two things—the production of milk by the mother, and the getting of that milk by the baby. It is a marvelous system. Although milk is made automatically in response to sucking, the breasts need to be emptied at each feeding to restore the supply. Nature has provided the mechanism to do both.

A *let-down reflex* is triggered by the pituitary or "master" gland, which produces a hormone called *oxytocin*. This hormone is secreted in response to the baby's sucking. As the baby sucks, he compresses the area around the nipple and the large sinuses or ducts around it. In response to the sensations received by the mother when her infant sucks, cells called "basket cells"—which are around the duct walls—contract, the little ducts in the breasts are compressed, the big ducts widen, the milk is pushed out with considerable force into the main sinuses under the nipple, and milk flows out. Mothers report feeling the let-down reflex in response to the baby's crying; thus, the reflex is actually conditioned to occur. Sometimes the milk is so profuse that the nursing baby may sputter and choke and have to stop feeding to catch a breath.

The let-down reflex is absolutely necessary for the best nourishment of the baby, for although a baby can get about one third of the milk without the reflex, the highest fat content of the milk is available only when the reflex is operating. The last bit of milk is the richest, and since 50 per cent of the calories in milk come from the fat, the baby will not be satisfied unless he gets this rich milk. It is interesting to note that the first milk of a feeding is thin and bluish and the last bit is creamy and white from the fat.

Difficulties in Nursing. There are many reasons why a mother who wants to nurse might not have a good let-down reflex. If she is tired, tense, overworked with other children, embarrassed about nursing, or anxious about how much the baby is getting or how long he is nursing on a side, the hormone that causes the reflex is not triggered by the pituitary gland. Subtle messages by physicians and hospital personnel that breast-feeding is somehow inappropriate will all have a negative impact on the reflex mechanism.

If the breasts get overfilled and the baby cannot grasp the whole area around the nipple to nurse, milk may pool in the breast and the chance of infection sets in; the nipples may also crack. New mothers must be made aware of the need to get lots of rest, to nurse in a quiet place, to plan the restructuring of household tasks, to get help with other children, and to develop a relaxed attitude about the whole process.

The ability to nurse has little to do with breast size. It depends on the mother's general body growth. If the hormones are in balance and the woman has had a normal body response to hormonal influences, then she can nurse. What prevents women from being "able" to nurse are complex cultural and emotional factors. Women whose physicians have not taken care of many nursing mothers are sometimes subtly urged to bottle feed. Mothers whose own mothers did not nurse are less likely to nurse. Women who feel uncomfortable about exposing their breasts or have husbands who feel embarrassed about their wives nursing will get the message that it is not appropriate to nurse.

There are always mothers who do not or cannot breast feed. Some must go back to work soon after delivery and cannot arrange an easy schedule for feeding. Some teenage mothers will be going back to school and will have to place their infants in a day care

Breastfeeding has become recognized as beneficial for both mother and child.

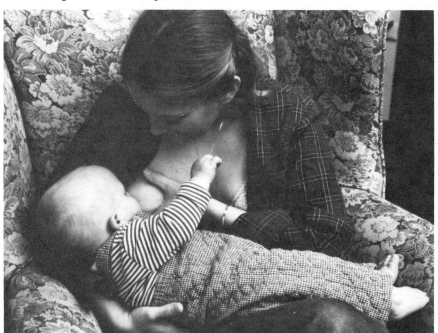

Judith Kruger Michalik

center. These mothers can have emotional contact with the baby through bottle feeding, just as with breastfeeding. The important aspect is to hold, touch, and rock the baby and to relax. When held close to be fed, babies feel secure and nurtured. Mothers should not prop a bottle when feeding the baby. Babies cannot control the rate of flow of the formula and might choke. Babies need to be held. They associate feeding with security, warmth, and comfort.

Infant Formulas. About 30 years ago, many mothers in the developed countries switched from breastfeeding to bottle feeding. Much time and energy were spent sterilizing bottles, making and then altering formulas, adjusting nipples, and making the middle-of-the-night run to the refrigerator. Later, companies developed prepared infant formulas, thus freeing mothers from this task. So persuasive were the manufacturers of prepared infant formulas in extolling their virtues, that mothers in poorer, less economically developed countries also frequently became convinced that bottle feeding was the fashionable, modern, and correct thing to do. Because of the unavailability of refrigeration and poor sanitation, more and more babies developed diarrhea, became dehydrated and malnourished, and, as a result, died. The connection between the increasing use of these formulas, together with the use of inadequately cleaned and inadequately refrigerated bottles of milk, and the subsequent intestinal infections was gradually understood (Pryor, 1974). This new information precipitated a campaign urging mothers in these countries to go back to breastfeeding. A concerted effort on the part of many women all over the

TABLE 4–7 NUTRITIONAL COMPONENTS OF MILK

Cow's Milk	Human Milk
Protein	
Twice as much as in human milk; milk must be diluted; produces large curds	Less protein, small curds that are easy to digest
Fewer amino acids	More amino acids, especially in first milk (colostrum)
Fifty per cent of protein excreted	All protein used; less total volume needed to meet dietary requirements
Fat	
High in saturated fats	Low in saturated fats
Diluted cow's milk has half the amount of fat of human milk	All fat available
Sugar	
Low in sugar; carbohydrates have to be added	Twice as much sugar
Less lactose; means more alkaline intestinal medium	Mostly lactose; helps in the absorption of calcium; more lactose means more acid intestinal medium and less risk of bacterial infection
Vitamins	
Few; some may be lost when formula is heated or sterilized; supplementary drops needed	Two to ten times as much essential vitamins as cow's milk
Iron	
More iron available	Less iron available; infant may need supplemental iron if mother is anemic; more readily available to the baby; digested easily
Immunity Factors	
Provide no immunity against disease	Provide many antibodies against viral diseases; particularly found in colostrum

world was made to encourage the manufacturers of the formulas to stop advertising and distributing them in less developed countries. A boycott of all products produced by the makers of the formulas ensued, with noticeable results for a brief period of time. Although it is difficult to predict the long-term effect of these pressures, it is an example of the power that consumers have in the marketplace. In this case, it was the concern of women for childbearing women around the world. The United Nations has formally protested against the aggressive promotion of infant formulas in countries where breastfeeding is more suitable economically.

Within the last several years, there has been a dramatic shift back to breastfeeding in the United States. Physicians have begun to recognize its advantages for both mother and baby and are more supportive and willing to help the mother over the rough spots that are inevitable when she is starting to nurse. A nutritional comparison of breast milk and cow's milk is shown in Table 4–7.

Bonding

The first few moments after birth are very important for the mother and baby. The uterus must contract to prevent further bleeding. It is common for the mother to be given a drug called *synthetic oxytocin* to facilitate these contractions. Sometimes, the

Contact between mother and baby is established very early and affects the infant's ability to respond throughout life.

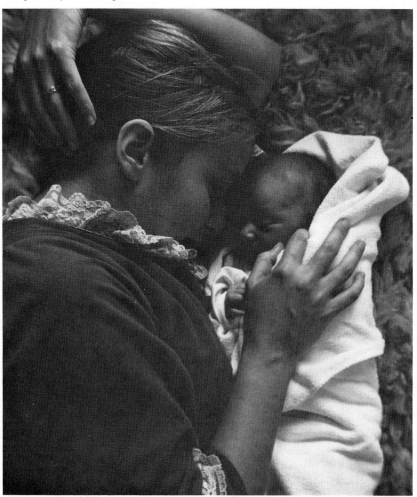

Judith Kruger Michalik

baby, if alert, will be given to the mother to nurse. The sucking action causes the natural secretion of oxytocin. This initial contact with her newborn is an important first step in establishing a good relationship.

We call this first relationship *bonding*. It is an almost indescribable, almost physical sensation to protect, nurture, and cherish the young. We believe it is as old as mammalian life itself. It is easy to see that if a mother is asleep, is heavily anesthetized or has had a cesarean section, she is less likely to be alert enough to participate in these first few moments. This does not mean that there will be no "bonding." It does mean that every effort must be made to enable the mother to have physical contact with her baby as soon as possible. For this reason, mothers are even encouraged to take care of their premature infants in the nursery.

Infant Responsiveness. Of particular interest is the recent knowledge that very young babies are capable of many responses that once were thought to apply only to older infants. Harth and Campos (1977) found that infants can track and follow movements at birth; they can differentiate colors, shapes, and familiar faces at 1 month, and by 2 months they can discriminate between flat and three-dimensional objects. In fact, some studies indicate that fetuses can "see" *in utero* if the mother stands in the bright sunlight.

Babies hear at birth, but because their ears may be filled with fluid that takes several days to be absorbed, they might not even respond to loud noises. First-time mothers are likely to be concerned by this, and it is helpful to her if questions are asked about the infant's behavior and response to stimuli, together with an explanation of what is happening. By 2 months, some babies are even responding to different syllables.

McChuish and Mills (1974) have noticed what they term "wariness" behavior in neonates as young as 4 weeks. Folk history describes the suspiciousness of strangers that occurs around 9 to 13 months. However, many mothers report babies who cry when picked up by a stranger as early as 4 months.

Because we now know much more about newborn potential and responsiveness, anyone working in a nursery for newborns should try to find the time to sit and rock and sing to new babies. Every nursery should have a rocking chair. It might also be suggested to parents that those midnight feedings at home are a lot more tolerable in a rocking chair.

Maternal Responsiveness. The advent of "rooming-in," the situation in which mothers and fathers take care of their babies in their own rooms within the hospital, either full time or just during the day, has increased the opportunities for more parent–infant interaction. These exchanges also become good observational experiences for hospital personnel. It is important to be alert for strained interactions, lack of responsiveness, tension, or depression, any of which could be indications of some current or potential difficulty in the bonding process.

Bonding, as we just described, is defined as "anything that binds or fastens; a uniting force; a tie or link; a binding covenant, obligation, or promise." In many ways, the bonding between mother and child fits all the above definitions, for the inner sense that we are indeed linked to, and obligated to protect and sustain, our infants becomes the force that enables infants to thrive. If the possibility of difficulty is noticed, it is essential to provide nonjudgmental support and encourage more frequent contact between the two.

Osofsky (1976) studied infant and maternal responsiveness as a way of determining interactional styles. In her study, 134 mothers and newborn babies were randomly sampled from the population born at Temple University Hospital in Philadelphia between September 1973 and June 1974. The patients were exclusively nonwhite and from a lower socioeconomic population. The infants, between 2 and 4 days old when included in the study, consisted of 73 boys and 61 girls. Ages of the mothers in the sample ranged from 13 to 37, with an average age of 19.9.

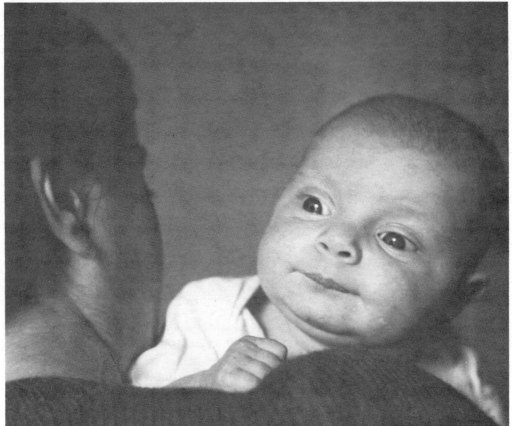

Wariness behavior may be evident as early as four months.

Leonard Hassol

The first observations were done for 15 minutes during feedings. All the babies were bottle fed. The mothers' behaviors that were rated were attentiveness, general sensitivity, frequency and quality of voice, eye contact, touch stimuli, and facial movement. Infant behaviors rated were alertness and changes in alertness, eye contact with the mother, and responsiveness to voice, eye, and touch stimuli.

The second observations (also 15 minutes) were done 1½ to 2 hours after the feeding. Babies were awakened and given to their mothers. Most babies were moderately alert at this time. The mothers were then asked to present a variety of stimuli to their babies, given some suggestions on how to go about this, and observed. Stimuli included shaking rattles at the baby, looking closely at the baby, and talking to and cuddling the infant.

Results showed that the mother–infant interactional style is established very early in life. Both mothers and babies contribute to this patterning. Babies consistently demonstrate responsive behavior toward mothers who stimulate them a great deal. Babies who registered a bit lower on the 5-minute Apgar scale tended to be less alert and responsive, eliciting less responsiveness from their mothers.

This evidence points to the necessity of helping mothers react to their babies even when the babies are not too responsive initially. Because persistent ways of dealing with infants start very early in life and have implications for many future interactions, assisting and encouraging the mother at this time are vitally important.

Weight Gain and Bonding. Other studies have also focused on the issues of bonding and early interactions. Even weight gain in infants appears to be a function not only of nutritional intake but also of the mother's behavior during feeding. Pollett and colleagues (1978) indicate that the behaviors of both mother and baby are predictors of weight gain during the first month. Their findings indicate that heavier babies tended to be more vigorous suckers. Mothers felt more competent and comfortable handling them. Those competent feelings seemed to be transmitted by "body language" to the baby. The babies then gained more rapidly.

It is possible that small babies might need help to establish vigorous feeding patterns. Mothers may have to be taught to respond appropriately to their small infants. It is not easy to accomplish this. Mothers frequently leave the hospital within 72 hours after delivery, having had little time to regain strength, to establish successful feeding patterns, and to learn how to handle their babies. Nor are there many grandmothers waiting at the front door for the new arrival any more. The support systems that were available "in the old days," when mothers spent a week in the hospital and then went home, are gone. We rarely see a baby nurse walking down the street wheeling a carriage. And yet, we expect new mothers to manage; to take care of other children, to be successful nursers, to develop positive feelings about their new babies, and to reestablish contact with a husband who might be feeling left out.

It is not hard to understand why so many new mothers feel overwhelmed and tired and irritable and have a difficult time "reading" their babies' signals. Babies cannot recognize a connection between their own signals and maternal reactions. It is the mother's response to these signals and the way in which she modifies her behavior that become vital. We now know that babies even recognize the smell of their own mother's breast milk as early as 6 to 10 days (MacFarlane, 1975). Other infants as young as 1 week have shown distress when fed by a mother wearing a surgical mask; they responded by avoiding eye contact, feeding poorly, and developing disruptive sleep cycles.

Sleep Cycles and Bonding. Newborns organize their sleep cycles more readily if exposed to a single caregiver. Rooming-in babies establish a day/night routine much more readily than babies in a traditional nursery who are cared for by many people on a more rigid 4-hour schedule (MacFarlane, 1975). When a caregiver responds to a crying infant within 90 seconds, the crying tends to cease within 5 seconds. If the caregiver waits more than a minute to respond, it requires an average of 50 seconds to quiet the baby (Losoff et al., 1977). Mothers and fathers need to know that it is important to comfort a crying infant even though many hours of holding and rocking may be required.

Child Abuse Potential and Bonding. Nursing personnel on a maternity floor have another important observational function. They must become aware of the possible implications for future child abuse, based on maternal behavior in the labor and delivery room.

Gray and co-workers (1976) studied 350 mothers at Colorado General Hospital in Denver. The babies of these mothers were all full-term infants who did not need any intensive care following birth. The first part of the two-part study included a screening procedure that scored parents for factors that might indicate later abuse. The second part studied the effectiveness of an intervention program designed to prevent abuse.

Parents were interviewed before the birth of their child and asked about their feelings toward the pregnancy, their expectations about the unborn child, and so forth. The investigators were particularly interested in such things as concern over the sex of the baby, pressure that the presence of a baby might put on an overburdened family, support available from relatives, family background (with particular attention to any history of parental abuse or neglect), living conditions, and appropriateness of planning for the baby.

The next observations were made during labor and delivery. Nurses were asked to observe four things: How the mother looked at the new baby, what she said, what she did, and the father's reaction. Again, notations were made of inappropriate or hostile comments. Eventually, 100 mothers were selected as being a "high risk," and 50 mothers were controls. All the high-risk mothers received routine interventions, such as well-baby clinic care, immunizations for the child, and other general care. In addition, 50 of these high-risk mothers received services organized to provide them more contact, more frequent clinic visitis, and more frequent telephone contact with a pediatrician, as well as home visits by a public health nurse.

The physician assigned to the baby in the nursery remained the primary physician, seeing the baby at all follow-up clinic visitis. The physician also monitored other aspects of family life, interceding with other agencies when necessary. When the babies were between 17 and 35 months of age, a random sample of the intervention, nonintervention, and control families were visited. Interactions between mother and child were observed. Investigators also obtained all child abuse reports filed with the local reporting registry.

Eight of the high-risk children had been reported as abused; none of the control group were. In the high-risk intervention group, there were no hospital admissions. In the high-risk, nonintervention group, there were five admissions for serious injuries. Although this intervention did not change parenting behavior, it did prevent serious injury to the child.

Child Abuse and Infant Health.   Hansen and associates (1977) discuss another aspect of potential difficulty. They studied low-birth-weight babies and the mother–child relationship. The study was done with children who had been separated from their mothers at birth as a result of low birth weight or sometimes for relatively minor problems. These infants who did not go home with their mothers were compared with other low-birth-weight babies who did go home. The follow-up, done when the children were 7 years old, showed that 18 of the 23 children in the first group had a variety of somatic symptoms ranging from sleep disturbances to gastrointestinal problems. In comparison, only 7 of the 23 children in the second group were identified as having problems. Mothers in the first group reported that their children were hard to manage. They also reported difficult pregnancies and deliveries, and they felt less able to cope.

This finding is important because we know that a higher proportion of premature, low-birth-weight babies become abused or neglected. These difficult-to-manage, frequently sickly, hard-to-comfort babies can cause great frustration and may require time-consuming care. They do not provide the new mother with the same sense of competence that a placid, healthy baby does. Observations of the interactions between mother and baby therefore take on more meaning. Members of health care teams need to be encouraged to trust their own trained instincts as an accurate barometer of difficulty and to act on these instincts.

Mothers also need to know ranges of normal behavior, as well as sleeping and eating patterns of the newborn. They will be getting advice from many friends and relatives and will be anxious to do everything perfectly. There is no "perfect" way, but new mothers can be reassured by remembering and being reminded that their own mothers were not perfect. Babies have their own timetables, which change from day to day. They eat when hungry, can be bathed any time it is convenient, will not suffer if the bath is skipped on occasion, and will have wakeful periods that differ from week to week. One new mother, anxious about sponge-bathing her new baby on a dressing table, put a heavy mat and clean towel on the floor and bathed the baby in this fashion until she felt more competent. Her own mother was available to help with the first real bath in a tub. The most important message is that babies need to be held, talked to, rocked, and, most of all, enjoyed!

Infants

The period of time between 1 month and 1 year is generally thought of as infancy. Staff members of a well-baby clinic may have only sporadic contact with an infant because not all mothers bring their children back on a regular basis. The total physical and developmental progress of that baby must be assessed from information offered by the mother, as well as on the basis of the health worker's observations of the infant.

Health Assessment

In many clinics, the policy is to have the infant checked every month for the first 6 months, every other month until the baby is 1 year old, and then every 6 months for the next year or two. Many mothers do not have access to a well-baby clinic and will utilize hospital emergency facilities only when the baby is ill. All this makes the task of establishing a good relationship with the mother difficult. The information received by the staff will be filtered through feelings and perceptions that the mother has about how babies grow, the role of the hospital or clinic personnel, and her own feelings concerning her competency. During the introductions, the mother should be told what kinds of information clinic staff members are interested in obtaining. The baby's name should always be used. If nurses do not take the time to learn the baby's name, the message is clear. That baby is just another "job" in a busy day. The nurse interacts with many mothers, some younger than the staff, who may feel uncomfortable in an institutional setting, as well as others who may have had many babies and to whom a clinic visit is not a top priority issue.

Although the physician is responsible for examining the infant, an understanding of the examination by the nurse helps in explaining to the mother what will happen. The examination covers all aspects of development from weight and height to the baby's responsiveness, together with eating and sleeping patterns.

Most babies double their birth weight by 6 months and triple it by a year.

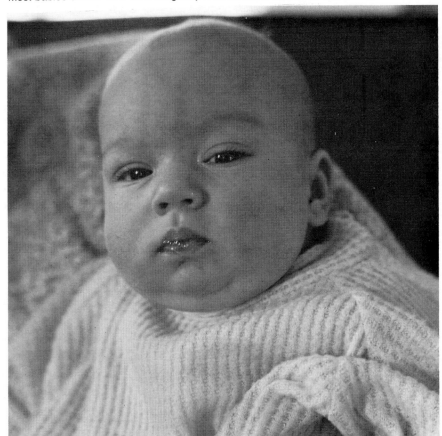

Judith Kruger Michalik

The actual amount of weight gained is not as important as its relation to birth weight. A baby who is not gaining well will be checked for gastrointestinal problems. Some babies suffer from a condition called "failure to thrive." Babies who do not thrive are often ones whose emotional and nurturing needs are not being met. They may be left alone for long periods of time, are not held warmly and closely, have their bottles propped for feedings, and may appear depressed, wan, and thin. Because most babies who display these signs have no physical abnormalities, the finding of a listless, deprived-looking child may signal that the infant is being neglected. A much more detailed account of family life will probably be requested, and information concerning family supports, whether the mother is working, the mother's feelings toward the baby, and any other potentially stressful situation will be explored.

Nutrition

Most babies double their birth weight by 6 months and triple it by a year. They increase in length by about 50 per cent in 6 months. The head grows so rapidly that by 1 year the brain is two thirds its adult size (Pillitteri, 1977). Babies should be weighed and measured nude.

For chubby babies with protruding abdomens, those slack abdominal muscles tighten up once the baby is on the run and need not cause concern. Mothers are being encouraged to postpone the start of feeding solid foods for several months and to nurse or use specially prepared formulas exclusively, which are easy for infants to digest. The first solid food is usually a bland cereal. Mothers should be taught to avoid baby foods that contain salt or sugar. New foods are added slowly, one at a time, both to allow the infant to get used to the new taste and to determine whether the baby has developed any allergic reaction to it. By the time of the first birthday, the infant can be eating solid foods, ground up or chopped in small pieces.

Immunization

At 2 months of age, normal children will be placed on an immunization schedule to protect them from a variety of childhood diseases such as diphtheria, tetanus, whooping cough, measles, mumps, poliomyelitis, and German measles. These immunizations and boosters will be repeated at various ages well into late childhood (Table 4–8). The vaccination for smallpox has been eliminated because the disease has been eradicated (Spock, 1974). Some children may run a slight fever and become fussy after an inoculation. The physician may prescribe a medication to keep the fever down. These procedures, and, in fact, vaccinations in general, may be resisted by people from other countries and cultures where preventive medicine is not practiced and where there may be a bias against giving "medicine" to supposedly well babies.

Day-Care Programs

In our economically stressed society, more mothers are returning to work within months of giving birth. Developing a resource list of good, supervised, home-centered day-care facilities might be an exceedingly helpful function for a well-baby clinic. Mothers need to be encouraged to talk about their feelings concerning the need to put their baby into a day-care center. Many mothers feel guilty about leaving a baby with someone other than a family member. State regulations should be checked so that the rules under which they operate can be discussed. Many home-based centers must have trained and certified workers and are regularly inspected. Many centers are flexible enough to allow parents to bring a baby occasionally or at different times during the day, depending on the parents' schedule. A checklist of items that mothers should look for in a day-care center could be developed by the clinic and should include the personality qualifications for a

TABLE 4–8 IMMUNIZATION SCHEDULE

Age	Inoculation	Booster	Protects against
2 months	DPT*	15–18 months 4–6 years	Diphtheria, whooping cough, tetanus
	Oral Sabin vaccine	18 months 4–5 years	Poliomyelitis
4 months	DPT Oral poliomyelitis vaccine		
6 months	DPT Oral poliomyelitis vaccine		
1 year	Measles vaccine Mumps vaccine German measles vaccine		Measles Mumps German measles
Booster Schedule			
15 months	DPT		
18 months	Oral poliomyelitis vaccine		
4–5 years	DPT Oral poliomyelitis vaccine		
15 years	DPT		

*Diphtheria-pertussis-tetanus (vaccine).

loving, caring person-in-charge, physical facilities, equipment, access to the outdoors with playground equipment, and caretaker–infant ratios. There are some studies that have been undertaken to determine the consequences of day care for an infant and that might be reassuring for a working mother to know about.

Newman and Newman (1978) found that, with a small number of caregivers (most often the case in a home-based center), a young infant was able to distinguish between them and learn the unique characteristics of each. The baby could then predict responses from each of these people. Many older infants were not distressed by many faces, enjoyed stimulation, and showed a highly developed social sense from being in contact with many adults. Thus, some babies, it appears, may do well in a setting that has several "mothers," lots of children, and more activity.

Some day-care centers that accept small infants are connected with large companies and are situated on the premises, enabling mothers to see and care for their children during the workday. These centers are likely to have highly trained staff and to adhere to the state requirements for staff–child ratios as well as space requirements. Day-care centers can also become social and outreach networks for families, providing assistance in other aspects of life.

Changing Roles in Parenthood

Some health care team members may be pleasantly surprised to find themselves explaining feeding schedules, immunizations, and diaper rash to fathers instead of mothers. A father may be ill at ease with his new, nontraditional role. If both parents are working, his might be the easiest schedule to work around, but he might not think that it is his job to dress, transport, and manage this squirming bundle. Sometimes it is the father who is unemployed, and this could add to his discomfort in not being the primary wage earner. On the other hand, these days, the father serving as primary caregiver may be absolutely delighted with himself and his new role. In some families, couples deliberately arrange their work schedules so that one parent is home with the baby at all times, thus avoiding the necessity of day care. Whatever the reason for his being at the clinic, a father needs to know that others regard him as an important part of his baby's life and development. What may have started out as a reluctant duty could turn into a positive experience, as the father realizes the complexity of childrearing and the importance of developing a close relationship with his baby. By assuming some of the work of child maintenance, he hopefully is also indicating to his wife that he supports the other dimensions of her life and the effort and energy she expends by both working and childrearing.

Assuming these new roles may not be easy for men or women. Traditionally, men have been socialized to leave baby raising to the mother. Men have also been taken care of by women, and that expectation often continues into marriage and parenthood; the man may assume that his wife will take care of him, clean his house, and raise his babies while he brings in the money. When events conspire to disrupt this lifestyle, there may be friction and tension in the family. Both parents can be encouraged to share their concerns and possibly signal potential trouble spots ahead for their own relationship and their relationship with their baby.

REFERENCES

Apgar, V., et al.: Evaluation of the newborn infant, second report. *Journal of the American Medical Association*, 168:1985, 1953.

Boston Women's Health Book Collective: *Our Bodies, Ourselves* (rev. ed.) New York: Simon and Schuster, 1979.

Brewer, T., Brewer, C.: *What Every Pregnant Woman Should Know: The Truth About Diet and Drugs in Pregnancy.* New York: Random House, 1977.

Chapman, M., Chapman, J.: *Behavior and Health Care: A Humanistic Helping Process.* St. Louis: C. V. Mosby Company, 1975.

Dick-Read, G.: *Childbirth Without Fear.* London: W. Heineman Ltd., 1968.

DiMasico, R., Gregori, C., Breen, J.: Smoking and pregnancy. *Journal of the Medical Society of New Jersey*, 75(2):124–135, 1978.

Falicov, C. T.: Sexual adjustment during pregnancy and postpartum. *American Journal of Obstetrics and Gynecology*, 117(991):345–352, 1973.

Ferreira, A. J.: The pregnant woman's emotional attitude and its reflection upon the newborn. *American Journal of Orthopsychiatry*, 30:553–561, 1960.

Fielding, J.: The pregnant smoker. *American Journal of Public Health*, 68(9):833–835, 1978a.

Fielding, J.: The pregnant drinker. *American Journal of Public Health*, 68(9):836–838, 1978b.

Flowers, C., Littlejohn, T., Wells, H.: Pharmacologic and hypnotic analgesia. *Obstetrics and Gynecology*, 16(210):210–212, 1960.

Gaskin, I.: *Spiritual Midwifery.* Tenn. The Book Publishing Company, 1978.

Gray, J., Cutler, C., Dean, J., Kempe, C. H.: Perinatal assessment of mother–baby interaction. In Helfer, R., Kempe, C. (eds.): *Child Abuse and Neglect* (vol 1.). Cambridge, Mass. Ballinger Publishing Company, 1976.

Hansen, L., et al.: Mother–child relationship in low birth weight. *Child care, health and development*, 3(2):92–103, 1977.

Harth, M., Campos, J.: Human infancy. *Annual Review of Psychology*, 28:251–293, 1977.

Healthy People: The Surgeon General's Report on Health Promotion and Disease Promotion. Background papers, 1979, US DHEW/Public Health Service, DHEW PHS 79-55071A.

Hinkers, H.: The influence of alcohol on the fetus. *Journal of Perinatal Medicine*, 6:3–10, 1978.

Jones, K., Smith, D., Ulleland, C., et al.: Pattern of malformation in offspring of chronic alcoholic mothers. *Lancet*, 1:977–998, 1973.

Josiah Macy Foundation: *The Midwife in the United States.* New York, 1968.

Leboyer, F.: Childbirth Without Violence. New York; Knopf, 1975.

Lewis, P.: Drugs, the bitter pill in pregnancy: Adverse effects on the developing brain. *Nursing Mirror*, 47(14):38–39, 1978.

Losoff, B., et al.: The mother–newborn relationship— limits of adaptability. *Journal of Pediatrics*, 91(1):1–12, 1977.

MacFarlane, A.: Olfaction in the development of social preference in the human neonate-parent-child interaction. *CIBA Foundation Symposium 33.* Amsterdam: Elsevier Publishing Company, 1975.

MacFarlane, A.: *The Psychology of Childbirth.* Cambridge, Mass.: Harvard University Press, 1977.

Macy, J.: Foundation. *The Midwife in the United States.* New York: Josiah Macy Foundation, 1968.

Masters, W., Johnson, V.: *Human Sexual Response.* Boston: Little, Brown & Company, 1966.

McCauley, C.: *Pregnancy After 35.* New York: E. P. Dutton, 1976.

McChuish, E., Mills, U.: Recognition of mother's voice in early infancy. *Nature*, 252:123–124, 1974.

Miller, A., Brooten, D.: *The Childbearing Family: A Nursing Perspective*, Boston: Little, Brown & Company, 1977.

Moore, M.: *Realities in Childbirth.* Philadelphia: W. B. Saunders Company, 1978.

Newman, B., Newman, P.: *Infancy and Childhood.* New York: John Wiley & Sons, 1978.

Osofsky, J.: Neonatal characteristics and mother-infant interactions in two observational situations. *Child Development*, 47:1138–1147, 1976.

Pillitteri, A. R. N.: *Nursing Care of the Growing Family.* Boston: Little, Brown & Company, 1977.

Piran, B.: Smoking during pregnancy. *Obstetrics and Gynecology Survey.* 33:1–13, 1978.

Pollett, E., Gilmore, M., Valcarcie, M.: Early mother–infant interaction and somatic growth. *Early Human Development*, 1(4):325–336, 1978.

Pryor, K.: *Nursing Your Baby*. New York: Harper & Row, 1974.

Rossett, H. Ouelette, E., Weiner, L.: A pilot prospective study of the fetal alcohol syndrome at Boston City Hospital. *Annals of the New York Academy of Science*, 273,115–122, 1976.

Sanders, R., James, A. (ed.): *Ultrasonics in Obstetrics and Gynecology*. New York: Appleton-Century/Crofts, 1977.

Scanlon, J.: Obstetric anesthesia as a neonatal risk factor in normal labor and delivery. *Clinics in Perinatology*, 1(2):465–482, 1974.

Smith, D., Stenchever, M.: Prenatal life and the pregnant woman. In *The Biologic Ages of Man*. Philadelphia: W. B. Saunders Company, 1978.

Solberg, D., Butler, J., Wagner, N.: Sexual behavior in pregnancy. *The New England Journal of Medicine*, 288(2):1098–1099, 1973.

Spert, M.: *Midwifery in Retrospect: The Midwife in the United States*. New York: Josiah Macy Foundation, 1968.

Spock, B.: *Baby and Child Care*. New York: Simon and Schuster, 1974.

Stevens, Cheryl J.: The fetal alcohol syndrome: Cause for concern. *Maternal Child Nursing*, Vol. 6, July/August 1981, p. 251.

Streissguth, A.: The fetal alcohol syndrome: An epidemiological perspective. *American Journal of Epidemiology*, 107:467–478, 1978.

Zabriskie, J.: Effect of cigarette smoking during pregnancy. *Journal of Obstetrics and Gynecology*, 21(405):734–735, 1963.

THE TODDLER:
Autonomy

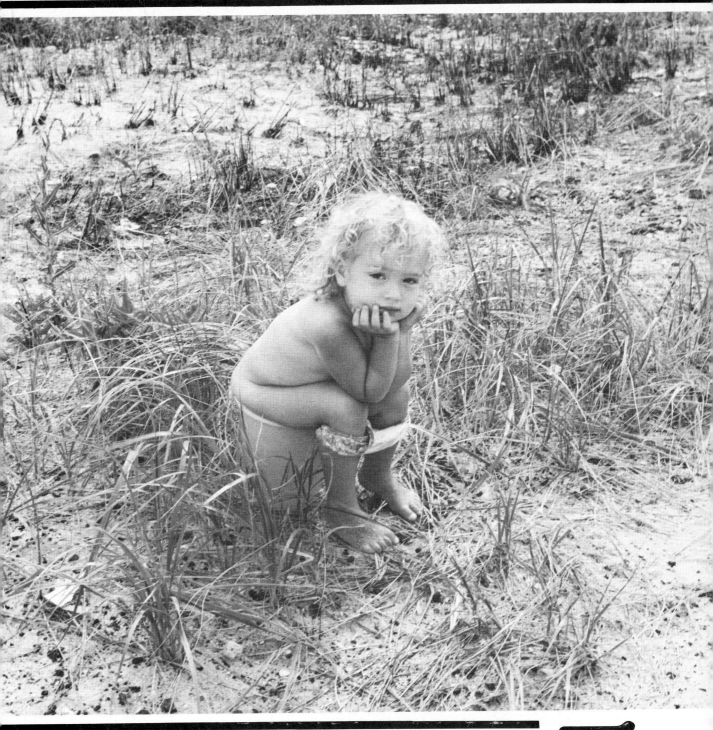

CHAPTER 5

There are many who do not regard the months between the time the infant begins to walk and the time of readiness for a typical nursery school (at age 3) as a distinct age period. Though some abilities beyond infancy are present (language, upright locomotion), the toddler still does not attain the self-assured competencies of the preschool child.

The age tends to be characterized by a kind of cherubic appearance, which, in fact, was the model for the dimpled baby angels of medieval art. The ties to infancy are still apparent; early in the period, if you touch the sleeping child gently near the mouth, it is possible to stimulate the old sucking response for a few seconds, even though the child has probably been getting liquids from a cup for a number of months.

The toddler's approach to objects will be more like that of a younger than an older child—the whole object tends to be used, first with banging, swinging, shaking, or waving. After the overall inspection is done, it may be possible for the toddler to settle down to pounding in the dowels, fitting the boxes together, or putting the disks on the ring, sometimes more haphazardly than parents might wish. But this is still a time for more global occupations; details will come later. Like the infant, the young toddler also understands more language than can be produced at this time.

That limitation is going to change, however, into one of the dramatic accomplishments of this age period. The child becomes a competent user of language in what is likely the most remarkable intellectual accomplishment he or she will ever make. But more of that later.

COGNITIVE DEVELOPMENT

If the toddler is fortunate, the world of sights and sounds, touch, tastes, and smells will expand just slightly ahead of the developing cognitive ability to manage the new "inputs." The growth of intelligence involves understanding the events in one's world—matching what is sensed to the cognitive unit, which Piaget (1952) calls a *schema* (see Chapter 3).

At this age, the event must actually occur in the child's immediate world in order to afford any possibility of its being understood. Events in Europe or even in the neighboring household cannot yet be part of awareness. Furthermore, for the toddler, personal experience is the only means of encountering the world. Experiences are "processed," systematized, and ordered by being fitted into an existing schema; or an existing scheme is altered somewhat to enable a better "fit" by means of the twin processes of *assimilation* and *accommodation*, which were described in Chapter 3.

When stimuli are too complex or too overwhelming, the child is unable to process, and much that happens in the environment is thus "lost." On the other hand, if the environment is barren, the sensory information will be minimal and not conducive to building schemata; then later events may be "lost" owing to the lack of any cognitive structure to which they might be fitted.

The vastly increased mobility of the toddler, under ordinary circumstances, will bring many more sensory and motor possibilities within range. The child will still be living in the present, with a past that can be invoked sometimes by signaling events (a coat, for example, means "going outside," a meaning derived from the past) and a future that involves only a vague similarly derived anticipation. During this period, however, the child will begin to develop the use of language, a feat so enormous in importance that we will devote a special section to it. Ability to use words brings entire new dimensions to experience. A word expands the concept of object permanence; the word "daddy" makes it possible to refer to daddy even though he is not there. This is termed "symbolic" processing, the symbol representing or standing for the object or event. To "have" a word vastly extends the possibilities for intellectual growth. Words ultimately free us from the necessity, characteristic of the sensory-motor period, of having to experience every event. Words can bring events within reach that are not experienced personally, and words can convey those experiences to others.

Piaget called the new cognitive period, initiated and marked by the developing mastery of language, *preoperational*. It begins during the toddler years and covers all of early childhood right into the first few grades of elementary school (approximately 18 months to 7 years of age).

One of the delights for parents and observers of toddlers is the beginning of what is described by Piaget (1972) as *symbolic play* or, as we commonly think of it, "pretend" play. It occurs when the child uses one object as if it were something else. Piaget describes his daughter Jacqueline at age 15 months, laying her cheek on the fringed washcloth and putting her thumb in her mouth (as she always did when going to sleep on her fringed pillow), laughing delightedly all the while. A few days later, she used the tail of her donkey, which seemed to have reminded her of the fringe on her pillow, in the same way, laughing again as if to indicate that she knew it to be ludicrous (a word derived from the Latin for "play"). An elaboration of this kind of pretended play is called *deferred imitation*. It often takes the form of role playing. Sally observes mother tucking the new baby into the crib. Later that afternoon she tucks her dolly into its bed in careful imitation of mother's behavior.

But for all the seemingly advanced stage of cognition of the preoperational child (compared with the sensory-motor period of infancy), the thinking process is still extremely limited and rudimentary. It is characterized by a quality called *egocentrism*, which refers to a naive assumption that one's own perceptions are exactly the same as those obtained by everyone else. This assumption ought not to be confused with the notion of selfishness or being preoccupied with the self. Rather, for the young child, it reflects the view of the world confined to one's own surroundings with the self at the center. Later, the child will be capable of understanding that other people have their own vantage points and views; for now, however, the toddler confidently offers mother a lick on the old sucker that has been located in the snowsuit pocket, sure that she will have the same appreciation of it that he does.

This also accounts for the fact that toddlers (frequently) treat each other as things, crawling over or bumping into other children as if they were not there. Parents are often dismayed when their little ones refuse to "share;" not only do children seem to hang on to the coveted toy, looking like grim death, but in the bargain, they'll make overtures toward a toy that another child has. Though this may seem "selfish," remembering that the egocentric quality of thinking simply characterizes the incapability of taking anyone else's desires or rights into consideration places it in an "ages and stages" perspective.

One of the advantages that some understanding of Piagetian principles can offer is the lightening of a parent's concern that the child might remain forever asocial; the transition from egocentrism to more mature orientations will take place normally and naturally as the child's own development and experiences promote growth and change. Piaget tended to insist that planned intervention or instruction would not accomplish any real hastening of the progression, though he did not disregard the overall influence of environment.

LANGUAGE DEVELOPMENT

How do babies learn to speak their language? "Oh, that is easy," is the usual answer. "Babies listen to the talk around them and soon begin to imitate it."

The baby hears the language and begins to make sounds that resemble those heard. Sooner or later, something happens when a sound is produced. Baby says "da," and the long-trousered one turns himself inside out with excitement. The effect of this is not lost on baby, nor is the fact that saying "ba" causes mother to scurry and get the bottle. The sounds uttered by the baby obtain dramatic results, especially in the beginning, and that encourages further sound production. This explanation of language development involves a "learning theory," as offered by Harvard psychologist Dr. B. F. Skinner (1957). He suggests that language is acquired quite like other forms of learning: a response that obtains a result or effect tends to be repeated. When a "da" is followed by father's pleasure and approval and "ba" brings the bottle, the child is reinforced and will use the sounds again.

This explanation sounds sensible, but there are some problems with it. The first has to do with the enormous amount of learning represented by language acquisition. The child proceeds from a state of no speech production to something on the order of 1000 words in about 2 years (Dale, 1976). Even more telling, the child also learns grammatical rules from the beginning, for instance, saying "big car" rather than "car big." To reinforce every "proper" sound combination appropriately would be an impossible task and no parent could accomplish it.

Another explanation of language acquisition included the idea that rules of language are learned right along with the words. Dr. Noam Chomsky (1968) believes that human beings are biologically equipped to "process" the language they hear according to a kind of universal set of rules. This "deep structure" is thought to be shared by all languages, even though languages differ vastly in their "surface structure." Some support for this position is obtained from observations of children's early utterances, which are remarkably similar in the order of appearance of expressions no matter what language the child is speaking. For example, many of the first two-word sentences are describing actions ("car go") or locating and naming ("there ball"). Possession and quantitative modifiers appear early ("baby hat," "pretty dress," "big house"). Negation ("no wash") comes a little later (Slobin, 1971).

The Acquisition of Language

The order in which all children acquire their linguistic behavior seems to follow a fixed sequence, with only minor deviations, among children speaking any language. The earliest noncrying sounds made by a baby occur during contented times and tend to consist of cooing and long vowels or of gurgling noises of various kinds. At about age 6 months, the sounds become more varied, more repetitive, and much more frequent. This is called the *babbling phase*. Babies produce similar sound patterns across different language groups and cultures. All the basic sounds of every language are present in these early babblings. A relationship between amount of babbling and later vocabulary, intelligence, and attentiveness has been found for girls but not for boys (McCall and Kagan, 1967). The explanation for this has not been discovered. Some suggestions have been made that the advanced maturity of girls over boys enables their early verbal behavior to be a better predictor of later cognitive ability.

Another suggestion has been offered by a study (Moss, 1967) indicating that mothers spend more time talking to their infant daughters than to infant sons. Kagan (1971) also found a relationship between the amount of vocal play engaged in by mother and child and the amount of vocalization in which the infant engages. He compared American infants whose mothers spoke to them about 25 to 30 per cent of the time when they were wide awake with Guatemalan infants, who are typically not spoken to by their mothers (because the mothers feel that there isn't much value in speaking to an infant who cannot speak back). The difference in behavior of the infants was significantly apparent. American infants tend to spend about 25 per cent of their waking time in vocal activity, whereas Guatemalan babies spend about 7 per cent of the time vocalizing when awake.

Deaf babies and those raised in unstimulating orphanage environments are often deficient in the frequency of vocalizations and the variation of sounds, though the infants begin to vocalize at about the same time as hearing and home-reared babies. This phenomenon suggests that babbling is, at first, an innate response that thereafter can be modified—increased or decreased—depending upon how much environmental stimulation is received. Deaf babies hear neither their own sounds nor those of parents responding, whereas institutionalized infants may be unlikely to obtain the attention of caretakers; therefore, the babbling of these children does not proceed at the normal rate (Brodbeck and Irwin, 1946).

At about 10 months of age, the child is likely to use a first word. Before this, however, a certain amount of understanding has already transpired. This is evident when the child responds to simple commands or phrases, such as "Where is your nose?" "Pat a cake." "Go bye bye?" This is often called *passive language*. The child's own speech production is termed *active language*. Most children begin with single words that are requests, commands, or names of objects. The words stand for entire sentences and are termed *holophrases*. "Up" can mean "pick me up," "put it up there," or "it is up there," for example. "Broke" can mean the doll "is broken" or even "fix it," depending on the context. Verbs and nouns predominate in this vocabulary. Missing are the pronouns, such as "I," "we," "you." The fact that "no" is learned before "yes" may be a commentary on the words we use to admonish the wandering toddler. Many children— having been scolded with an emphatic "no! no!"— will solemnly reproach themselves while engaging in the forbidden activity.

Once the toddler acquires a basic stock of words, the next great revolution occurs as the child begins to combine words into two- and three-word sentences. Because a relatively small supply of words can be combined into a great number of ideas, this new progression vastly expands the possibilities for expression. This is the period of "cute sayings," which families treasure and repeat many times to the delight of the now older and more fluent child.

An issue that arises in this regard has to do with some folklore still being passed around. This has it that one must not speak "baby talk" to young children. Like most prescriptions for childrearing, it contains only a sand grain of truth, in that this notion might apply in the very special case of a parent who wished to retain a child in infant status. On the other hand, to attempt to speak to a small child as one would to another adult would be ridiculous.

There seems to be a common pattern of interaction with infants that is very different from behavior with older children or adults. "Baby talk" is only one aspect of this specific set of reactions, which includes a kind of "surprise" face, an exaggerated amount of head bobbing and shaking, and a special form of speech that consists of shortened sentences, simplified sentences, some nonsense sounds, and some sound transformations (pretty rabbit may become "pitty wabbit") (Ferguson, 1964). Early in the child's life, the mother is quite likely to hold "conversations" with baby and provide a pause for the imaginary answers. A feature of this kind of "dialogue" is that the timing is approximately what it would be if the interchange were actually taking place. For example:

> Are you my pretty baby?
> Yes, I am (imagined response).
> Yes, you are. You sure are.

Stern (1977), who has analyzed the exchange, suggests that this provides a kind of time frame for dialogue that the child will fit into later.

As the child begins to use two- and three-word sentences, the parent's sentences grow longer, forming combinations that the child will be using within the next year or so. The toddler's exchange is still short (*telegraphic*—because it omits all but the most crucial words in the sentence), but it maintains the word order and meaning.

Factors Affecting Language Development

The difference between middle-class children and those in lower socioeconomic classes with regard to language development is clear and troubling. Lower-class children score less well on all measures of language, including articulation, sound discrimination, vocabulary size, and sentence length. The differences appear as early as the second year (Lichtenberg and Norton, 1972).

A number of investigators have pointed to differences in the amount of speech to which the child is exposed (Nelson, 1973). Not only are children with advanced language development spoken to more often by the significant adults in their lives, but they are also likely to have had more experiences outside the home—outings and trips to the park, zoo, and supermarket—and mothers who are relatively uncritical and unintrusive. Children who watch a lot of television and who spend considerable time in the company of other children do not develop either vocabulary or grammatical competence.

Concern about language development and differences among children with regard to fluency, vocabulary size, and understanding stems from the fact that progress in school is significantly related to the child's language level. If language usage can be enhanced, the child's chances in school are tremendously augmented.

In the 1960s and early 1970s a number of programs were started that aimed at increasing children's language capabilities. Some of these attempted to teach mothers how to play with their babies and talk to them long before they would be able to reply. Others intervened directly, sending graduate students and social workers into the household to play with the baby. Still others adopted various means of teaching words and concepts to preschoolers in such programs as Head Start.

All of the programs have been less successful than the investigators hoped, but more successful then their detractors claimed. The major problem seems to be that learning language is not a 1- or 2-year project, even though the chief capabilities may be acquired during that time. However, children who demonstrate superior language ability tend to live in a superior language environment in which language is reinforced, reading is considered important and exciting, adults take time to engage children in conversation and listen to what the children have to say, and everyone expects the child to do well in school. It seems to be the combination of these factors, rather than language usage per se, that correlates with school success (Gordon, 1972).

But these are practical considerations of adults, in no way comprehended by the child who is learning to speak. Whether the child eventually learns an academically acceptable vocabulary or whether language usage remains on the level of the functional, dealing primarily with immediate needs, we need only reflect on the enormity of the task to obtain a hearty respect for the accomplishment at whatever level. If you were suddenly transported to a strange land and had to learn the language from the beginning, it is doubtful that you could obtain the fluency equal to that of an ordinary 3-year-old by the end of 2 years, even though you would have had the advantage of previous language experience to provide a model with regard to how words "go together" and how words are used. Remember, baby begins "from scratch," so that even the concept of a designation for plural, past tense of verbs, and prepositional forms must be acquired. It is very disconcerting to an adult attempting to master a new language to realize that even the young children of the land speak the language better.

Language in Animals

One of the most intriguing questions about language concerns the possibility of its use by other species. There is a good deal of evidence that animals communicate threats or fear to one another. It is known that honeybees inform other workers about the location of honey with a kind of wing-dance at the entrance to the hive. More recently, there has been interest in the more complex sound patterns of dolphins and whales (Frisch, 1967).

J. C. Lilly (1963) has suggested that dolphins can imitate human speech. He recorded sounds made by dolphins in response to his speech and used a tape recorder to play back the sounds at a slower speed. The noises then sounded much like the words Lilly had used. Jane Goodall (1963) reported that chimpanzees in the wild use a·rich and varied vocal and nonvocal communication; they have a great many different calls, each prompted by a different emotion, and these are understood by the others.

A remarkable group of investigators equipped some chimpanzees with several "unspoken" forms of the English language—unspoken because chimpanzees lack the vocal apparatus necessary to form audible words. One young female named Washoe was taught the American Sign Language (ASL), the hand signs used by the deaf. She acquired a substantial working vocabulary and, even more impressively, was able to generalize meaning. For example, after she had acquired the word "open" to refer to a door, Washoe used it for a drawer, a soda-pop bottle, and a faucet. After creating some flagrant mischief, she acknowledged that she had been naughty, signing "come-hug-love-sorry-sorry" (Gardner and Gardner, 1969, 1977).

Washoe was transferred from the University of Nevada, where she was trained, to the University of Oklahoma to join a small group of chimpanzees who are also being taught ASL. The research focuses on the kinds of interactions among chimpanzees who can use ASL. Of special interest is the question of whether the chimpanzees will teach their children to sign. There is no answer yet available, though the adults have been observed signing to each other (Fouts and Couch, 1976).

Another chimpanzee named Sarah learned the symbolic meaning attached to small plastic forms and was able to arrange these forms to communicate such simple phrases as "Mary give apple Sarah" (Premack, 1970). Koko, a gorilla, had learned more than 200 signs by the age of 4 years, according to her trainer at Stanford University (Patterson, 1977).

Though it should be noted that questions have been raised about the claims for the capabilities of these primates (Limber, 1977), there can be little doubt that the research opens up fascinating possibilities for studying acquisition and function of language. It is quite accurate to point out that none of the animals has begun to approach the accomplishment of an ordinary human 3-year-old with regard to language development, but there had been no expectation that the animals would approximate human language competence. On the other hand, when the group of Oklahoma chimpanzees was startled by a snake in their midst, most of them screamed with fear. Not Washoe, however. She signed "Come-come-hurry-hurry." Did her ability to "verbalize" help prevent the typical screeching that signals stress for chimpanzees? (Fouts and Couch, 1976).

AUTONOMY

Along with the expanding language capability, there arrives a new developmental task. The toddler has grown out of the passive, receptive infancy and has become, overnight as it were, a small adventuring dynamo. Leave her unattended for a few minutes and she is off, exploring: emptying the lower kitchen cupboards, unwinding the toilet tissue, diving into the wastebasket, and sampling from the puppy's dish.

The toddler has changed, and so has the environment. The doting adults who had been such loyal servants now begin to make demands. The child is likely to encounter "No! No!" upon making a shambles of the Sunday paper or creating interesting marks with mother's lipstick. The household schedule, which formerly revolved around the feeding and sleeping schedule of infancy, swings back to normal. The toddler must start to adapt to the family and its practices, rather than the reverse. The process of *socialization*—of training the child to live in society—has begun.

However, the child has actually changed from a receptive little being into a self-propelled person with definite, self-initiated desires and ideas. Now, building upon the earlier-established sense of trust, the toddler insistently asserts the right to make independent decisions: to come or not to come, to eat or push away the plate, to nap or remain awake, to use the potty or refuse, to give up the plaything or defiantly retain it. The stage is set for the development of the second important ingredient of the healthy personality, the quality Erikson terms *autonomy*—the sense of being someone who can decide for one's self, of standing on one's own two feet—a quality of sturdy, steadfast independence.

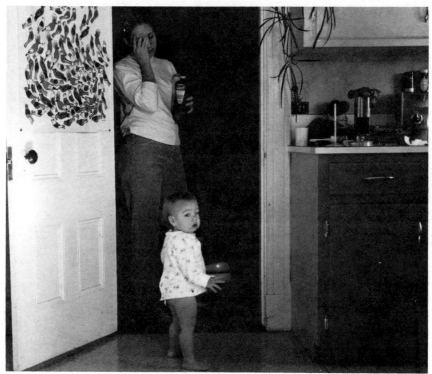

Judith Kruger Michalik

The toddler is a small adventuresome dynamo who can try the patience of any adult. Though toddlers need the freedom to "get into" things, they also need protection from the very real dangers they are unable to comprehend.

Parents become aware of this step in personality development when the placid 1-year-old becomes the fiercely rebellious 2-year-old whose favorite word is "No!" This is the "negative stage." Because of its similarity to the renewed bid for independence that takes place later on, some psychologists call it the "first adolescence."

It is a difficult age, certainly for the parents and probably for the child. The toddler's experience is still too small for understanding the routines and regulations that must seem so arbitrary. There are real dangers that children are incapable of comprehending and from which they must be protected. They cannot be permitted to run into a busy street or to sample contents of the detergent bottle. Furthermore, toddlers must begin to abide by some of the rules that make it possible for us all to live together in society. And yet, the budding struggle for autonomy needs to be accepted and encouraged so that it can blossom into wholesome confidence in making their own decisions while, at the same time, learning to heed advice and good counsel on important issues.

This, it can be seen, creates a fine and precarious balance between independence and conformity that each of us must work out, over and over again throughout all of our lives. Indeed, some psychologists see it as a balance that has crucial influence on psychological well-being. Erich Fromm (1955) calls it the conflict between the "need to think" (for one's self) and the "need to be loved." He describes the fact that the family (and, later on, the group) tends to reward for compliance—for giving in. The reward is approval, being accepted. But there is, in all of us, an inner need for freedom to be ourselves. And so each of us must decide, over and over, whether to stand by our own choice or whether to go along with the wishes of another.

Erikson (1963) suggests that the basic pattern for this balance is determined during the critical period for acquiring autonomy. Although the child proclaims his resistance from the roof tops, he is still terribly aware of his utter dependence upon the very adults he defies. This dependence makes him so vulnerable to the potent weapons adults have at their disposal—ridicule, shame, withdrawal of love—weapons well contrived to make the child doubt himself and his capacity for self-determination.

The successful outcome of the negative stage is the independence of spirit that we Americans prize so highly, embodied in literature by our frontier heroes, explorers, inventors, and others who persevered against great odds, especially when most people were counseling "give it up!" The unsuccessful outcome, self-doubt, takes many forms. Among these is a too-heavy reliance upon approval and commendation in order to feel confidence in one's decisions.

It happens that in our culture, men are generally more independent and less influenced by concern for what someone may think about their behavior. Women tend to be much more dependent upon the opinions of other people. It seems very possible that this difference has some origins during the period in which autonomy is developing. The difference is likely to begin with the expectations of parents for appropriate behavior in a small boy compared with that in a small girl.

In either case, the child has changed from a passive baby to a little-being-in-perpetual-motion with a definite mind of his or her own. Furthermore, the child's desires often run counter to parental demands. It is not known whether the male toddler is actually more physically active at the motor level than the female, though there is some evidence that points in that direction. It is known, however, that little boys are punished more severely and more frequently than little girls—presumably for their impulsive, noisy motor activity that "gets on parents' nerves." The evidence does support the fact that the small boy is more aggressive than his female age-mate. This too could get him "into trouble" more often (Bardwick, 1971).

The result seems to have led to the folk-sense that girls are "easier to raise." Add to this the expectation of more dependence for girls and the encouragement of independent action for small sons. The differing parental demands are subtle but, it seems, exceedingly effective. The results show up in different play behavior by the age of 13 months (Lewis and Goldberg, 1972), with boys being twice as willing to leave their mothers to investigate playthings at the other end of the room and more vigorous in attacking a barrier that was placed in front of the toys. Although it could be argued that these differences are present from the beginning—are genetic, built into the orginal nature of the organism—it seems more likely that parents are more protective of little girls and less restrictive for little boys.

When mothers bring their toddlers to a room with toys at one end and a chair for herself at the other, it is possible to predict with maximum accuracy whether the child is a boy or girl by observing the mother's behavior. If it is a boy, she is likely to give him a little shove in the direction of the toys. If it is a girl, she will be most likely to take the lass by the hand and accompany her to the toys (Lewis and Goldberg, 1969).

The outcome has long-range consequences, especially for the lives of girls. To be more dependent on the approval of parents translates into being more compliant and having a less well-developed sense of one's own needs and desires—in Erikson's words, less autonomy. It is a serious gap because, according to Erikson, the remaining stages, built on a faulty foundation, will also be flawed and can be compensated for eventually only with great effort and risk of some deficiency.

The problem of less self-reliant girls (and women) is not an academic one. Insofar as it is possible to predict from present trends, it appears that girls are being reared for a life that they are not likely to lead. Girls are still being taught that they will spend the major share of their adult lives as wives and mothers and that it is the choice of a husband that will most strongly influence their future (Angrist and Almquist, 1975). A vocation and career for a girl are still seen as secondary, with the implication that she will be supported by a husband; even years of preparation for a career are often discounted as a "good way to spend the time" between her dependence upon parents and her later dependence upon a spouse (Bernard, 1981).

When a new baby arrives, parents typically envision a shining bride and radiant mother if the child is a girl. But few parents first picture husbanding and fatherhood for their newborn son. So deeply entrenched are the traditional views of sex roles that girls are encouraged to think of any choice of work as provisional and temporary, something to "fall back on," and unconnected with any goal of future economic security (Lowenthal et al., 1975), whereas a boy is made aware of the importance of his vocational decision from the moment he can respond to the question, "What are you going to be when you grow up?"

However, the current statistics need to be impressed upon our consciousness and should be required reading for everyone with responsibility for influencing and guiding young children. To begin with, women constituted 52 per cent of the labor force in 1979 (Women's Equity Action League, 1980). Of this number, almost one half were working because of economic necessity. They were single, widowed, divorced, or separated, or they had husbands earning less than $3000 per year (Vetter, 1978). In large measure, because so few of these women had prepared for their work-force entry, the gap between women's earnings and men's earnings has actually increased over the years. Today women earn 59 cents for every $1 earned by men; 25 years ago, it was 64 cents for every $1 (Levy, 1980).

Jane Roberts Chapman, writing for the Foundation for Equal Rights (1976, p. 20) sums the case for assisting girls to become more independent and realistic about their future:

> One cannot help but feel, however, that if the economic implication of sex-differentiated practices of child-rearing and the resulting dependency of women were better understood, it would not be encouraged by anyone. If parents knew of the disproportionate number of women in poverty; if they knew not only of the high and increasing divorce rate but also that current statistics show that after four years only 33 per cent of court-awarded child support payments are made, and after 10 years practically none—if parents were to comprehend these facts, perhaps they would not encourage their daughters' expectations of marriage as a lifetime guarantee of "a loving husband who is able to take care of me" or educate their daughters without regard to occupational goals.

The toddler period, with its developmental task of acquiring a sense of ability to decide some things for one's self, would seem to be the place to begin encouraging *both* boys and girls to be self-reliant. Parents need to reexamine their idea of a "good little girl" as one who sits quietly, stays clean, and does not assert her own wishes. Parents need to applaud the explorations and discoveries of the small daughter as well as those of her spunky brother.

There is a corollary to this enlisting of parental support for daughters who come to think of themselves as competent and able to solve their own problems. It would suggest that sons be afforded training in nurture and the household arts. Men, almost as frequently as women, may have to "go it alone" for a period of time. Just as important, men ought to be capable and comfortable with shouldering an equitable half of the home-making responsibilities in fair share with a career-engaged mate.

By the same token, as future partners and parents, small boys need to be permitted some expressive aspects of their nature. They should not be told that it is unmanly to cry or that men do not feel hurts. Small male toddlers need dolls to cuddle and love as well as ample hugging and snuggling from warm adults.

Even without the new prescription that daughters be encouraged to be less dependent and that tenderheartedness be valued in sons, the toddler period is not one for which there are easy recipes. The parent must steer a hazardous course between extremes in the effort to enable the child to trust an inner gyroscope on many occasions and yet heed guidance and follow directions on others.

Toilet training, nap time, play time, eating—almost anything can become the focus for a problem. However, it is almost never the particular issue that is causing the trouble; rather, the issue is joined in terms of the relationship between parent and child, and most especially in terms of parent expectancies. It is the picture-in-the-head of what childhood should be that will influence the parent's interpretation of a situation. Some parents are threatened and offended by the challenge from a small character standing less than 3 feet tall. Some parents regard the child's defiant "no" as a test of wills, indicating that the time has arrived when the child must learn "who is boss." (Recall that

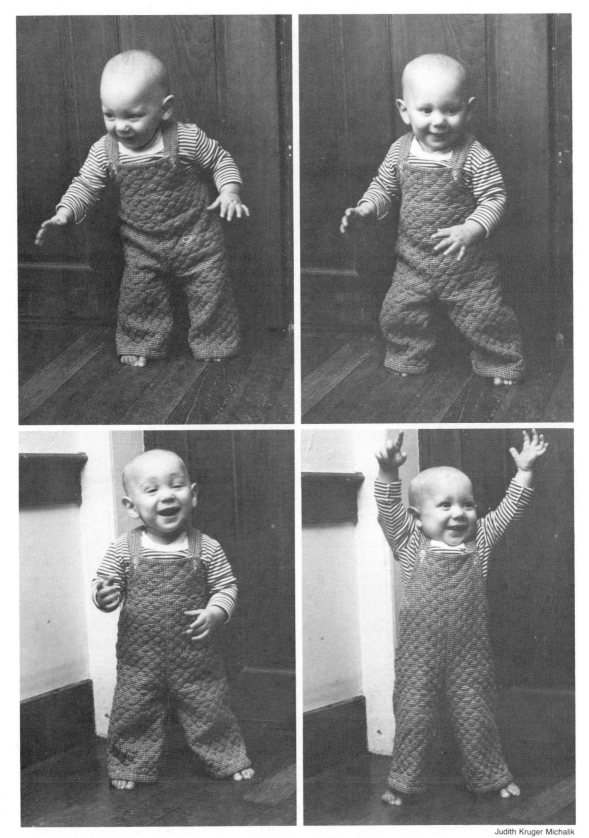

Judith Kruger Michalik

The steps are wobbly, but parents watch the toddler try and be delighted in his own success. Throughout the growing years, parents need to remember not to overprotect and not to intervene too quickly.

the old term for toilet training was "breaking," and that it was considered a contest between civilized parent and untamed child.)

On the other hand, it is possible to think of the toddler's demands for self-determination as an opportunity to glimpse the emerging personality and a chance for parents to gain some sense of the child's individual characteristics. In any case, parental responses and practices will be fashioned in terms of how they see the roles of parent and child. Thus, it is not what the parent does in any one instance that affects the quality of a parent-child relationship, but rather the day-in and day-out "back-and-forths" of the interactions that are absorbed by the child and transformed into the deepest attitudes about self and the self's capacity for decision making.

Although this may sound as if it were all laid upon the shoulders of parents, such an implication is not intended. The transactional nature of the parent-child relationship needs to be noted and underscored (Bell, 1968.) The child brings a unique set of dispositional and behavioral tendencies to the family setting. Some children are more vigorous in their self-assertion, so that "crossing" them precipitates a major crisis every time. Others are more placid, even reasonable, often accepting parental explanations and dictums with good grace. The self-assertive child will be on a perpetual collision course in a household where the parent's words are law and questioning is not tolerated. On the other hand, an easy-going child may be totally "washed out" in such circumstances, never daring a mite of self-expression.

This is surely an argument for parent education. Both the strong and "stubborn" child and the one who is more retiring would benefit by parents' understanding and acceptance of the "negative stage" as the time when children need to test themselves to discover their powers and the necessary limits.

Parents can be taught how to stand by "in the wings," unobtrusive but available. It involves permitting the child to engage in as many "me do it!" accomplishments as possible, even when it means making a mess or when the adult could manage so much more efficiently. It means refraining from overprotecting and not intervening too quickly to help. Parents can also learn confidence in their own judgments, becoming secure enough to set up rules and guidelines that children are expected to follow.

The objective for this toddler age is for both girls and boys to develop a buoyant sense of autonomy and a sturdy self-respect that will be essential in acquiring respect for the rights of others. In addition, they should have learned some boundaries and restrictions, in that while portions of the world can be commanded or mastered, other portions do not yield. Finally, they should have learned first lessons in cooperation and the fact that it is possible to give in on occasion without being forever diminished. These are large lessons for ones so small, and there is such a short time in which to learn. Look away for what seems only a moment, and they are off and joining the tricycle brigade.

GLOSSARY

ACCOMMODATION   Piaget's term for the process by which a schema is adjusted to fit changing information and circumstances.

ACTIVE LANGUAGE   The child's own speech production.

ASSIMILATION   Piaget's term for taking in, processing, and incorporating information.

AUTONOMY   Erikson's term for the second developmental task—gaining the sense of being someone who can decide for one's self and who can stand on one's own two feet.

EGOCENTRISM   Piaget's description of the naive assumption in young children that their own perceptions are exactly the same as those obtained by everyone else.

HOLOPHRASES   Single words used by the child in initial speech production to evoke the meaning of an entire sentence.

PASSIVE LANGUAGE   Early understanding of language that cannot yet be produced by the child.

SCHEMA   For Piaget, the cognitive unit that comprises the comprehension of environmental events.

SOCIALIZATION   Training of children to live in society.

SYMBOLIC PLAY   Imaginative or pretend play.

TELEGRAPHIC SPEECH   An early-childhood form of speech that omits all but the most essential words in a sentence.

REFERENCES

Angrist, S. S., Almquist, E.: *Careers and Contingencies: How College Women Juggle with Gender.* New York: Kunellen, 1975.

Bardwick, J.: *Psychology of Women.* New York: Harper & Row, 1971.

Bell, R. Q.: A reinterpretation of the direction of effects in studies of socialization. *Psychology Review,* 75:81–95, 1968.

Bernard, J.: *The Female World.* New York: The Free Press, 1981.

Brodbeck, A. J., Irwin, O. C.: The speech behavior of infants and families. *Child Development,* 17:149–160, 1946.

Chapman, J. R.: Introduction. In Chapman, J. R. (ed.): *Economic Independence for Women.* Beverly Hills, Cal.: Sage Publications, 1976.

Chomsky, N.: *Language and the Mind.* New York: Harcourt Brace & World, 1968.

Dale, P. S.: *Language Development: Structure and Function,* 2nd ed. New York: Holt, Rinehart & Winston, 1976.

Erikson, E.: *Children and Society,* 2nd ed.: New York: W. W. Norton & Company, 1963.

Ferguson, C. A.: Baby talk in six languages. In Gumperz, J., Hymes, D. (eds.): *The Ethography of Communication,* New York: Holt, Rinehart & Winston, 1972.

Fouts, R. S., Couch, J. B.: Cultural evolution of learned language in chimpanzees. In Hahn, M. E., Simmel, E. C. (eds.): *Communicative Behavior and Evolution.* New York: Academic Press, 1976.

Frisch, K. von: *The Dance Language and Orientation of Bees.* Cambridge, Mass.: Harvard University Press, 1967.

Fromm, E.: *The Sane Society.* New York: Rinehart, 1955.

Gardner, R. A., Gardner, B. T.: Teaching sign language to a chimpanzee. *Science,* 165:664–672, 1969.

Gardner, R. A., Gardner, B. T.: Comparative psychology and language acquisition. In Salzinger, K., Denmark, F. (eds.): *Psychology: The State of the Art.* New York: Annals of the New York Academy of Sciences, 1977.

Goodall, J.: My life among the chimpanzees. *National Geographic Magazine,* 124:272–308, 1963.

Gordon, I. J.: What do we know about parents as teachers? *Theory into Practice,* 11:146–149, 1972.

Kagan, J.: *Change and Continuity in Infancy.* New York: John Wiley & Sons, 1971.

Levy, C.: Women pushing to close wage gap. *Providence (R. I.) Journal,* Oct. 26, 1980, business section, F1, p. 13.

Lewis, M., Goldberg, S.: Perceptual-cognitive development in infancy: A generalized expectancy model of mother-infant interaction. *Merrill-Palmer Quarterly,*15:81–100, 1969.

Lewis, M., Goldberg, S.: Play behavior in the year-old infant: Early sex differences. In Bardwick, J. (ed.): *Readings on the Psychology of Women.* New York: Harper & Row, 1972.

Lichtenberg, P., Norton, D. G.: *Cognitive and Mental Development in the First Five Years of Life.* Rockville, Md: National Institute of Mental Health, 1972.

Lilly, J. C.: Productive and creative research with man and dolphin. *Archives of General Psychiatry,* 2:111–116, 1963.

Limber, J.: Language in child and chimp? *American Psychologist,* 32:280–285, 1977.

Lowenthal, M. F., Thurnher, M., Chiriboga, D.: *Four Stages of Life: A Comparative Study of Men and Women Facing Transitions.* San Francisco: Jossey-Bass, 1975.

McCall, R. B., Kagan, J.: Attention in the infant: Effects of complexity, contour and familiarity. *Child Development,* 38:939–952, 1967.

Moss, H. A.: Sex, age and state as determinants of mother-infant interaction. *Merrill-Palmer Quarterly,* 13:19–36, 1967.

Nelson, K.: Structure and strategy in learning to talk. *Monographs of the Society for Research in Child Development,* 38:1–149, 1973.

Patterson, P.: Linguistic capabilities of a young lowland gorilla. In *An Account of the Visual Mode: Man versus Ape.* Washington, D.C.: American Association for the Advancement of Science, 1977.

Piaget, J., Inhelder, B.: *The Origins of Intelligence in Children.* New York: International Universities Press, 1952.

Piaget, J.: *Play, Dreams and Imitation in Childhood.* New York: W. W. Norton & Company, 1962.

Premack, D.: The education of Sarah. *Psychology Today,* 4:54–58, 1970.

Skinner, B. F.: *Verbal Behavior.* New York: Appleton-Century-Crofts, 1957.

Slobin, D. I.: *Psycholinguistics.* Glenview, Ill.: Scott, Foresman and Company, 1971.

Stern, D.: The first relationship: Infant and mother. In Bruner, G., Cole, M., Lloyd, B. (eds.): *The Developing Child.* Cambridge, Mass.: Harvard University Press, 1977.

Vetter, L.: Career counseling for women. In Harmon, L. W., Birk, J. M., Fitzgerald, L. E., Tanney, M. F. (eds.): *Counseling Women.* Monterey, Cal.: Brooks/Cole Publishing Company, 1978.

Women's Equity Action League: Legislation briefs. *NAFE Network News,* November 1980, vol. 1, p. 3.

THE PRESCHOOL YEARS: Initiative

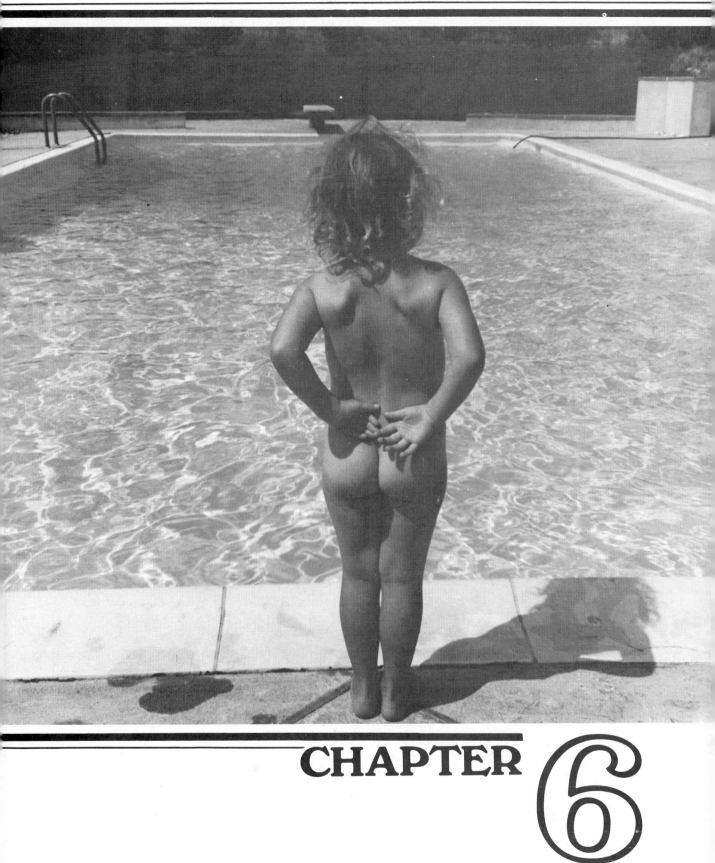

CHAPTER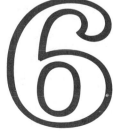

Ages 3, 4, and 5, the "preschool years," unfold with a whole new set of challenges. Having gained some confidence in the ability to decide certain matters independently, the child turns attention to the larger world. Erikson (1963) describes this period as the search to find out "what he will become." In imagination and play, roles are tried on, tested, and doffed. The tricycle brigade speeds up and down the sidewalk, pretending to be riding motorbuses, huge dump trucks, and cargo carriers. The early use of simple, one-theme symbolic play in toddlerhood now explodes into exuberant self-expression in finger-paint smearings of color, using mud and sand, and through action and sound, provided the environment encourages such activity.

Probably never again is it possible for the child to be so intensely creative, unrestrained (as yet) by reality. For Piaget (1962a), this is a salient feature of the preschool period—the fact that, for the child, reality is very easily distorted to suit demands of the moment. "I am sailing around the world!" announces Tom, sitting in a little tub on the lawn. And for him it is quite, quite true, believed, according to Piaget, "spontaneously, without effort" (1962a, p. 168).

It is difficult for adults to capture in memory the magic of that time in childhood when it seems possible for *anything* to happen. One can sometimes regain a fleeting glimpse of how it was in the experience of heightened expectations and excitement, often in connection with a family ritual or celebration. For the fortunate child, the witchery is everywhere—awakening to discover the pictures drawn by Jack Frost on the window, sailing little "boats" down the gutter to the storm sewer, watching the ants trudge off with crumbs, learning how to make a first snow-angel, sitting behind the steering wheel of the family car and pretending to be the skillful driver.

Less happy children with survival concerns will have fewer opportunities for carefree experience and will have bleaker childhood lives as a consequence. They may be missing more than idle pastimes, it appears. There is increasing evidence (Bruner, 1975; Singer, 1973; Sutton-Smith, 1967) that play, especially pretend play, is vitally important to the developing cognitive skills during preschool years. We will discuss this in more detail in the forthcoming sections.

By preschool age, the various motor skills have progressed to the point where running, jumping, climbing, and similar feats no longer demand the intense concentration needed in earlier years. The advances in language ability and ever-widening circles of experience help to create a marvelously fresh perception of events and the world, repeated in the family circle during later years to the enjoyment or discomfiture of the originator. Chukovsky (1963) reports some delightful comments on life and its wonders by Russian preschool children:

"Mother, who gave birth to me? You? I knew it! If daddy had, I would have a mustache."
"Why do they put a pit in every cherry? We just have to throw the pit away."
"Mothers give birth to boys too? Then what are fathers for?"

It is the language explosion that sets this age apart. From its modest beginning of some 50-or-so functional words at age 2, the preschooler will literally learn several words a day, gaining a vocabulary of up to 10,000 words by the time of first grade (Carey, 1977). Much of what we know about the cognitive development of this period is mirrored in the child's use of language, revealing the quality of thinking by means of the questions and comments.

COGNITIVE DEVELOPMENT

The preschool child is still *preoperational* in thinking. The preoperational period, according to Piaget (1952), is an extensive one, beginning in toddlerhood and lasting into the early school years. The child's thinking, though now more sophisticated as befits expanded experience, continues to demonstrate the *egocentrism* described in Chapter 5. The ability to comprehend that another's point of view is not the same as one's own is still missing.

Egocentrism

Egocentrism is manifested in a number of ways—for example, in the young preschooler's conversation with another child. The two children are likely to "take turns" in speaking, first one and then the other, after the manner of polite conversations they have heard. However, the content of the conversation will sound bizarre because neither child responds or even seems to listen to what the other is saying. Thus:

Brian: I am going to build a bird house out of this wood.
Debbi: These dolls are having a picnic.
Brian: Then I will put it in a tree and the birds will build their nestes (sic) in it.
Debbi: Maybe we will go to the beach.
Brian: I am going to paint it, too.
Debbi: I think we will have weiners and chocolate cake.

Egocentrism prompts the exasperation of young children when parents or babysitters do not understand the neologisms that are part of the preschooler vocabulary. Tom asked his father to turn on the "dinken" while in the car, and though father had to translate this into "turn signal," Tom himself was serenely confident that he would be understood.

Similarly, preschool children do not understand that a parent cannot know what is in their minds. One of the predications of the Oedipal conflict, you will remember, was that the small boy becomes convinced that father *knows* about those hostile wishes. Another manifestation of the egocentric "same-mind" presumption is the conversation that children initiate without any explanation of previous connection, for example, "Do you remember when Grandma dropped the pancake?" to a nursery school teacher who does not know Grandma and can have no idea that the event occurred during summer vacation.

During family crises, egocentrism shows in the child's preoccupation with what is going to happen *to him*. Parents who are divorcing, unaware of the level of preschool thinking, often attempt explanations that are far too elaborate for the youngster of this age. Explanations can come later, when the child's questions indicate a quest for more complete information. Now, however, what is needed is reassurance on three counts:

1. That *nothing* the child did or said or thought has caused the family troubles.

2. That the child will be cared for, all the time, and that there will be a specific person responsible for this task.

3. That the noncustodial parent is nevertheless still a loving parent and that there will be visits at specified times that will be spelled out.

Egocentrism also brings anxious questions about people who are maimed or crippled. The inquirer is really asking, "Will that happen to me?" The answers ought to be directed at soothing the alarm.

A well-intentioned parent or Sunday School teacher may attempt to impress preschool children with the Easter story by vividly detailing the Crucifixion agony. A recounting of the Holocaust suffering can produce the same effect, as can television programs that depict cruelty to children, killing of parents, or any kind of hurt to a character (even an animal) with whom the child identifies a loved one. The child cannot yet cognitively place events in time or assess the probability of an actual occurrence. Television dramas are seen as real, and egocentrism leads to the presumption that the event is personally imminent; that any day now, he will be crucified or sent to a gas chamber or see mother shot by thugs.

Though it is all very well to suggest that the world does hold tragedy and danger, it does not follow that these should be deliberately thrust on the child who is without cognitive resources for adequate defense. We are, all of us, in terrible danger every minute of our lives, from war, assailant, stroke, accident, or other horror. But if we were to live actually expecting the worst at every moment, it would be the psychological equivalent of living under a state of siege. Unhappy necessity may force this upon human beings at times, but it is certainly not recommended as the life most likely to promote well-being and self-confidence in children.

But remember that children do not remain egocentric in their thinking all their life. There will be ample time for full appreciation of the Easter story, for sorrowful grief over those broken bodies of Auschwitz, and for fierce anger toward anyone who hurts another. The message of Piaget's ideas, at base, is an optimistic one. All in good time, parents. All in good time!

Phenomenalism

The thinking of preoperational children has other characteristics that seem to give their outlook and comments a special clear-eyed charm. One of these is the quality termed *phenomenalism,* the unquestioning acceptance of extraordinary events as without wonder. Adults show some of this too: think how often you have flicked a light switch without once ever contemplating what accounts for the remarkable, instantaneous flood of light, or how often you have started the engine of your car without giving it a second thought. In just the same fashion, Brian, having his first experience with a big-city hotel elevator, accepted it matter-of-factly as "the little room where you go in and shut the door and then they quick run around and change the rugs."

Phenomenalism means that the "ordinary" cause-and-effect connections between events are not only absent from the child's thinking, but are not even missed. A young child who swallowed an entire vial of carelessly mislaid thyroid tablets is discovered in time and is whisked off to the hospital for emergency procedures, including stomach pump. Returned home, white and wan but out of danger, he is placed on the sofa with some toys. Suddenly, to her horror, mother finds him on the floor, in the process of retrieving and eating a thyroid pill that had apparently rolled out of the bottle in the first episode. It was clear that the meaning of the day's events, the wild dash to the hospital, the tubes, the stomach pump, and the blood pressure checks, had bypassed him completely. His mother wonders, "Does he think I just took it into my head to put him through all of that?" The answer to her question is probably "yes."

In the same manner, questions of right or wrong do not have the significance for preschool children that is accorded by adults. Parents who are outraged by "lies" or "stealing" need help in understanding that the child cannot (which is quite different from "will not") understand anything more than the fact of the parent's anger. The child will be uncertain as to which behavior triggers the parental explosion. Frequent parental outbursts can lead to the child's bewilderment and a kind of general conclusion "everything I do is bad."

Phenomenalism also underscores the concerns raised about the widespread American practice of physical punishment for misbehaving children (Gil, 1970). Doubtless, preschool children are often exasperating. They make messes, spill things, break precious bric-a-brac, put dirty shoes on clean chairs, sometimes have toileting accidents, explore forbidden territory, and engage in a thousand kinds of irritating mischief that any parent can list. For many parents, the behavior is a deliberate transgression and the physical punishment is intended to "teach" what the child "needs to learn."

The problem is, of course, that the connection between the parental wrath and the misbehavior is not likely to be comprehended by the child. Nor does physical punishment teach the child what to do to gain approval. Instead, it provides a model of how adults deal with anger and a pattern that tends to be repeated when children grow up and have children of their own (Kempe and Helfer, 1971).

Connections between behavior and consequences seem to be more readily fashioned if pleasant events are forthcoming. This merely involves the psychological principle of positive *reinforcement,* a powerful instrument for encouraging repetition of the behavior. In contrast to punishment, reinforcement does inform the child—"do this again." So, a smile or a kiss, a hug, a "good," or a pat all tell the child she is doing fine. A child who is doing fine in her own mind will be more confident and secure than one who lives under a threat of punishment that can occur at any time (or so it seems) without warning.

To understand the characteristics of preoperational cognition, then, means assuming that the child's thinking encompasses only the most primitive of consequential relationships and that what seems so patently evident to an adult is not likely to be apparent at all to the child. "When I get big, will you be little?" asks Debbi in another expression of the child's blissful acceptance of all sorts of earthly phenomena, including growth and, perhaps, a quite-as-possible undoing of the process.

The thinking of the preoperational child, according to Piaget (1962b), is not yet capable of taking in several aspects of an event at one time, but rather tends to focus on global sensory impressions for problem solving and reasoning. For example, the preschool child is shown two equal balls of clay and affirms that they are "the same." Then one ball is rolled out into a sausage shape and the child is asked whether the pieces of clay are still the same. The preoperational child will be trapped by perception of the length of the sausage, failing to take the narrow width into consideration and will be confident that the two are no longer the same. It is not possible for the child of this age to mentally comprehend the possibility of restoring the sausage to its original shape and thus to see that the amount of clay has not changed.

The problem just described and similar ones have been used by Piaget and his colleagues to ascertain the child's level of thinking. It is often suggested that children might be instructed and trained in the specifics of the problem. Wouldn't it be possible to demonstrate how the sausage can be squeezed together, back into its original shape? Wouldn't the child then understand that it is, indeed, still "the same"?

Piaget did not believe that this kind of "acceleration" is true learning. He granted that the child may learn the "correct answer" in rote fashion by such means, but will forget it quickly and be unable to apply the principle to other situations (Pulaski, 1971). Piaget believed that the child will acquire the appropriate mental development in the normal course of events and will be best off engaging in the normal activities of childhood.

What are the ordinary occupations of the preschool child? Much depends upon the location of activities—big city, small town, or country area. Much depends on the kinds of activities encouraged by parents, since the preschool child is typically still under some type of caretaking supervision. Swinging, sliding, chasing, splashing, climbing, coloring, cutting, pasting, hiding, digging, watching and listening, building, pretending: these are the usual childhood pursuits called play. We will take a look at the significant role accorded to play in cognitive development.

Play, Fantasy, and Symbols

Play has been given rather belated recognition as worthy of adult notice (Stone, 1971). A work-oriented society had tended to consider play as of no consequence, merely idle amusements of children who have nothing better to do. Pestalozzi and Froebal, two European educators of the late 18th and early 19th centuries, were influential in countering the prevailing ideas ("the devil finds work for idle hands") with an emphasis upon "natural" activities for the young. Their teachings became incorporated into the first American kindergartens (literally, in German, "children's gardens"), and play materials were considered vital to the child's natural development (Maxim, 1980).

Functions of Play

However, it is only within the past two decades that the notion of "play is the child's work" has received serious research support (Pulaski, 1974; Singer, 1973; Sutton-Smith, 1967). One example is the work of Sutton-Smith (1967), in which three different functions for play are suggested.

Consolidation. One type of play, he believes, serves to consolidate the mental operations

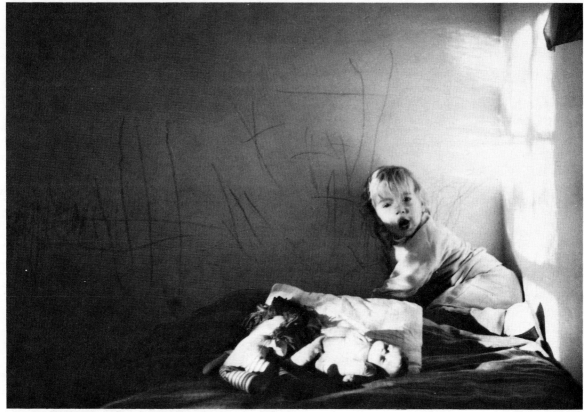

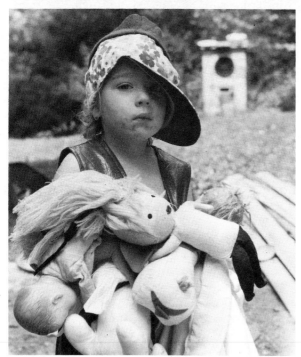

Today we realize that play is a child's work.

that have already been developed cognitively. So we see the preschoolers setting up the doll corner for a tea party. All the participants are poised and self-confident in their knowledge of what to do. A newcomer to the play time will be given directions, instructed in a role, corrected, cajoled, and tolerated as long as she "fits in."

Limits. A second function for play, according to Sutton-Smith's classification, enables children to test the limits of what they can do, discovering the boundaries of competencies and what they are "good at," finding out what and how things work, enduring the stings of other children's rejection and disapproval, and basking in the glory of other children's acceptance. This is clearly visible on the playground as children compete for attention. "Look at this!" "Hey, watch me!" Having mastered the climbing of monkey bars, some daring one will hang by the knees—and then others will try it too. Or two will set off on tricycles, racing down the sidewalk, pedaling as furiously as legs can turn the wheel. Or the jigsaw puzzle will be turned in for a more elaborate one. Or the sand castle is crushed—to be replaced with another, larger and fancier.

Imagination.   The third kind of play is believed to stabilize and expand competencies into new forms and organizations. Sutton-Smith suggests that the child uses present cognitive and motor skills in novel combinations, often involving marvelous flights of imagination.

The world of fantasy and imagination opens up entire new vistas and possibilities. Though many parents remember their world of make-believe during childhood with fondness and tend to encourage their own children's fantasy play, other parents are uneasy about children's imaginings (Dennis, 1976). The most frequent response to the question of attitude toward children's pretending was "Well, it's all right, provided he doesn't do it too much." Some parents were uneasy about the possibility of "living in a dream world" (Dennis, 1976).

However, imagination means the ability to create a mental image of some aspect of the outer world. This kind of representation makes language possible. The word is not the thing: it just "stands for" the thing. Without the symbol, the inner picture, there would be no object permanence, no ability to plan ahead or look back. It is the basis for memory, for problem solving, for judging and making comparisons, and for goal setting (Pulaski, 1974).

The link between imagination and verbal ability was given early empirical support by the work of Smilansky (1968) in Israel. The problem arose because of great difficulties in school experienced by children of nomadic Jews who were extremely poor. Smilansky discovered that the meager existence of these people precluded toys or even time for play for the children. Brought to a room with a number of toys, the children literally did not know what to do. They wandered about aimlessly, showing little interest and certainly no inclination to use any of the toys in play.

Smilansky suggested that the lack of ability to play, especially the lack of imaginative play, accounted for the language difficulties, the inability to sustain attention, and the lack of persistent focus that put the children at a large disadvantage in school classrooms. She set about teaching them to pretend, beginning with concrete objects such as a comb, a cup, and a pencil. The child would first be taught how to use the actual object, then how to pretend to use the object, and, finally, how to pretend without the object. Then the children were introduced to pretend games, "socio-dramatic play," becoming doctors, airplane pilots, mothers, storekeepers, and teachers in fantasy play. Smilansky reported substantial gains in vocabulary level and language usage, as well as longer attention span, lessened impulsivity and aimlessness, and greatly enhanced ability to follow a sequence of directions.

A series of similar studies in America (Freyberg, 1973; Pulaski, 1970; Saltz and Johnson, 1973) have followed the same line of thinking, the association of imaginative play with good language abilities and powers of attention. The relationship seems to be well supported in each instance.

Imagination can serve another purpose in addition to its function as a builder of intellectual competence for symbolic processes. Imagination is akin to planning, a process in which one envisions what will happen next and what will happen after that, or what will happen if the initial circumstances are changed. It is possible to test solutions to problems in imagination and to construct alternatives from which to select the best. This kind of foresight in imagination can save many foolish mistakes.

It is also possible, by means of imagination, to "work through" many a feared or traumatic event in fantasy. It can be a means of obtaining mastery over dread, reassuring oneself that the situation need no longer be feared. This aspect of pretend play can be used by parents to help children over unwished for, but inevitable, life difficulties (Peller, 1952). A frightening experience with a large barking dog, for example, could be recreated with the parents taking the role of the dog. The "dog" might "growl" to himself, "Oh gosh, I was only barking to say 'hello!' I really didn't mean to frighten you. I am so sorry. Please give me another chance."

Parents can use these kinds of dramatics to prepare the child for a forthcoming hospitalization or a move to another city, or to deal with a death in the family. It is often enlightening for parents and children to play with simple role reversals so that the parent becomes the child and the child acts out being mamma or daddy. Now and again, the portrait of you, as parent, is unflattering and therefore a little unsettling. But the situation can also be used to enact child behaviors that are irritating or undesirable. Seeing yourself as others see you in the context of play may be more instructive than many sessions of scolding and nagging.

This "cathartic" use of dramatic play can also serve within the hospital. A small investment in some dolls dressed as doctors and nurses and play-time medical kits will pay handsome emotional dividends as small patients subject the dolls to the procedures. Though the children may often be too ill to play for a sustained period of time, it is often possible for an imaginative caregiver to brighten the day with even a short fantasy excursion while tending the child. "Let's take a pretend walk in the woods, just you and I. Close your eyes and I will tell you what we see." Then it is possible to do all sorts of marvelous things—climb tall trees, swing from vines, talk with a lion, have lunch with the wise old owl.

Imaginary companions often turn up at this age, most frequently for first-born children, only children, or later-born children with an age gap between themselves and siblings (Manosevits et al., 1973). The same study found that children with imaginary companions tend to be those who are capable of initiating their own play situations and have the capacity to become engrossed in the activity. They also tend to be gregarious and to enjoy engaging in activities with other members of the household; thus, the stereotype of the child with an imaginary companion as an isolated "loner" was not upheld.

Another study (Schafer, 1969) found that creative adolescents report having had imaginary companions during early childhood more often than do adolescents who are not considered creative. Parents and other adults might well regard most imaginary playmates as evidence of the child's developing ability to enjoy a rich fantasy life—a gift and a blessing!

Television

The question of television's influence on play is not one for which there are clear answers. There is little doubt that it supplies a stock of ready-made characters for role taking, but it also seems possible that it encourages a passivity that is quite different from the activities that occupied leisure time of boys and girls in earlier decades. The fast-paced, rapid shifts of scene are thought to be especially detrimental to imposing one's own private imagery on the material (Singer and Singer, 1979).

Inveighing against television, however, is pretty fruitless. Television, for good or bad, has become an integral part of our lives. More beneficial would be a concerted effort to help children (and their parents) to become discriminating viewers. Parent groups and individuals should be encouraged to applaud good programs and to protest bad ones. Parents need to be helped to become self-confident and firm about restricting the amount of time children are permitted to watch television and about monitoring the quality of the programs. Parents might also consider the question of what other kinds of activities would be available to children if the set were not turned on. Would there be opportunities for reading, playing vigorous outdoor games, constructing, or creating?

One of the recommendations offered by Rue (1974), in conjunction with the National Association for Better Broadcasting, urges parents to watch at least some of the programs with their children, communicating judgments and attitudes toward the situations depicted and tempering the hard-sell commercials. An added suggestion might be a review of parents' own viewing habits. Just as parents who never open a book can hardly expect their children to be avid readers, so parents who are glued to the television set, no matter what the program, can hardly expect their children to be selective in what they watch.

Interaction Between Child and Adult

Birth Order.   It is a recurring theme of this textbook that sharing and interchange between child and adult are exceedingly important in the developmental process. One source of documentation for this proposition has been the birth-order studies, which regularly point to the first-born child as advantaged in intelligence and verbal ability. The implication is that parents have more time for the first child, are more interested, and therefore interact more frequently and for longer periods of time. It has also been suggested that first-born (and only) children spend a longer time in an atmosphere "undiluted" by other childish minds (Zajonc, 1976).

Other indicators of the same direction are the Florida parent-educator studies, which focused on teaching poverty-level mothers to play with their babies. The idea was that the kind of attention usually given to first-born children would be advantageous for other children as well, and that the verbal and playful interaction would be especially beneficial in settings that do not usually encourage mothers to play with their infants. The findings not only pointed to substantial developmental gains for the infants, but also for siblings of these babies—for older children who joined in the games and for younger ones coming later who gained from the mother's previous experiences (Gordon, 1969).

Reading.   Of all the occupations a parent or caretaker can share with the child, reading promises the greatest gifts for the child's future. It should start early, long before the child understands the word, with picture books, the adult identifying objects and helping to turn the page.

The chief pleasure of being read to is likely the full attention of a beloved adult. First, there is the warmth and comfort of being snuggled securely against the adult body. The story itself becomes important later. But all the time, the child is receiving messages about reading—that grown-ups regard it as important; that the reading material is a source of delight and information. As soon as children discover that reading can be fun, they are captured by the pastime for the rest of their lives.

Furthermore, it is an activity that parents can promote for later-born as well as first-born children. If it is a one-to-one adult-child contact that seems to enhance first-born development, special attention to later children may serve to close the gap.

Sex Roles

A last word regarding play. There is a general tendency to regard the boisterous, rough-and-tumble play of boys as appropriate to their sex, whereas girls are more often directed into quieter, less active pursuits. Although the question of innate differences in activity level between boys and girls has not been resolved (Maccoby and Jacklin, 1974), there can be little doubt that the full body movement of so many boys' games offers remarkable dividends, not only in terms of agility and coordination but also in psychological well-being. There is an exhilarating sense of self that comes of knowing that your body will do your bidding. There is daring and risk taking that can be ventured into only if you are confident in the motor skills to see you through. When girls are discouraged from testing themselves in vigorous physical endeavors, another area is established in which they consider themselves "not able" and permit boys to take the lead. Though it is true that the world needs both leaders and followers, the new message for our time is one of hope that these behaviors will come about by reason of the individual's own inclinations rather than assignment by gender. It is hoped that the future will see men and women assuming both leadership and follower roles without anyone finding the sex of the role-taker at all unusual. This should in no way be thought of as a plea for training girls to be exactly like boys. Rather, the suggestion with regard to team sports and active physical pursuits (which would, of course, include dancing) is made primarily in terms of gaining self-confidence, strength, and control.

Physical skill is not the only means to achieve this, but the emphasis of the ancient Greeks on a sound body as a first requisite is difficult to refute. Parental support and approval for achievement-oriented rather than docile daughters will be necessary. The Chinese have an expression for the notion of women assuming shoulder-to-shoulder partnerships with men in order to accomplish the requirements of adulthood. It is:

> Women must achieve equality in order that they may hold up their half of the sky.

If women are, indeed, to hold up their half of the sky, the training must be well begun during the preschool years for both boys and girls. It will be as necessary for men to welcome equal partners as for women to gain the capabilities for partner or team effort. Erikson described the developmental task of this age as that of initiative, the earliest comprehension of one's expected role in the adult world.

INITIATIVE

The child of preschool years, if all has gone well, will have acquired a fundamental concept of the world as a pretty good place and as peopled with individuals who are dependable; the child will also have confidence in the ability to decide a number of matters autonomously and yet be comfortable on occasion with bowing to the decision of others. To have become fairly sure of one's self as a person here and now leads to a new question: What kind of a person will one become in the future?

The search for "what kind of a person one can be" begins with the discovery that boys are different from girls and that women and men are grown-up versions of girls and boys. This is really a very profound discovery in the child's life and often leads to some exploratory activity on the child's part. This is the time for the sporadic "sex play," occurring more frequently when children are unusually curious about genital differences (Mace, 1970), but common even for normal children who may be verifying and confirming their information. Parents need to remember that it is the adult concerns that load "sex play" with such high emotion (Gagnon, 1977). For the child, it is not likely to be any more or less marvelous than any other fascinating, newly discovered phenomenon.

Erikson (1963) calls the search for the kind of person one might become "the age of initiative" because, he explains, this quality is necessary to embark upon an imaginative thrust into the unknown. As the child tries out same-sex adult roles in the sandbox, with building blocks, or in the doll corner, we call it "play," but it is a serious kind of play. It is a way of acquiring, as a deeply integrated part of the very being, the conviction that one will become, someday, a full-grown man or woman as fine as the good adults who are important in the child's life. It is a way of getting a feel not only for one's own role in the future scheme of things, but also for the relationship of that role to others, especially the opposite sex. Little girls play at being mother, scold doll children, and, these days, perhaps bid doll children good-bye as they go off to work, all in careful mimicry of mother's habitual tones and practices. Little boys, likewise, lower their voices in imitation of the adult male, read the paper, drive the tricycle, and interact with "mother" using father's characteristic gestures and manner.

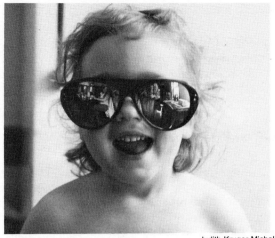
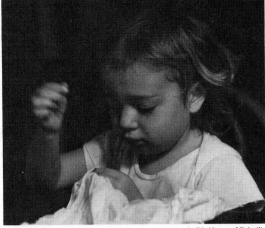

Wearing mommy's sunglasses and trying a needle and thread just like mommy are an important part of trying out roles.

The Single-Parent Home

We have been speaking as if the child comes from a traditional family with both mother and father present. In matter of fact, the current divorce rate dictates that about one in every six children lives in a one-parent family (*Boston Sunday Globe*, August 17, 1980). In such a case, *identification* with the appropriate parent role model will be a lttle more complicated—not impossible, but somewhat different. The primary requisite seems to be that the child have access to an adult of the same sex who has a well-established sense of personal worth and who carries out the gender role with a feeling of purpose and value. The single parent can help all the children by encouraging positive interaction with the other parent if at all possible. There should be wholesome, close associations with other adults also—grandparents, uncles and aunts, teachers, and friends. Various adult possibilities can be deliberately pointed out to children: "Look, there is a man who knows how to build houses." "That woman is a lawyer." "Men can be nurses and women can be doctors, too." "Some people think that only girls should be dancers, but you see that boys can be great dancers just as well!"

The most important message, however, for single parents or for a mother and father together to convey in clear, unambiguous terms is that whatever the child's sex, it is fine and the child has something important to do in the world. This attitude then becomes an integral part of the youngster's own concept of self as male or female.

Lack of Role Models

It is easy to see how this process can be detoured. The primary model might be harsh and rejecting or weak and ineffective. In some instances, a family may value one sex more than the other. The underrated one is likely to bear deep psychological scars that prohibit comfortable acceptance of one's own sex as "O.K."

There is also the fact that many fathers in the modern world tend to be too removed for close contact with their offspring. This can be as true of fathers who come home every evening as of fathers who are divorced and have arranged visits only. Before the industrialization of our society, most fathers worked close to home, in the fields of the family farm or in small business establishments just down the street. Under such conditions, it was relatively easy to see and comprehend "what men do." Under present-day conditions, the majority of fathers work at a distance from home. Often, the youngster is left completely in a mother's or a female caregiver's charge. The female person comes to seem to be the chief arbitrator of life's rewards and punishments. The father's part in the household is more difficult to perceive.

It is true that the more recent emphasis upon the importance of "fathering" (Lewis, 1972) has helped young fathers realize the necessity of making a special effort to interact warmly and frequently with their children. But until our society begins to demand a "humanization" of the marketplace, the work-a-day world will continue to require long hours from its participants and it will take a determined juggling of priorities to include children into busy lives.

The Working Mother

The same injunction needs to be applied to mothers of preschool children who are employed outside the home. Although the research does not report adverse effects on children that can be attributed specifically to the mother's working (Hoffman, 1974), and although children in well-run day-care programs seem to fare as well or better than those at home (Caldwell et al., 1970), this is not the same as saying there is no effect whatsoever. Rogers (1977) points out that it is probably more important for the mother to spend "quality time" with the child than "quantity time"—which means that just having mother physically present in the environment is not as positive as having mother spend sufficient one-on-one, attention-focused time with the child. This is a difficult prescription for most working mothers who tend, in reality, to be holding two positions. One involves the career or job, and the other frequently includes all of the responsibilities of the home (Frieze and Sales, 1978). Surveys of dual-career or two-income families clearly indicate that household tasks are not divided evenly between parents (Gauger, 1973), and if the mother is heading the family, her time has even more demands upon it. So, modern mothers, too, need to try to be sure that somewhere, somehow, there is time left over for sharing with the child. Children will never remember fondly how many floors were scrubbed or how clean the bathroom was. But they will recall the time spent baking gingerbread men together, the walk in the park, or the quiet talk just before bed.

Androgyny

All of this acknowledges a rapidly changing society. It is no longer as clear, as it once seemed to be exactly what kind of sex-role identity the child should acquire. It seems evident that we no longer want to socialize either sex for a rigid, boxed-in, stereotyped role. Boys as well as girls can be encouraged to show warmth and compassion, to express emotions, and to be supportive rather than competitive in interpersonal relations. Girls as well as boys can be encouraged to display daring, self-confidence, assertiveness, and objectivity (Combs, 1981).

The easy assumption of characteristics suitable to a situation rather than those that are assigned to a specific sex has been called *androgyny* (Bem, 1975). The term describes persons who are neither strongly feminine nor strongly masculine in behavior and role taking, but rather tend to keep open for themselves the full range of human emotions and the ability to respond appropriately when any kind of problem arises. Forisha (1978), in reviewing the research on androgynous individuals, suggests that they tend to be more mature, self-confident, self-reliant, warm and accepting, self-accepting, and self-assured than individuals who are heavily identified with the traditional sex roles. The idea of an androgynous role taking is one that is likely to achieve increasing prominence in a world that has every indication of continuing its rapid changes and therefore calls for a high degree of adjustment flexibility (Bem, 1975).

Ages 4, 5, and 6, then, seem to be the crucial time for acquiring the cheerful conviction that what one is, male or female, is simply great and that there are important things for one to do in the world. It is also the time to understand, with deep unspoken certainty, that the opposite sex is also splendid, with a comparative set of tasks to undertake. Above all, it is necessary for the child to gain faith in his or her own *initiative*, the serene inner assurance that it will be quite possible to grow up and become a highly regarded man or woman.

SEX EDUCATION

The first specific questions regarding reproduction are likely to arise during these preschool years. Usually, the youngster's interest is triggered by the sight of a pregnant woman, and the question is straightforward. "Why is she so fat?" It provides a perfect time for a straightforward answer. "She is big because there is a baby inside, growing where it is safe and warm, until it is big enough to be born and live outside."

Ordinarily, these days, such questions do not give parents much of a problem. Parents have become rather well aware that this kind of "sex education" is important and should be accomplished early, without any bypasses through "babies are brought by storks" mythology. There is general understanding that the child's specific question should be answered without a great deal of elaborating detail. If the child needs more information, this can be supplied in response to the questions. The main goals are that children should feel free to ask the questions and that communications between parent and child are kept open.

The problem for parents tends to come up somewhat later when it would be important to convey information about sexual activity and sexual response. Here, parents struggle with conflicting values and their own background of missing information and misinformation. Gagnon (1977) points out that until recently the primary means by which adults attempted to control sexual activity was to keep sex a secret. Most parents feel that their own information with regard to sex was sadly deficient, and they resolutely intend to do better with their own children. On the other hand, they are uncertain regarding exactly what should be told to children, and, most especially, they do not want their children engaging in sexual experimentation (Gordon and Dickman, 1977).

Several suggestions might help with these anxieties. First, there is no evidence whatsoever indicating that children who are familiar and comfortable with the sexual facts of life tend to engage in earlier sexual activity. As a matter of fact, it is much more likely to be the insistently curious child who, finding no sanctioned way for obtaining answers, embarks on some forbidden explorations (Spanier, 1976).

Second, the question is not one of whether or not the child should be informed. Rather, the question that the parents answer, possibly by default, is who will inform the child. If it is not to be the parent, it most assuredly will be someone else, not necessarily of the parents' choosing. In matter of fact, the principal informants are the popular media and peers (Sandler et al., 1980). Furthermore, these authors also indicate that despite heightened public awareness of sexuality and an apparent increase in certain types of sexual activity, there remains widespread confusion, ignorance, and lack of responsible

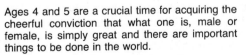

Ages 4 and 5 are a crucial time for acquiring the cheerful conviction that what one is, male or female, is simply great and there are important things to be done in the world.

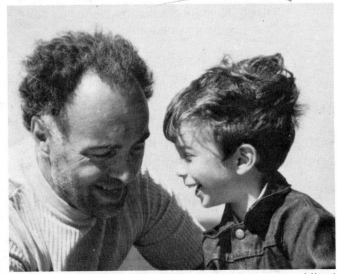

J. Hassol

sexual decision making among today's adolescents; thus, it does not appear that good sex education for children has progressed very far as yet.

Third, the fact is that every parent and care-giving adult *is* providing a quantity of information about sex without ever saying a word. Each time father gives mother a playful pat on the fanny, every time adults hold hands under the table, every time the adults intereact (conversing, quarreling, supporting, deprecating, or complimenting each other) the child is instructed about sexual relationships. A muttered "woman driver!" relays a whole block of scorn toward women to tuck away in memory banks for future attitudes toward the self or toward the opposite sex. Warm or cold, accepting or rejecting, delighted or hostile, mischievous or boring: the quality of parental interaction provides the picture-in-the-head of how men and women behave toward each other, the prototype of everything to come.

The pervasive influence of home life on small children has been acknowledged and documented for well over half a century. It comes about because the child is so limited, still, in knowledge of the rest of the world, and cannot recognize or compare other ways, cannot yet judge, cannot yet even be objective. The characteristics of the preschool child's thinking, described earlier, promote acceptance and assimilation of particular family patterns as "the way it is, everywhere." It becomes a built-in, deeply rooted aspect of the personality—unquestioned, unexamined, unarticulated, truly corresponding to what Sigmund Freud termed "unconscious." These are the attitudes toward the self and others that will ultimately influence sexuality more importantly than an understanding of the "facts of life."

Parents who fear that their own background and feelings about sex might transfer something they have no wish to impose upon children might well consider joining a Community College or Evening Division class in human sexuality. Sometimes there are seminars or workshops sponsored by local mental health organizations that are very effective, serving to desensitize old attitudes and to encourage new, more understanding outlooks. Parents' own sexual interactions are often improved as a result of the new understandings forming a happy byproduct of such a venture.

There is no known society that has not regulated and prescribed sexual behavior for its members, a fact that attests to the recognized power of sex for creating bonds or for disrupting society's relationships (Katchadourian and Lunde, 1975). Such a power ought to be harnessed for human good, used to bridge the gap that separates each human from one another and making bearable the loneliness of each existence. Sex combined with love, ideally, to form a circle of protection around the vulnerable young. This is the view of sex that, it is hoped, can be passed on to our children. We would hope that they come to experience their own sexuality as both gift and responsibility through which each partner undertakes the wonderful "pleasuring for self and another" that the human body and psyche make possible.

GLOSSARY

EGOCENTRISM Piaget's description of the naive assumption in young children that their own perceptions are exactly the same as those obtained by everyone else.

INITIATIVE Erikson's term for the third developmental task, which brings about the inner assurance that it will be possible to grow up and become a highly regarded man or woman.

PHENOMENALISM Described by Piaget as the quality in a young child's thought that unquestioningly accepts extraordinary events without wonder or further inquiry.

PREOPERATIONAL PERIOD For Piaget, this is the second period of intellectual development, lasting roughly from ages 2 to 7. It is characterized chiefly by increasing mastery of language and by the ability to use symbols, especially engaging in pretend play.

REINFORCEMENT Anything that, following behavior, increases the probability of repetition of that behavior.

REFERENCES

Bem, S.: Sex role adaptability: One consequence of psychological androgyny. *Journal of Personality and Social Psychology*, 4:634–643, 1975.

Bruner, J.: Play is serious business. *Psychology Today*, 8(8):81–83, 1975.

Caldwell, B. M., Wright, C. M., Honig, A. S., Tannenbaum, J.: Infant day care and attachment. *American Journal of Orthopsychiatry*, 40:397–412, 1970.

Carey, S.: The child as word learner. In Halle, M., Bresman, J., Miller G. A. (eds.): *Linguistic Theory and Psychological Reality*. Cambridge, Mass.: The MIT Press, 1977.

Chukovsky, K.: *From Two to Five*. Berkeley, Cal.: University of California Press, 1963.

Combs, A. W.; What the future demands of education. *Phi Delta Kappman*, 62(5):369–382, 1981.

Dennis, L. B.: Individual and Familial Correlates of Children's Fantasy Play. Unpublished doctoral dissertation, University of Florida, 1976.

Erikson, E.: *Childhood and Society*, 2nd ed. New York: W. W. Norton & Company, 1963.

Forisha, B. L.: *Sex Roles and Personal Awareness*. Morristown, N.J.: General Learning Press, 1978.

Freyberg, J. T. Increasing the imaginative play of urban disadvantaged kindergarten children through systematic training. In J. L. Singer (ed.): *The Child's World of Make Believe*. New York: Academic Press, 1973.

Frieze, I. H., Sales, E.: Making life decisions. In Frieze, I. H., Parsons, J. E., Johnson, P. B., Ruble, D. N., Zellman, G. L. (eds.): *Women and Sex Roles: A Psychological Perspective*. New York: W. W. Norton & Company, 1978.

Gagnon, J. H.: *Human Sexualities*. Glenview, Ill.; Scott, Foresman, 1977.

Gauger, W.: Household work: Can we add it to the GNP? *Journal of Home Economics*, October 1973, pp. 12–23.

Gil, D. G.: *Violence Against Children: Physical Child Abuse in the United States*. Cambridge, Mass.: Harvard University Press, 1970.

Gordon, I. J.: *Early Childhood Stimulation Through Parent Education*. Final Report to the United States Children's Bureau. Gainesville: University of Florida, College of Education, 1969.

Gordon, S., Dickman, I. R.: *Sex Education: The Parents' Role*. New York: Public Affairs Pamphlets, 1977.

Hoffman, L. W. The effects of maternal employment on the child—A review of the research. *Developmental Psychology*, 10:204–228, 1974.

Katchadourian, H., Lunde, D. *Fundamentals of Human Sexuality*. New York. Holt, Rinehart & Winston, 1975.

Kempe, H., Helfer, R. E.: *Helping the Battered Child and His Family*. Philadelphia: J. B. Lippincott Company, 1971.

Lewis, M.: Parents and children: Sex role development. *School Review*, 80:229–240, 1972.

Maccoby, E., Jacklin, C.: *The Psychology of Sex Differences*. Stanford, Cal.: Stanford University Press, 1974.

Mace, D. R.: The danger of sex innocence. *Sexology*, November 1970, pp. 50–52.

Manosevits, M., Prentice, N., Wilson, F.: Individual and family correlates of imaginary companions in preschool children. *Developmental Psychology*, 8:72–73, 1973.

Maxim, G.: *The Very Young: Guiding Children from Infancy Through the Early Years*. Belmont, Cal.: Wadsworth, Inc., 1980.

Peller, L.: Models of children's play. *Mental Hygiene*, 36:66–83, 1952.

Piaget, J. *The Origins of Inteligence in Children*. New York: International Universities Press, 1952.

Piaget, J.: *Play, Dreams and Imitation in Childhood*. New York: W. W. Norton & Company, 1962a.

Piaget, J. *The Psychology of Intelligence*. New York: W. W. Norton & Company, 1962b.

Piaget, J.: *Six Psychological Studies*. New York: Random House, 1967.

Piaget, J.: *The Child and Reality: Problems of Genetic Psychology*. New York: Grossman Publishers, Inc., 1973.

Pulaski, M. A. Play as a function of toy structure and fantasy predisposition. *Child Development*, 41:531–537, 1970.

Pulaski, M. A.: *Understanding Piaget: An Introduction to Children's Cognitive Development*. New York: Harper & Row, 1971.

Pulaski, M. A.: The rich rewards of make-believe. *Psychology Today*, 7(1):68–76, 1974.

Rogers, D.: Maternal deprivation. In Rogers, D. (ed.): *Issues in Child Psychology*, 2nd ed. Belmont, Cal.: Wadsworth Inc., 1977.

Rue, V. M. Television and the family: The question of control. In D. Rogers (ed.) *Issues in Child Psychology*. 2nd ed. Monterey, Calif.: Brooks/Cole, 1977.

Saltz, E., Johnson, J. Training for thematic-fantasy play in culturally disadvantaged children. In *Studies in Intellectual Development*. Detroit: Wayne State University, 1973.

Sandler, J., Myerson, M., Kinder, B. N.: *Human Sexuality: Current Perspectives*. Tampa, Fla.: Mariner, 1980.

Schafer, C. E.: Imaginary companions and creative adolescents. *Developmental Psychology*, 1:747–749, 1969.

Singer, D., Singer, J.: Is human imagination going down the tube? *The Chronicle of Higher Education*, 18(9):56, 1979.

Singer, J.: *The Child's World of Make Believe*. New York: Academic Press, 1973.

Single-parent families increase 79% since 1970. *Boston Sunday Globe*, August 17, 1980, p. 19.

Smilansky, S. *The Effects of Sociodramatic Play on Disadvantged Children*. New York: John W. Wiley & Sons, 1968.

Spanier, G. B.: Formal and informal sex education as determinants of premarital sexual behavior. *Archives of Sexual Behavior*, 5, 39–67, 1976.

Stone, G. P.: The play of little children. In Herron, R. E., Sutton-Smith, B (eds.): *Child's Play*. New York: John Wiley & Sons, 1971.

Sutton-Smith, B.: The role of play in cognitive development. *Young Children*, 6:202–214, 1967.

Zajonc, R. V.: Family configuration and intelligence. *Science*, 185:227–236, 1976.

HEALTH CONCERNS IN EARLY CHILDHOOD

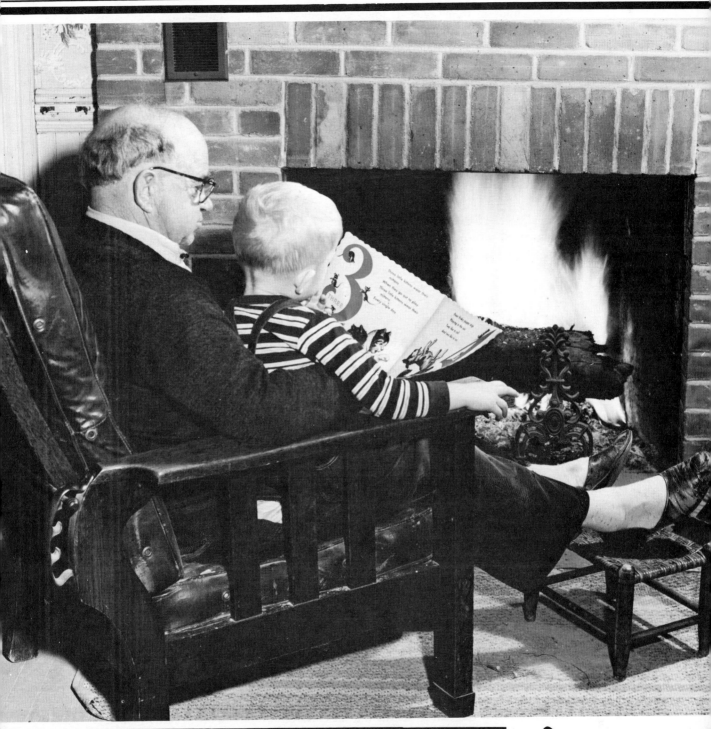

CHAPTER 7

Children from ages 1 to 3 are called *toddlers* and those from ages 3 to 5 *preschoolers*. Parents tend to have differing reactions to this period. On one hand are those who relish watching the "person" emerge, who delight in playing, teaching, and exploring with their child. There are others who miss the warm, clean-smelling, dependent infant who ate and slept and whose demands for attention focused around a full belly.

Toddlers are bundles of inconsistencies. Pot belly forward, spine curved, the toddler walks with a wide-based, unsteady gait. Napping schedules change just as they are getting established; food preferences and active food dislikes develop; tempers peek out from angelic faces. What is going on is called autonomy—the need to determine the who, what, and why of the world and to explore and manipulate it.

HEALTH ASSESSMENT

Compared with infants, toddlers are more wary of people and the whole idea of going to the physician. They are much less willing to be undressed, poked, and weighed. Brazelton (1974) describes this experience:

> Being examined is an intrusive and frightening experience for most people, most of their lives. To a small person who has had a bad experience and who is the midst of normal concerns about his body and its integrity, it is especially threatening to be exposed and undressed.

Mothers should allow the child to bring a security blanket or doll. Showing how the medical instruments work and demonstrating their use on a toy or on one of the parents will help prepare the child for the examination. Parents should be urged *not* to remind their child that there won't be pain; the toddler is not concentrating on pain, but on the examination. By constantly mentioning pain, a parent only instills more anxiety in the youngster.

MEDICAL ISSUES

Skin Care

Some physical signs and symptoms show up fairly consistently in work with inner-city toddlers and preschoolers. Jordan and associates (1978) conducted physical examinations on 1094 children in day-care centers in Washington, D.C., over a 3-year period. Among the most common findings were skin complaints, particularly dry skin. In many instances, parents had been putting detergents in the bathtub to prevent dirt rings. When urged to stop the practice and to oil the child's skin, the dry skin cleared up.

Dental Care

Another common finding in Jordan's study was the incidence of dental caries. In 50 per cent of all the children checked, there was evidence of unattended dental decay. Parents need to help children establish good dental hygiene habits during the preschool years. Even a 2-year-old can brush his or her own teeth. In the beginning, the parents will have to brush the child's teeth, but all children are delighted to have their own brush and to do the same thing they see their parents doing. Flossing can also be taught to preschoolers, but it is hard for most of them to do alone and a parent should help. By age 3, a visit to the dentist or dental clinic is a good idea. If a child is initiated into this routine before difficulty occurs, the dentist's office becomes an intriguing place to visit, with levers to push and chairs that move up and down.

Bathing

From time to time, almost every mother adds bubble bath to the bath water. Girls are particularly sensitive to bubble bath because it may be irritating to tender vaginal tissue.

In addition, the use of bubble bath with the resulting irritation may mask other underlying causes of that irritation, such as vaginitis, urethral infections, and even gonorrhea. It is a practice that mothers should be urged to cease.

Nutrition

One of the most common complaints verbalized by parents of toddlers and preschoolers is the frustration of watching a baby who earlier ate everything suddenly become what they describe as a "picky" eater. Somewhere around 1 year of age, many babies change their eating habits. They become more choosy and less hungry. If babies kept on eating at the same pace they did as infants, they would be tremendously overweight, and contrary to popular folk wisdom, a heavy baby is not a healthy one.

There are many reasons for this sudden shift besides the slowing down of the growth curve. Some babies may become cranky and irritable when teething; some just begin to realize that they have some choice and are prepared to exercise it when it comes to mealtime. Others develop some real likes and dislikes in the food department. As adults' tastes vary, so do young children's. What looked very appetizing one day looks totally distasteful the next. When given a variety of foods to choose from, children will eat a surprisingly well-balanced diet. A typical selection of foods to be included in the daily diet is shown in Table 7–1.

In discussions of food with parents, there is an ideal opportunity to stress nutrition practices that will be important throughout life. In the United States, many of us have developed some eating habits that are contradictory to the maintenance of health. Far too many people, young and old, are swayed by the advertising on television, in the newspapers, and on the radio. The era of "fast foods," prepared meals, and preprocessed ingredients have all combined to make the American diet potentially unhealthy. There is even some evidence that the use of refined grains and flour, reducing the amount of roughage in the diet, is suspect in the increase in intestinal cancer.

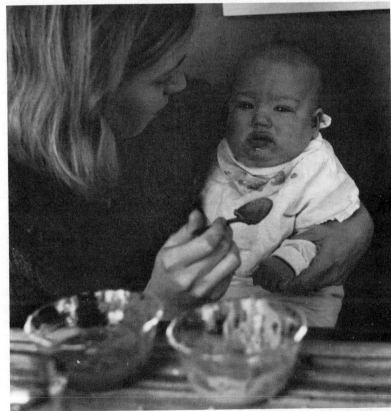

Babies have likes and dislikes when it comes to food, and they assert their taste preferences.

Judith Kruger Michalik

TABLE 7–1 DAILY DIET FOR TODDLERS AND PRESCHOOLERS*

Food	Quantity
Milk (in any form)	1½ pints
Meat, fish, or poultry	1 serving
Eggs	1
Vegetables	1 or 2 times a day; some raw; either green or yellow
Fruit	2 to 3 times, mostly raw, including orange juice; cooked fruit prepared without sugar
Starchy vegetable	1 or 2 times a day
Bread, crackers, or cereals	Whole grain, 1 to 3 times a day

*Adapted from Spock, B.: *Baby and Child Care.* New York: Simon and Schuster, 1974.

It is possible to avoid all prepared foods, including commercial "baby" or "toddler" foods, when planning a menu for a small child. It is actually less expensive and more convenient to feed them what the rest of the family is eating, provided those foods are wholesome and unprocessed. For the infant, the family can purchase a small food grinder. It is easy to demonstrate how easily and cheaply food can be prepared, how waste is eliminated because only the amount the baby will be eating at one time is prepared, and how the baby can eat a portion of what the rest of the family is eating.

Parents should eliminate salt and sugar from their baby's diet. When babies get used to sweetened and salted foods at an early age, they are much less interested in eating "natural" foods without flavor enhancers. High salt intake has been recognized as a health hazard for all ages. There is no need for food to be prepared with salt; when the manufacturers of baby food use salt, it is to make the food taste better to the parents, not the children. Recognition of the hazards and public and government pressure have influenced manufacturers to greatly reduce or eliminate additives to baby and toddler food.

Toddlers can become very fussy about what particular foods are eaten. If a child refuses a certain food, other foods can be substituted that contain the same nutrients. Some alternatives are listed in Table 7–2.

Some children will drink vegetable juice. Others will eat raw vegetables eagerly. Fish and chicken make excellent low-cost substitutes for beef and are lower in cholesterol. Parents should avoid feeding toddlers "luncheon" meats, frankfurters, and sausage, because they are too fatty and very salty and are not wholesome meats for young children.

If the child has really decided not to eat a vegetable, vegetable soup or a mixture of vegetables might be more acceptable. Mothers may find that their children get into ruts about eating and insist on one food for every meal. Some children will eat peanut butter and jelly sandwiches until their mothers begin to worry. However, whole wheat bread and peanut butter, accompanied by fruit and milk, is an adequate meal. Generally, young children will eat a balanced diet if given a chance to sample a wide variety of healthy foods without many sweets. Any temporary deviance from what a mother considers to be a well-balanced diet is nothing to worry about. What is more important is allowing the child the chance to pick up the food, manipulate spoons, try out foods with different textures and tastes, and learn to enjoy the process of eating independently. It is a messy process. The ability to use a spoon can develop as early as 12 to 14 months if the child is given a chance to practice. By 18 months, a toddler may be using a spoon quite well.

TABLE 7–2 MENU SUBSTITUTIONS

Food	Substitutes
Milk	Puddings, yogurt, cottage cheese, processed and natural cheeses
Meat, poultry, fish	Peanut butter, other nuts, beans, eggs
Vegetables	Substitute fruits for a while if the child refuses vegetables. Vegetable juice, vegetable soup; raw vegetables rather than cooked.
Bread	Unsalted whole wheat crackers, graham crackers, whole-grain cereal

If the parents are concerned about the amount of food that ends up on the floor, a plastic tablecloth placed under the highchair will make the clean-up easier.

Respiratory Illness

Often a parent is concerned about the number of colds the child has. The common cold is not avoidable. Most children have many colds from being in contact with other children and family members.

Sometimes using a vaporizer or humidifier in the child's bedroom will make him more comfortable. The vaporizer should be out of reach of the child and the water level checked often to be sure the water hasn't run out. Some vaporizers are manufactured with an automatic shutoff when the water level gets low. They are relatively inexpensive and very useful in our dry, desertlike, winter-heated homes.

Motor Skills

As the first birthday approaches, the infant's world and awareness will have expanded by leaps and bounds. Good health maintenance demands continued monitoring of the baby's progress in many areas: physical, mental, emotional, and nutritional. Signs of normal development include muscular dexterity, crawling, walking, the ability to respond to and use a variety of toys, and ability to relate to others. Mothers compare notes and babies, even as they sit in the waiting room of a clinic or physician's office. One mother may notice that her baby does not crawl as well as another, still another that her baby has no discernible vocabulary. The role of the health worker as teacher will be important in reassuring families that babies develop according to their own internal timetables. If the baby is physically and mentally sound and has a warm, accepting, and stimulating environment, the appropriate skills should appear in due time.

SAFETY

Small children need to have a safe, danger-free, but nonconfining environment that allows a chance to explore their world. Parents need to know about the many hazards that are in every home. They cannot prevent all accidents, but they can try to make the home as safe as possible.

Car Safety

The most common cause of death in small children is car accidents. Holding a child on a parent's lap is not enough protection; in fact, in an accident it may even make the child's injury worse. When a car is traveling only 20 miles an hour, a 15-pound baby is thrown at a force of 300 pounds in a car crash. Such a force will tear the child from the parent's arms and throw him against the window or dashboard. If the parent is not wearing a seat belt, he or she could be thrown against the dashboard, crushing the child in between. All children riding in cars should be strapped into car seats approved for their age. There are specially designed infant car seats that can be used from birth. Some can be reversed as the child gets bigger. These car seats should be used until the child weighs about 40 pounds. By then, the child is able to use an adult restraining belt. Children will quickly accept the belt if it is used consistently.

Precautions at Home

Parents also need to remember that all children explore their world through their mouths. All small objects, such as beads, buttons, nuts, popcorn kernels, and so on should be put out of reach. Highchairs ought to have a broad base, and the baby should be secured by straps when sitting in one. Latches should be placed high enough on doors so that small fingers will not be able to reach them. Gates should be set up in front of doorways to rooms that the parents do not want the baby to enter. Parents can be taught to look at the house through a baby's eyes. Families must be reminded that plastic bags are easy for a baby to put over the head and can lead to suffocation. Another source of lethal danger is the practice of tying a pacifier on a string around the baby's neck; the child might be strangled.

The ways of "babyproofing" a house might be listed as follows: Removing ash trays; putting pots and pans in low cupboards and dishes in high ones; changing furniture around so that tables with sharp corners are temporarily put away. Babies do not know what "no" means. It is safer and wiser to remove unsafe objects first than to try to remove the baby from unsafe objects that he grabs. A year-old baby can easily be detracted from an unsafe situation. Finally, parents need to know the phone number of the nearest local poison center in case of an emergency. Table 7–3 lists common causes of accidents and how to prevent them.

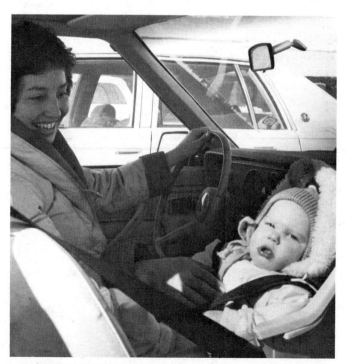

A car seat suited to the child's size and properly strapped into the car is essential to health promotion. More children in the United States under 5 years of age die from car accidents than from any other cause. In some communities, health professionals are helping parents protect their children by sponsoring rental programs to encourage low-income families to use car seats.

Courtesy of the Public Health Nursing Association for Burlington County, N.J.

TABLE 7–3 ACCIDENT PREVENTION

Hazard	Prevention
Fire	Use fire-retardant clothing
	Have a dry chemical extinguisher in the kitchen
	Turn pot handles in so that they don't protrude from the stove
	Don't use tablecloths or mats that can be pulled off by a small child
	Don't use open heaters
	Put outlet covers on all unused electrical outlets
	Put gates or screens around wood or coal stoves
Drowning	Put fences around large pools
	Make children wear life preservers near or in water
	Don't leave children in tubs or sinks alone, even for a minute
Poisoning	Put large labels on all medicines
	Lock up all medicines in a box
	Keep locked boxes on a high shelf
	Don't put any substance in a bottle that was labeled for another (putting cleaning fluid in a soft drink bottle)
	Throw away unused medicines
Poisonous plants	Keep the following out of reach: Apple seeds, caladium, dumbcane, foxglove, rhubarb leaves, lantana, mistletoe, potato stems, oleander, rhododendron, jimsonweed, yellow jessamine, hemlock berries

Lead Paint

One safety issue deserves special attention: The problem of lead paint poisoning. Until fairly recently, most paint used for interior as well as exterior painting contained lead. In older homes and apartments that have not been maintained, the paint chips away, exposing underlying layers. Small children, exploring windows, frequently chew on the sills and ingest the paint. Because paint with lead has a sweet taste, they eat more. The level of lead gradually builds up in the blood, causing lead poisoning.

Lead poisoning can produce irreversible brain damage. In addition, it can cause kidney damage, anemia, or seizures. The level of lead in the blood can be detected by a simple blood test.

About 200 childhood deaths a year are attributed to lead poisoning. According to the National Center for Health Statistics, 675,000 preschool children—about 40 per cent of the age group—have levels of lead in the blood that exceed government standards. Six times as many black children have excessive levels as white children. This is attributed to differences in socioeconomic class and living conditions.

Many cities have instituted lead screening programs at no cost to the parent. If there are any suspicions or indications that the child may be chewing on the woodwork, parents should have their child tested for possible lead poisoning.

The only prevention for lead poisoning is the elimination of lead paint from the house. This may mean scraping the woodwork down to the original wood in areas extending up to and including the window sills and repainting with lead-free paint. In some locations, landlords are required by law to repaint; in others, funds may be available to help do the job.

CHILD ABUSE AND NEGLECT

This is one area in which accurate observations concerning the health status of a child may be life-saving and in which nurses, aides, pediatricians, and all others involved in the care of children should feel a deep responsibility. As mentioned in Chapter 4, there are many subtle indicators that all might not be well in the family. Kempe (1978) suggests that all medical personnel be alert for the mother who comes into the emergency room or physician's office complaining of a variety of vague symptoms, such as insomnia, confusion, or anxiety. She may be trying to cope with feelings that even she does not understand; feelings of despair, uncontrollable anger, and the fear that she will unwittingly harm her baby. The mother who repeatedly brings her well baby into the emergency room claiming that he is ill may also be pleading for help, signaling that she can't control her angry feelings and is afraid of what might happen if she does not get some assistance.

Families with a record of child abuse are frequently isolated, with few contacts among their own families or friends. They try to protect themselves by going from one hospital to another when their child has been injured. A parent who comes in with an injured child and lives a considerable distance away must be regarded with suspicion. The hospitals in their home area should be checked to determine if the child has been seen there.

Helfer and Kempe (1974) point out that the physician has a legal as well as a moral responsibility to respond in suspected cases of child abuse or neglect. The physician is a mandated reporter in every state, as are nurses, social workers, teachers, dentists, day-care workers, and all others who, as part of their work, come in regular contact with children. As such, all are obligated to report to their local child abuse registry or other agency responsible for the monitoring of such cases.

All medical records, notes, and pertinent reports must be signed by a physician so that if a case comes to court, medical records may be submitted as evidence. A nurse who obtains information or makes observations that suggest child abuse or neglect has a responsibility to report to the senior medical officer qualified to act in an official capacity.

Common signs of abuse or neglect may include extreme filth, unexplained bruises, pain when limbs are moved, persistent vomiting (which may indicate intestinal obstruction due to a blood clot), malnutrition, severe or widespread diaper rash that has not been attended to, burns on the buttocks, round lesions that could be cigarette burns, a variety of fractures of the upper arms and skull, and marks on a baby's body that suggest a beating (an electric cord makes a classic curved abrasion from the loop of the cord).

We must all be concerned about the relationship a teen-age mother has with her infant. Many times, women who themselves have been neglected and feel unwanted in their own families marry at a very young age and find themselves pregnant. They equate babies with love and look forward to having someone "love" them. Often deserted when the marriage fails, they are left alone to cope with a new infant. When the baby demands attention, cries, or does not sleep; when old friends are no longer accessible; when boredom, isolation, and poverty become grinding realities—the potential for despair is high and child abuse may occur.

It is necessary for teams to work on cases of abuse and neglect, to gather information, and to obtain support. In all cases, the family of the child has to be informed of the team's findings. The pediatrician who has established a relationship with the family should be the one to maintain contact with them in a helpful, nonjudgmental fashion. If the physician does not control the chain of events, and if law enforcement or social agencies rush in before trust is established, the family will flee, and the child will be further victimized. It is in such cases that the same child is almost certain to reappear in an emergency room at some later date with more severe injuries. Helfer (1974) also suggests that if the physician does not assume the responsibility of coordinating the case, there is a 30 per cent chance that the child may be permanently injured or killed within the next several months.

The reactions of medical personnel to cases of child abuse are frequently anger and frustration. Kliot (1977) notes that if a child is hospitalized (often the best option for ensuring a complete examination and a cooling-off period), hospital personnel are likely to be both covertly and overtly hostile toward the parents and their ability to parent. The staff, in an effort to compensate for what they perceive as a lack of parental affection, may resort to excessive affection for and attention to the baby, making it difficult for both child and parents when the child is discharged. Often dramatic gains will be made during hospitalization and staff members will again feel anger and frustration about an order to discharge the baby, knowing that the family will probably not return for a follow-up examination and will go to another hospital the next time the child is injured.

It is of utmost importance that the baby be kept in the hospital long enough for the physician in charge to develop contact with the family and appropriate agency to monitor the initial interventions. The goal is not punishment: It is to initiate supportive help. Working within a team framework can help dissipate the feelings of helplessness, as well as coordinate future planning.

Davoren (1974) feels that social workers dealing with abusive families need to know all the family dynamics. What kind of mothering did the battering mother receive? Was the abusive father an abused child himself? We know that children are sometimes abused by parents who were themselves beaten. What are the expectations of the parents toward the baby? In many families, babies are viewed as little adults, capable of adult responses and able to understand orders about toilet training and other behavior. These questions provide the cues for parent education in child development that ought to be part of every clinic program.

Many parents realize that they need help desperately and will accept that help if they understand that they have the capacity to change. Social workers and other professionals, who are available—but not to rescue—and who are supportive—but not accusing—will be more successful in diffusing the hostility and suspiciousness of such a family. The best hope for the abused child lies within the family. Unless it is necessary to protect the life of the child, children should remain in their own home and not be placed in foster care. It is the role of all members of the health team to facilitate the goal of steady and reliable help for these families so that eventually the child can be safe with the parents.

Throughout this chapter, we have focused on some of the health maintenance issues involved in bringing up toddlers and preschoolers. Children of this age are essentially healthy. Many of the health issues in early childhood center on what is appropriate behavior for the age of the child. An understanding of normal child development enhances the ability of parents and health care professionals to promote health in early childhood.

REFERENCES

Brazelton, T. B.: *Toddlers and Infants.* New York: Delacorte Press, 1974.

Davoren, E.: The role of the social worker. In Helfer, R., Kempe, C. H. (eds.): *The Battered Child,* 2nd ed. Chicago: University of Chicago Press, 1974.

Helfer, R., Kempe, C. H. (eds.): *The Battered Child:* Chicago: University of Chicago Press, 1974.

Jordan, W., et al.: Physical exams in inner-city preschools. *Journal of the National Medical Association,* 70(8):563–567, 1978.

Kempe, C. H.: The pediatrician's role in child advocacy and preventive pediatrics. *American Journal of the Disabled Child,* 132(3):255–260, 1978.

Kempe, C. H., Kempe, R.: *Child Abuse.* Cambridge, Mass: Harvard University Press, 1978.

Kliot, C.: How to cope with feelings towards parents and children in child abuse cases in the hospital. In *Child Abuse and Neglect,* Vol 1. New York: Pergamon Press, 1977.

THE SCHOOL-AGE CHILD:
Industry

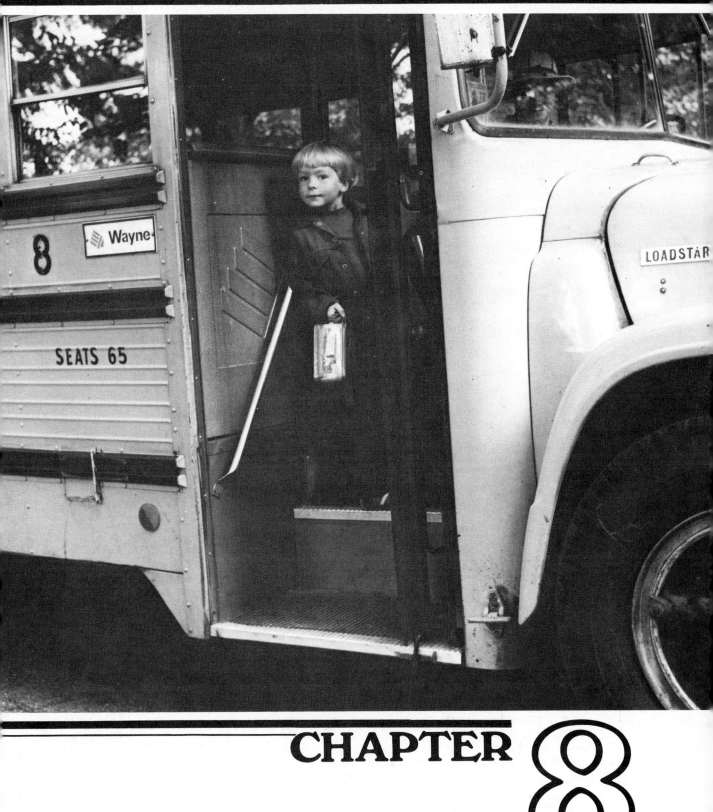

CHAPTER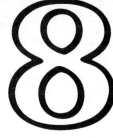

"School days, school days, dear old golden rule days." The very mention of this refrain brings a flood of memories to an adult mind. It is during these school days that one's own sustained, continual memories of childhood are fashioned. When an adult thinks of childhood, the recollection tends to be of the ages stretching between 6 and 12. Interestingly, these are not the years that a parent thinks of in remembering the childhood of family children. The clearest memories parents have will be of the preschool years.

There is a reason, of course. With the school years, the child moves up and out of the household. Long stretches are lived outside of the parents' view. Whereas the preschooler is housebound, the school-age child seems hardly able to wait to leave it. Whereas contact with friends is not central to the preschool child's main existence, the school-age child lives for friends and is tremendously influenced by them. Though still clearly dependent on parents, especially in moments of special vulnerability, the school-age child loses no opportunity to challenge their reasons, methods, and endurance. These are the days of the vehement **KEEP OUT** on the bedroom door. These are the days of an "OH, Mother, *nobody*. . . (wears that kind of lipstick, those jeans, that shirt, serves that kind of food, lives like that)" in scathing tones that every mother will recognize; the days when a peanut butter sandwich at the home of a friend takes on the aura of a banquet and of the regular pronouncement that "our family is dumb!"

The 6-to-12's are sometimes called "the Society of Children" (Berger, 1980, p. 436) because of age-group cohesion and more importantly, because children initiate other children into the rites and rules. One generation of children informs another of the school principal's spanking machine in his office and of the proper configuration for a hopscotch layout. Because the myths and lore are transmitted by word of mouth, parents are startled to hear a chant or riddle from their children that they hadn't thought about for years.

"Adam and Eve and Pinch-Me went out in a boat. Adam and Eve fell overboard; who was left?"

"What is black and white and red (read) all over?" (A modern-day response to this one is "an embarrassed zebra.")

"A plane crashed on the border between the United States and Canada. On which side of the border were the survivors buried?" (Only the dead are buried)

"It's raining, it's pouring, the old man is snoring. He went to bed with a cold in his head and didn't get up until morning."

It is known that many children's games have been played for thousands of years. Ball courts much like our own have been uncovered in ancient Mexican ruins, and the game of tic-tac-toe was inscribed in the roof of an Egyptian temple dated 1400 B.C.

References to hopscotch and blind man's buff occur in Shakespeare. Homer alludes to a game similar to backgammon in the *Iliad*. There are early Sanskrit records (dating from about 800 B.C.) that describe games known to be the forerunners of chess. A 16th-century painting by Pieter Breughel, appropriately titled "Children's Games," depicts more than 80 games of the time, many of which are clearly recognizable to players today (Avedon and Sutton-Smith, 1971).

During this period, most schoolchildren will thin out, losing the rounded, "all tummy and fanny" look of the preschool child, and become more like beanpoles, straight up and down. Physical growth is slower, though, than it had been during earlier years and than it will be during adolescence. The chubby cheeks of early childhood are lost, and the comparatively lean features of these years give some forecast of how the child will look as an adult. Most notable are the loss of baby teeth and the arrival of new replacements: the gap-toothed grin is a sure sign of a first- or second-grader, with the typical 8-year-old having a chipmunk appearance as those huge front teeth erupt. The face and jaws will catch up in the coming years so that everything matches by adolescence.

Though by implication these middle years are being treated as if they comprised an age-grouping of similar children, it is necessary to note that not only are there great

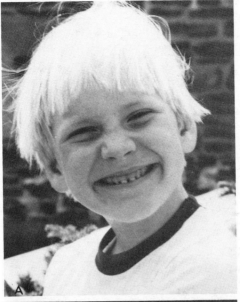
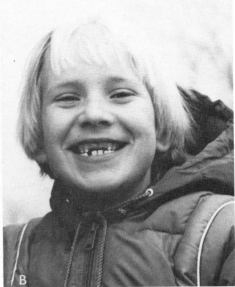

L. Newman

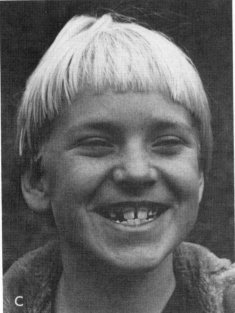

(*A*) Age 6 years. (*B*) Age 6½ years. (*C*) Age 8 years. Two years make a big change in the grin of the school-age child.

physical differences among normal children of the same age, with some who are much larger or smaller than average, but that the years 6 to 12 encompass large personality and social differences as well. The early portion of these years finds children still retaining a remnant of preschool immaturity, still relatively dependent, still enjoying cuddling and snuggling, probably on the fringes of neighborhood play groups, willing chasers of balls and wholly overcome with joy to be included in a game. Only a few years later, the child grimly tolerates an adult caress, escaping as soon as possible to the more comfortable presence of age-mates. By the end of the period, both boys and girls are likely to have set one foot in adolescence with a more assured independence, a scorn for things childish, and a kind of sophistication that many adults find positively unnerving, especially as girls (approximately 2 years ahead of their male contemporaries in rate of maturation) take on the contours and mannerisms of young women.

COGNITIVE DEVELOPMENT

The thinking of the middle-years child undergoes a qualitative change, which is sometimes very dramatic. The fact has been marked for centuries, with 7 years of age termed the Age of Reason by early church and law. Seven was the age at which children were apprenticed and the age at which children of the well-to-do were sent off to boarding school.

The characteristics of this change have been described by Flavell (1977) as especially including a new appreciation of reality (and therefore relinquishing belief in magical events), an ability to think through a process and then mentally undo it and reverse the operation, and an ability to keep account of more than one thing at a time (and therefore not be deceived by appearances).

These abilities are all characteristics of the cognitive period that Piaget termed *concrete operations*, during which the thinking of the child is much more flexible, more logical, and more objective. Though there are differences in development rate, especially in instances of poor nutrition and emotional deprivation, most children are ready for the academic tasks of school.

One of the changes involves shedding some of the egocentricity that kept the younger child's thinking closely tied to the self and to personal perceptions. Now the broadening of experience, plus the actual maturing of abilities, enables the youngster to take another's point of view and, in so doing, to obtain some sense of self as a separate entity: a doer and thinker in relation to others. In this way, the world does not seem so mysteriously changeable. The line between make-believe and reality is relatively clear. Some kinds of events are seen as predictable, offering stability and even the possibility of influence or control. Just as the concept of object permanence creates a more constant world for the infant (so that objects don't forever appear and disappear in bewildering succession like the cat in *Alice in Wonderland*), so this new thinking prowess frees up learning capacity. The child will be able to turn attention to obtaining information, discovering, and knowing.

The description so far may seem as if all this happens overnight, but such an implication is not intended. The process takes years, all of the years of middle childhood. One of its hallmarks is the ability to *conserve*. Remember the description of the preschooler and the two balls of clay? (See Chapter 6.) The preschool child will assent to their equality, but if one is flattened into a pancake or rolled into a long weiner, the preschooler becomes bemused by the change in shape. Flatter or longer appears bigger, and to the preoperational child, the two are no longer the same. But you can't fool a concrete operational child that way! Now the child is able to report the line of thinking that undergirds the answer. "Squeeze it together again and you'll see that they are just the same."

The ability to "squeeze it together again" mentally, understanding that it has not changed, is called *reversibility*. The child obtains the capacity to perceive entire sequences that have a beginning and an end and that can be "run through" again, after the fashion of a movie film. No longer limited by the one-perception-at-a-time competence of the preoperational period, the middle-years child also achieves a sense of order. It becomes possible for the child to classify, to group objects on the basis of one or two common characteristics (more complicated classifications must wait a few more years), or to arrange items according to some sort of order of size (called *seriation*).

CONSCIENCE DEVELOPMENT

The remarkable change in cognitive ability is sometimes termed the "5-to-7 shift," referring to the new possibilities for the solving of complex problems that occur during those years. One of the noticeable areas of change is in the realm of judgments about "good" or "bad" behavior, often called *moral judgment* or *conscience development*. For an understanding of the development of moral judgment in the school-age child, it will be helpful to first go back to the beginning and proceed forward.

The toddler had to be watched all the time. Every mother knows the deafening silence that precedes some mischief. However, the preschool child begins to be able to maintain "desirable" behavior in a number of different situations. The question of how children learn right from wrong has always seemed self-evident. Children learn right from wrong from parents, it has been believed, and later, from church and school. But for Piaget (1965), the self-evident answer had not been enough. His invention of methods for understanding what children are thinking and why they think that way also led him to consider the problem of children's views on right and wrong.

Piaget's Experiments with Young Children

Piaget used a series of little stories, each posing a kind of moral dilemma. He asked children of various ages to decide about the amount of blame that ought to be attached to the wrongdoer, what kind of punishment would be justified, and what kind of punishment would best keep the child from repeating the offense. Responses to the questions about the stories convinced Piaget that moral judgments, like other cognitive functions, progress from a relatively simple, egocentric consideration of wrongful acts to one that is more objective, takes motivation into account, and advocates restoring things to the way they were, if at all possible, rather than one that recommends severe punishment.

Piaget discovered that the very young child decides how "bad" an act is in terms of its consequences. According to this level of thinking, the child who broke 12 cups accidentally should be punished more severely than one who broke a single cup while snitching a forbidden cookie. Notice the preoperational mode that can focus on only one thing at a time, the preoccupation with the enormity of 12 broken cups, and the motivation ignored altogether.

Furthermore, the very young child, accustomed to punishments that must often seem to follow deeds that have not been understood as being forbidden, is convinced that the act of misbehavior itself will provide its own punishment. Therefore, you would get a bad stomachache from apples stolen out of Farmer Brown's orchard, but no such stomachache would come from apples purchased at the store. Piaget's contribution to our thinking about all this is to remind us again that the world does not look the same to a child as it does to an adult and that the factor governing that outlook is the child's own level of development. It is not inferior, just as one does not think of an infant as inferior. But it is different.

Kohlberg's Studies on the Development of Moral Judgment

Kohlberg (1969) picked up on the Piagetian formulations and elaborated further. He, too, points to a gradually developing capacity of the child to understand the world and how it works. In Kohlberg's view, the very young child judges whether an act is good or bad on the basis of how angry the parents would be, and the child's perception is that parents are most angry when a deed has some unthinkable outcome (like breaking 12 cups!). As time goes on, however, the child becomes increasingly capable of comprehending the ways of the world and more knowledgeable in cause-and-effect sequences. Kohlberg also uses a story technique to test the level of thinking that forms the child's judgments; on the basis of the response, he can identify the stage of the child's

TABLE 8–1 DEVELOPMENT OF MORAL JUDGMENT*

Level and Stage	What Is Right	Why One Should Do Right
Level I—Preconventional		
Stage 1. Punishment and obedience orientation	Do not do anything for which you might be punished.	To avoid being punished.
Stage 2. Concern with satisfying own needs	Right doing is when you get something out of it. It is also when there is an equal exchange so that both gain.	It helps get you what you want in a world where everyone has needs and wants that need to be recognized.
Level II—Conventional		
Stage 3. "Good boy, good girl" orientation	"Being good" is the goal for right behavior. Living up to what is expected of you is necessary.	You are a good person both in your own eyes and in the eyes of others.
Stage 4. The law-and-order orientation	Right behavior is obeying the law and the rules.	Laws and rules are necessary to the social system to avoid its breakdown
Level III—Postconventional†		
Stage 5. The social contract	Right conduct is what results in the greatest amount of good for the greatest number of people in the society. Good is therefore this type of general consensus . . . a social contract.	To live in a society is to undertake the obligation for abiding by the laws that offer greatest welfare and protection of everyone's rights.
Stage 6. The universal "good"	There are certain universal principles that transcend even what a given society may have designated as right. The individual is obligated to live by these principles, which include justice and equality of human rights.	To be a truly rational human being, it is necessary to believe in and abide by universal principles according to one's own conscience.

*Adapted from Kohlberg, L. The development of children's orientation toward a moral order: 1. Sequence in the development of moral thought. *Vita Humana*, 6:11–33, 1963.
†Stages 5 and 6 are described in Chapter 10.

development. Like Piaget, Kohlberg is uneasy about attempts to pinpoint the exact age that ought to have reached a certain level of moral development, preferring to call attention to the necessity of passing along the levels in order, without skipping and without regressing.

We will discuss the first four of Kohlberg's six stages here (Table 8–1), although the first two predate the school-age years now under consideration. The final two of the six stages will be reviewed in the discussion on adolescence in Chapter 10.

Early in life, according to Kohlberg, the small child judges right and wrong wholly in terms of himself and his egocentric view of the world. The ideas he gathers are built on the punishments and disapprovals of parents, and there is absolutely no concept of morality or of conformity to the larger world. Therefore, the level is termed *preconventional morality*.

Stage 1. The first stage of preconventional morality is that of simply judging acts in terms of consequences. "If I don't get punished, it must be good, and if I do get punished, it must be bad." The child begins the process of conforming to the dictates of family, religion, and society by obedience, to avoid being chastised. The first lessons are taught in the family in terms of particular prohibitions. Although the "No! No!" of toddlerhood must be enforced by parental presence, the preschooler can usually be counted on to abide by the rules the family has emphasized most heavily: "Do not hit the baby; do not pull kitty's tail; do not dump the wastebasket on the floor; do not go anywhere without asking mother." The child has no idea of the adult reasoning behind these regulations. Kohlberg suggests that the child carries them out to avoid punishment and considers a violation to be "bad." It is strictly a "what-keeps-you-out-of-trouble" outlook.

Stage 2. Just a little later, though, the child's ideas on right or wrong take on a quality of personal righteousness, the bare beginning of a value system. This is stage 2, still within the preconventional morality level. There are still many ideas about punishment mixed into the thinking, but there is also a slightly more elaborate concept of being good because it gets you something. It is a pragmatic approach, directed at obtaining one's own needs. As is evident, it is also egocentric in its basic orientation. This stage usually marks the end of the preschool period and the beginning of the school-age years.

The child's world expands to include more views and influences. There is contact with the rules for school, rules for church, rules for behavior in stores. There is gathering awareness that the world contains many social rules, and the stage is set for the second level, which Kohlberg calls *conventional morality*.

Stage 3. The first stage of the conventional morality level finds the child striving to be a "good girl" or "good boy" in order to win approval from other people. The new awareness of rules makes the child intensely legalistic, and cries of "that's not fair" ring out over the playground. Games with rules, especially those that invoke penalties for small infractions (such as red light; mother, may I?; hopscotch; and kick the can), become popular.

As this stage proceeds, the rules (as the child perceives them) are increasingly internalized. Now the stubborn facts of having been bad (hitting a sibling, taking something that doesn't belong to you) cannot be glossed over as easily as earlier. Some of the "senseless" rituals used by this middle-years child arise out of the need to neutralize the jabs of guilt for having violated a rule.

The chant "Step on a crack and you'll break your mother's back" is an example. Most of us remember a time of believing it and being very careful not to step on a crack and inflict harm on mother—even though we may have been furious with her earlier that very day. This provides the cue to the dynamics of the ritual. If you were very careful not to violate the procedure, mother would be unharmed and the earlier hostility (and therefore the guilty feelings about it) would be wiped out.

Children of this age are often trying so hard to be good that they are not even clear as to what they feel guilty about. The rituals, carried out with meticulous exactness, just make one feel better. Perhaps you can recall some of your own rituals. Common ones include the necessity of many arrangements before going to bed (shoes set just so, closet door shut, window shade adjusted to some proper height), racing up the cellar steps to escape an unnamed fate, or making bargains with the Creator ("Okay, God, if that cloud catches up with the other one, it's a sign that I can . . .").

None of this is far removed from the adult behavior of knocking on wood or throwing salt over the shoulder to avert bad luck. It placates "fate" or the "powers that be" and permits one to feel that everything is all right again. The school-age child in stage 3 is very aware of dependence on all of the powerful figures in the environment. The rituals augment the efforts to please, helping the child to feel better about herself, even knowing that she often falls far short of what she expects of herself.

Now and again, a 7- or 8-year-old is seen who has become too preoccupied with these kinds of rituals, fearfully making life miserable for herself and for everyone around with a multitude of precise formulas that need to be followed for every endeavor. In such an instance, parents ought to look at the demands they are making on the child and see if these might be excessive, creating inner furies that the child is frantically attempting to appease. If the burden does not seem to lighten within a reasonable length of time, it would be well to seek professional help to see what can be done to reduce the immoderate load of guilt.

Stage 4. By the end of the middle years, the child is likely to have reached a more objective, realistic view of the world and can understand rules that are set down by governments and how these are enforced. Stage 4, under conventional morality, is often called the "law-and-order" stage. Now the thinking emphasizes good citizenship, shows respect for authority, and promotes severe penalties for offense. The law-and-order stage is a self-righteous, eye-for-an-eye and tooth-for-a-tooth orientation, without consideration of motivation or mitigating circumstances. Kohlberg has suggested that many individuals never move beyond this stage, always calling for larger and stronger prisons, more enforcing powers for police and FBI, and reinstitution of the death penalty (Kohlberg and Elfenbein, 1975).

An interesting, related idea would place an entire society on the developmental scale, discerning its level of maturity from various indices, including how the society as a whole regards punishment. Our own society no longer engages in public floggings and hangings; it does attempt to segregate youthful violators, shows some concern for intent, and does not inflict the barbaric punishments that mutilate or prolong physical suffering. However, we are certainly ambivalent about the proper function of prisons, and we tend to believe that severe punishment is the best deterrent. We will discuss this further, when the final stages of Kohlberg's moral judgment sequence are described in Chapter 10.

THE PEER GROUP

We have spoken of the use of ritual to allay inner anxieties for children of school age. There is another use of ritual that needs mention—the sharing of rituals among same-age groups, which serves a powerfully supportive, social function.

Rituals and Belonging

Do you remember the secret handshake of your gang? Or dragging a branch behind to obliterate the path to a hidden clubhouse? Passwords? Messages in code? Taking part in these group rituals confers membership and belonging. Whether transitory and without specific goals or more permanent and purposeful, each group tends to maintain a we-against-them solidarity by its policy of exclusion. Typically, these are same-sex groups, so that it is chiefly those of the opposite sex who are to be shunned as if they carried the plague. Often, too, in the effervescence of moods and interests, today's outcast becomes tomorrow's favorite.

However, parents and teachers, though staying in the background, need to keep a watchful eye to see that the rejection is not always visited upon the same child or children. The gangs or clubs serve good developmental ends in fostering self-confidence, building independence, and teaching social skills. But those who are regularly shut out suffer in their feelings about themselves in ways that will be very hard to heal. One's concept of one's self as likable, acceptable to others, and worthwhile is at stake. Because peer groups are extremely important to self-esteem, it becomes a matter of some urgency to attempt to help the isolated ones be incorporated by one group or another.

There is evidence that some children simply do not know how to gain the approval and friendship of others. They must be instructed in ways of communication and cooperation (Oden and Asher, 1977). They need to learn to be sensitive to the behavior that makes other children dislike them—whining, tattletaling, being a poor sport, always wanting one's own way. It has been demonstrated, also, that actual coaching in social skills can be effective. When Oden and Asher (1977) undertook deliberate supervision of the children who had been unaccepted by their classmates, a month of the special

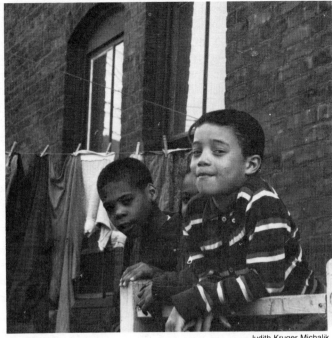

Peers serve an important supportive social function for the school-age child.

Judith Kruger Michalik

instruction was sufficient to enable low-rated children to be chosen as friends and seat-mates.

Shyness

The shy child is another who is often closed out of peer groups and who can benefit from special attention and help. Zimbardo's work on shyness (1977) suggests that the shy person anguishes a good deal in that "silent prison," missing out on the easy give-and-take of companionship and often losing credit in school situations because of inability to ask questions or offer answers, even when the material is really known. Shyness is characterized by extreme self-consciousness, concern about one's effect on others, and low self-esteem.

According to Zimbardo (1977), there are some child-rearing practices that tend to prevent shyness. Noting that the present-day Chinese seem to be raising children who are amazingly without shyness, he suggests that a society that minimizes competition among children, that emphasizes group goals, and that does not regard failure as a personal defect is apparently able to turn around the age-old Oriental use of shame, which produces virulent shyness (*i.e.*, in Japanese and Taiwanese), and to promote marked widespread sociability instead.

The Israelis have accomplished encouragement of a similar social poise for their children with methods that are quite different. In that land, which has been very conscious of the struggles of its people throughout history, children are seen as the hope of the future. Children are treated as very special and privileged beings. They are included in adult conversations, receive unstinting praise, and expect to be supported and reinforced by others for almost any endeavor. Furthermore, they absorb the society's commitment to toughness, to confrontation, and to the avoidance of passivity. All of this appears to have given the Israeli child protection from social anxiety and a sense of self-esteem that effectively averts shyness.

Shyness clinics have been established in many communities, following the success of Zimbardo's first one at Stanford University. Based on the experiences of these clinics, it is possible to gather suggestions for helping children with their shyness. First and foremost, every adult needs to become aware of the ways in which shyness is promoted, often unwittingly. All children have powerful needs for adult approval and affirmation. The adult who is quick to demean and criticize, who is grudging with praise and impossible to please is undercutting the possibility of the child's thinking favorably about herself. Often, an adult is reluctant to compliment, for fear the child will not try to improve, but actually an approval promotes trying harder. Zimbardo insists, "It is your task to make your children, your neighbors' children and your students feel good about themselves. Help them discover everything that is attractive about themselves." Compliments, sharing feelings, teaching the child to use mistakes for learning, encouraging self-reliance—all of these adult expressions of belief in the child's intrinsic worth will assist the child's self-acceptance and help to prevent shyness.

The Value of Peer Groups

Peer groups offer potent sources of information about the self for the school-age child. Children endure a great deal just to be noticed, as parents know who hear their child tagged with an unflattering nickname—Fatso, Rat Face, Four Eyes, Stinky (Harre, 1980). The gang also provides roles: leaders, followers, strategists, clowns. The most popular children tend to be leaders. Studies of leadership show these children to be less anxious, better adjusted, more intelligent, and possessing more skills than their less popular peers. It is also a fact that physical attractiveness counts, even though we might wish it were not so important (Clifford and Cohn, 1964). But there is no doubt of the significance of good looks, attractiveness, handsomeness, and beauty in adult society, so how can we expect the society of children to judge otherwise? A less well-known attribute of popularity, however, is a conventional name. A child baptized Bradbury or Wendall or Theron will have to have some special attributes to compensate for having an untypical name (McDavid and Harari, 1966).

Gangs begin as play groups during the early part of the school years, forming and re-forming, with proximity of the group members and the game of the moment serving as the main cohesive factor. As children grow older and become more mobile, the group tends to include members from beyond the immediate neighborhood. Regardless of composition, groups exert considerable influence over the lives of members. Parents sense this and inveigh against it, but the battle has been lost before it is joined. The time of life of the child dictates the first shrugging loose of parental ties, which will be replaced by the bonds of peers.

Peer Group and Parental Pressures

It is a rare child who can resist peer pressure, and most show a high degree of conformity during these school years. This is a continuing source of worry for many parents, aware that a number of undesirable practices can be initiated by gangs and carried out by children without any comprehension of long-term harmful effects. Glue sniffing, experiments with various drugs or alcohol, vandalism, and other forms of delinquency and sexual activity can all appear several years before parents are aware of the need to deal with these possibilities.

Parents may be surprised and horrified to learn of widespread drug use and other illicit activity in junior high schools, though the fact that sophistication with these illegal substances is being acquired by children who are younger and younger is well known to police and social workers. There is no simple answer to this problem. It calls for a community effort from the leaders, elected officials, church groups, schools, and families to mount a sustained program of activities that will engage youngsters in physical and psychological challenges.

Unfortunately, the concert of efforts also needs money at a time when competition for community resources is extreme. Furthermore, once a program with broad-based outreach, properly funded, is in place, the community must stay with it. Often the best-intentioned community program falters and dies for lack of sustained adult participation.

There is a paradox here, because there are other kinds of youth activities that suffer from too much adult interest. The most notable example is Little League; another activity rapidly gaining in the fervor of the parental cheering section is hockey. The profession-alization of what ought to be children's games, played for fun, unorganized, unsponsored, and uncoached, is a bizarre phenomenon that is totally contrary to children's best interests. It is the adult emphasis upon competitive child performance that needs rethinking. The fiercely hostile character of Little League and ice hockey competition is reflected in the faces of parents viewing the game and in the taunts and imprecations they hurl. The pressure on the children is too great, calling for unnatural effort and promoting too heavy a fear of failure (Elkind, 1982).

What is needed during these grade-school years is a sensible mix of adult-sponsored possibilities (with maximum child cooperation in planning these) that offer many oppor-tunities for stretching and learning, together with ample time for self-initiated pursuits. Erikson (1963) describes this as the "age of industry and accomplishment," with its developmental task—learning to work hard at something and to experience the satisfaction of having done it well.

INDUSTRY AND ACCOMPLISHMENT

These years of childhood have not always been designated as separate and special. Indeed, for most of the centuries during the rise of Western civilization there was no time of childhood (Aries, 1962). Infants were attached to their mothers or caretakers. But as soon as the infant was no longer a lap-child, he joined the society of adults in their taverns, marketplaces, fields, and fairs. Life was hard, and life expectancy was less than half of what it is today, with the mortality rate highest for children. There may have been some self-protective mechanism involved in not permitting oneself to become too attached to a child whose survival to adulthood was extremely problematic. Even more important, however, was the fact that every pair of hands was necessary for eking out a rude survival. Babies were nursed as long as possible; as soon as possible thereafter, they had to begin to contribute to their own livelihood.

Even during the last few centuries, children's efforts were required and necessary to the household, so that after-school chores and summertime labors were taken for granted. As a matter of fact, the present-day school calendar still marks the precedent of using children to help in fields during summer and releasing them for school when they could be spared. Under such conditions, "industry" did not have to be specified as a requisite for optimal development. Industry was vital for the well-being of the family.

The late years of the 20th century, however, have tended to remove meaningful work from the middle years of childhood. Child labor laws, instituted to prevent exploitation of children, inadvertently prevented the existence of many of the after-school jobs that children had once held. There aren't eggs to be gathered or cows to be brought home and milked. Few families have gardens to be weeded, clothes to be hung out or gathered in, or kindling to be split. Food preparation does not require the hulling, shucking, peeling, or long cooking it once did. Home-canning is not a likely enterprise. Even looking after younger brothers and sisters tends to be given over to the television set.

There isn't much that a child of school years can do that will really visibly matter for the family's welfare. This is probably the root cause of the battles waged over mundane chores such as keeping one's room clean and carrying out the garbage. It is "make-work" and the child knows it.

What, then, can the child of this age work at, hard and successfully? Some fortunate ones with good and enthusiastic teachers will learn to devote themselves to the various academic challenges. Some will give single-minded attention to rock collecting, model building, astronomy, and other kinds of hobbies. Some will perfect a talent for music or art or dance or writing. Some will work alongside father or mother in the patience-demanding skills of furniture refinishing, motor overhauling, or household carpentry. These are the lucky ones, according to Erikson. So are all those who learn to do something they can survey with pride. However, it is a fact that opportunities for these kinds of significant efforts are diffiult to uncover for the child of middle years.

The difficulty in finding meaningful industry probably accounts for the problem described earlier—too much parental intrusion or too little. Some children are pushed by parents into lessons, clubs, and activities in dizzying array, leaving little time for focus or concentration. But others are left to their own devices so completely that, if tragedy occurs, parents can only wring their hands in bewilderment.

Parents need to be aware of the need for close contact with their school-age children and yet be sensitive to the fact that the child needs to pull away and that too heavy a hand will impede growth and development.

A study of parental styles by Diana Baumrind (1971) has been instructive in this regard. Results showed that both permissive and authoritarian parents fail to offer the child the firm and steady support needed for optimal self-determination. The *permissive parent* is apparently deficient in offering guidelines, leaving the child too unprotected and lessening the child's ability to discipline the self for sustained attention and effort. The *authoritarian parent*, on the other hand, sets up too many strictures and regulations, permitting the child almost no practice in decision making and engendering a hostility from the child that, in itself, blocks the kind of concentration that "industry" demands.

The third parenting style described by Baumrind—the *authoritative*—seems to be a happy combination, avoiding the problems and capitalizing on the strengths of the other two. Rather than abdicating, as the permissive parent seems to do, the authoritative parent offers a firm set of limits and rules. However, these are reasonable and children are free to state a case if a rule seems too heavy. In contrast to the authoritarian parent's, "Do as you are told because I said so," the authoritative parent respects the child's right to autonomy—within limits—and the limits are not "fixed in concrete." Children are given ample opportunity to try their wings, but with the security of knowing the parents are ready and able to provide a "landing net" if necessary. Consequently, children from authoritative households seem to exhibit a kind of self-reliance and competence that apparently make accomplishment of the developmental task posed by Erikson much easier.

Neither too much nor too little parental intervention should be the watchword, and this calls for the walking of a tightrope with the same agility and sense of balance that a circus performer displays high above the heads of the audience.

In a slightly different but related vein, Elkind (1979) attends to the pressures on the child from ages 6 to 12, suggesting that "the hurried child" is a troubling phenomenon in American life. This child is urged to succeed and excel; extraordinary models of achievers are held up as norms that anyone who tries might reach. Consequently, ordinary children feel themselves to be complete failures. School becomes a place where grades are all-important and joy in learning disappears. As Elkind warns, hurried children become anxious adults. Somewhere along the line, childhood ought to offer a time for growing gradually, testing without fear of risking the total self, and having sure knowledge of parental regard and basic approval.

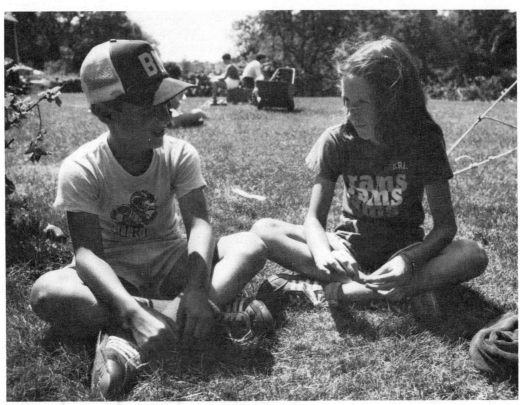

J. V. Barry

The 11- to 12-year-old differs greatly from the 6-year-old who first went off to school. The older school-age child needs space and time for growing before the intense pressures of adolescence and sexual maturity arrive.

Erikson's suggestion that industry and accomplishment are important self-perceptions that need to be acquired during this period points up a dimension of character that will be vital to the whole emerging person. The idea of the self as one who "can do," as one who is not afraid to tackle something demanding, one who can take a risk, and one who is not wholly devastated by failure—these are attributes of the developing self-concept, which can thrive only in a relaxed and tolerant atmosphere. Of all of the age levels, this one seems to be most vulnerable to unthinking neglect or unhelpful intrusion. Though parents can never solve all of their children's problems of development, during these years they will assist best by standing aside, without backing entirely out of the children's lives.

CHILDREN OF DIVORCE

The single most common major crisis in the lives of today's children is a divorce in the family. The incidence of divorce almost doubled in the decade between 1965 and 1975. Though the rate of increase has slowed somewhat, statistics show the number of divorces granted in 1980 to be 65.3 per cent higher than in 1970. Under these circumstances, an estimated one third of all American children will have experienced a family divorce by age 18 (*U.S. News and World Report*, June 16, 1980).

The discussion of the impact of divorce on a child's life has been reserved for this section because there is some indication that the school-age child has the most difficulty with coping. According to a longitudinal study by Wallerstein and Kelly (1976, 1980*a*) preschoolers reacted to family disruption with regression, but also used a number of expressive behaviors that were relatively adaptive. Tears, whining, and irritability succeeded in gaining them some attention that, under the circumstances, is better than nothing. Adolescents grieved but tended to reestablish teen-age preoccupations that helped defend against prolonged despair. But the school-age child suffered a great deal of sadness, entertaining fantasies of reconciliation between the parents and maintaining a fierce loyalty to the predivorce family, which persisted, in some instances, during the entire 5-year span of the study. Some 30 per cent of the children were still disapproving of the divorce that had occurred 5 years in the past. These children spoke of their anger and their loneliness. A significant number exhibited moderate to severe degrees of depression.

On the other hand, the same investigators found a third of the children doing very well at the 5-year mark. In a small proportion of the cases, the divorce had brought escape from a cruel and abusive parent. But the most significant factor in determining a successful outcome appeared to be continued contact with the noncustodial parent, including frequent, dependable visits and relations between the parents that were relatively free of rancor. For the child, the need for a sense of caring-that-endures seems clear.

The first year after divorce appears to be the hardest on all counts. Hetherington and associates (1978) found that households of divorced parents were more disorganized than those of intact families during this first year; mealtimes and bedtimes were more erratic, there were fewer sit-down meals with everyone together, there was less reading to the child at bedtime, and children were more likely to arrive at school late. Also, during the first year, relationships between parents and children were particularly stressful. Divorced parents communicated with the children less effectively, were less consistent in disciplining, offered less affection, and had less control than married parents. Custodial mothers were more restrictive than noncustodial fathers. In contrast, these fathers, especially in the beginning, attempted to create what was described as an "every-day-is-Christmas" situation. Neither the restrictiveness nor the showering with favors was effective in obtaining compliance from the children. The father could expect obedience only about 25 per cent of the time, even under the most favorable of circumstances; for the custodial mother, the compliance with her requests, in the case of a son, was down to 14 per cent. Daughters were only slightly more yielding to their mothers, obeying 23 per cent of the time.

It might appear that the parents were handling children rather poorly. However, it is necessary to remember that behavior is a two-way street. There do not seem to be clear-cut answers to the question of "who does what to whom." The Hetherington study reported high rates and duration of negative exchanges between custodial mothers and their children, but the data do not identify whether a distraught parent was initiating the incident or was reacting to undesirable behavior in the child. The investigators note that the children, especially the boys, "harassed" their mother. Both sons and daughters were resistant and defiant. The boys tended to be aggressive, and the girls were whining and complaining. The children nagged, withheld affection, and actively ignored instructions. One wonders if there is much else that might have been done to make a bad situation worse.

In most instances, however, substantial improvement took place during the second year. Two years after the divorce, households had settled into a much more organized pattern. Parents were demanding and obtaining more mature behavior from the children (who, of course, were 2 years older), were communicating better, and were more positive and consistent. Noncustodial fathers, it should be noted, had tended to become less available by the end of the 2 years, but they were no longer as indulgent. Both parents were able to use reasoning and explanation more effectively.

The discussion has focused on the still-typical arrangement of a divorced family with the mother having custody of children. It is estimated that fathers gain custody in only

10 per cent of the instances, though the number may be slowly increasing (Keniston, 1977). There are so few documented studies of this arrangement that almost nothing is known of how it is working out. An early British investigation (George and Wilding, 1972) indicated that a number of fathers have trouble coping with the dual demands of children and career, but this may also be said of mothers who are carrying custodial responsibility.

Neither is there much information available regarding the relatively new joint-custody plans by which children spend approximately equal time with each parent and both parents share in decisions affecting children's lives. It is obvious that this would require parents to communicate with a degree of cordiality and objectivity in order that decisions not become a repeated battleground. Because it ensures continued, regular, and substantial contacts with both parents (often involving a set of clothes and possessions at each home), joint custody may offer some advantages to children and to parents as well. Assessment will have to wait, however, until the evidence begins to accumulate.

Even in this day of widespread divorce, the rupture of a family traumatizes its members in ways that may not become recognized until the present generation of children grows to adulthood. There are too few supportive services to cushion the shock and to help sustain the one-parent family, which is often stretched thin in terms of financial and psychological security. Counseling of parents and children, even when brief, has been used with long-lasting advantages (Wallerstein and Kelly, 1980*b*). Communities urgently need to invest in a network of assistance in economic, educational, psychological, and child-rearing concerns. Good child-care facilities must become available for both preschool children and older children after school hours.

Divorce is one of the most serious social crises in present-day family life. So far, there have been no studies indicating that children (or parents) can come through wholly unaffected. However, a conflict-filled household also affects children in alarming ways. It is evident that our society is faced with unprecedented changes in traditional family structures and will have to discover ways of easing the distress for both the adults and childen involved.

SCHOOL IS FOR LEARNING

It would be derelict to discuss the development of the school-age child without considering the setting for much of that development—school. Although most adults acknowledge the importance of schooling, there exists a large amount of ambivalence regarding the school system. Parents have been impressed with numerous magazine and newpaper accounts that suggest Johnny can neither read nor write. They have been unnerved by "new math" and made fearful by the reports of rampant violence and vandalism. Every survey asking parents to rank-order characteristics of a "good school" finds *discipline* rated first. The startling rise of tax-cutting propositions indicates that the community has little respect for its school system. With teachers-on-strike arrayed on the opposite line, the unfortunate school children are caught in the crossfire. The imprudence of both teachers and community is likely to have far-reaching effects. Today's children are tomorrow's workers and citizens. The future of the United States depends upon their present education, health, and welfare.

Schools are for learning, but the process is being short-circuited for many children. Children who detect the underlying parental view that school is a "necessary evil" will faithfully reflect the disaffection, no matter what lip service is being paid to good learning. For others, the homogenization of teaching with regulations on curriculum, textbooks, and specifics of instruction so that teachers become almost interchangeable (a process, unhappily, intensified by unionization) results in a rapid deadening of the zest with which the typical first-grader approaches the first day of school.

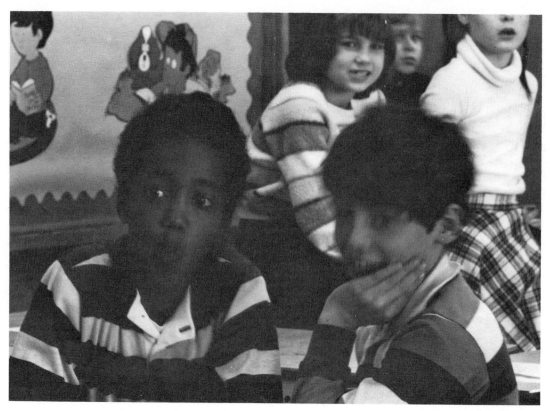

Judith Kruger Michalik

Today's children are tomorrow's citizens, and we all depend on what happens daily in our schools. With enthusiastic parents and teachers, the joy of learning can be present in our classrooms.

Furthermore, schools teach the values and skills that are safe and established. Therefore, no boat rocking: Do not raise unsettling questions about poverty, war, sex, prejudice, oppression, hunger, pollution, overpopulation, corruption, waste, or other social problems. The result, therefore, is a curriculum that is dreary and impossible to relate to real life. Television, with which the child spends most of the rest of the day, is likely to seem more relevant.

The problems of a stultifying school system and the unflattering public perception of its worth are not going to lend themselves to simple solutions. It will take enormous effort and good will from all the protagonists. Interestingly, one possible catalyst is already in place—asleep, but it could be revived. There was a time when the Parent-Teachers Association (PTA) was a powerful alliance for better schooling. Through the years, it has deteriorated into a sterile social exchange. But it could be given fresh life and its first purpose could be renewed! Teachers might also consider calling upon their unions for positive action and for looking farther than the paycheck. A concerted effort could unlock the dead hand of overregularization from the teaching profession. Standards of quality are necessary, but they have been permitted to take the individuality—and joy—out of teaching. With enthusiastic parents and teachers who want to teach, schools can again be for learning.

IN SUM: THE MIDDLE YEARS OF CHILDHOOD

Freud called these years the period of latency, suggesting that the intense psychosexual conflicts of earlier years became quieted. It was thought of as a happy time, before the

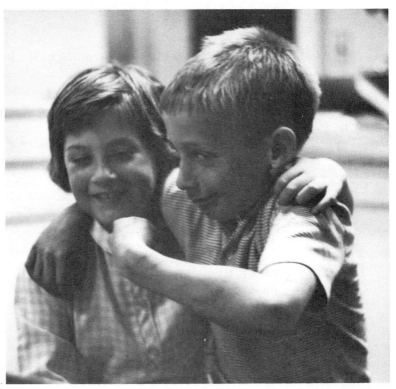

The middle years of childhood have been thought of as a happy time, free of psychosocial conflicts. Same-sex peer groups are of primary importance. Preadolescent relationships between boys and girls tend to include a lot of horseplay and showing off, precursors of the adolescent's discovery of the opposite sex.

Judith Kruger Michalik

"sturm und drang" (storm and stress) of adolescence. It has not been accorded much attention, either by development theorists or researchers. Other periods of life have seemed to play a more important role in determining adult outcomes.

Yet it can be suggested that this is neither a quiet time nor one without developmental significance. As a matter of fact, the newly emerging cognitive possibilities, the diminishing egocentrisim, the more accurate perception of reality, and the increasing independence all combine to make it a period of testing abilities and powers, with great risks to self-esteem, status, and security. Many stumble and fall. But the stakes are high. The stage is being set for what comes next.

GLOSSARY

AUTHORITARIAN PARENT   Baumrind's term for the parent whose word is law, who does not permit questioning of injunctions, and who punishes misconduct severely.

AUTHORITATIVE PARENT   Baumrind's term for the parent who sets firm but reasonable limits and combines judicious guidance with warmth, receptivity, and much child support.

CONCRETE OPERATIONAL PERIOD   The period of cognitive development taking place from about ages 7 to 12. During this time, the child begins to use mental operations that result in the understanding that if, for example, you pour lemonade from a short, wide beaker into a tall, thin one, the amount does not change. However, the child still needs to manipulate the actual objects and is still tied to concrete reality and unable to deal with abstractions.

CONSERVATION   The ability that, according to Piaget, develops over a period of time to comprehend that quantities such as mass, volume, and weight do not change even when their appearance changes. This understanding marks the concrete operational period.

CONVENTIONAL MORALITY According to Kohlberg, the second category of moral development. At this level, the child is impressed by society's punishments administered by teachers, police, prisons, and other adult forms; thus, "good" is obeying the rules and laws.

INDUSTRY AND ACCOMPLISHMENT Erikson's fourth developmental task, encompassing the school-age years. It is the time during which the child should learn to work hard at something and feel the thrill of satisfaction that comes from finally doing it well.

MORAL JUDGMENT Judgment regarding whether an act is right or wrong. According to Piaget and Kohlberg, the kind of judgment that an individual makes is a function of the level of cognitive development.

PERMISSIVE PARENT Baumrind's term for the parent who has abdicated control, is nonpunitive, and gives positive support to a child's decisions but does not offer much guidance or direction.

PRECONVENTIONAL MORALITY According to Kohlberg, the first category of moral development during which the child's conduct is controlled by punishments and rewards; therefore, to the child's mind, an act that is punished is "bad."

REVERSIBILITY The concrete operational child's ability to mentally "undo" a transformational sequence and thus account for a change in appearance.

SERIATION The ability to arrange events or objects along a continuum, going from smallest to largest or most to least.

REFERENCES

Avedon, E. M., Sutton-Smith, B.: *The Study of Games.* New York: John Wiley & Sons, 1971.

Baumrind, D.: Current patterns of parental authority. *Developmental Psychology* (Monograph 1) 4:1–103, 1971.

Berger, K. S.: *The Developing Person,* New York: Worth, 1980.

Clifford, C., Cohn, T. S.: The relationships between leadership and personality attributes of second grade children. *Journal of Social Psychology,* 64:57–64, 1964.

Elkind, D.: Growing up faster. *Psychology Today,* 12(9):38–42, 1979.

Elkind, D.: *The Hurried Child.* Reviewed in *The Lexington Minute Man,* May 6, 1982, p. 13.

Erikson, E.: *Childhood and Society,* 2nd ed. New York: W. W. Norton & Company, 1963.

Flavell, J. H.: *Cognitive Development.* Englewood Cliffs, N.J.: Prentice-Hall, 1977.

George, V., Wilding, P.: *Motherless Families.* London: Routledge & Gegan, 1972.

Harre, R.: What's in a nickname? *Psychology Today,* 13(8):78–84, 1980.

Hetherington, M., Cox, M., Cox, R.: The aftermath of divorce. In Stevens, J., Mathews, M. (eds.): *Mother/Child, Father/Child Relationships.* Washington, D.C.: National Association for the Education of Young Children, 1978.

Keniston, K.: *All Our Children. The American Family Under Pressure.* New York: Harcourt, 1977.

Kohlberg, L.: The development of children's orientation toward a moral order: 1. Sequence in the development of moral thought. *Vita Humana,* 6:11–33, 1963.

Kohlberg, L.: *Stages in the Development of Moral Thought and Action.* New York: Holt, 1969.

Kohlberg, L., Elfenbein, D.: The development of moral judgments concerning capital punishment. *American Journal of Orthopsychiatry,* 45:614–640, 1975.

McDavid, J. W., Harari, H.: Stereotyping of names and popularity in grade school. *Child Development,* 37:453–457, 1966.

Oden, S. L., Asher, S. R.: Coaching children in social skills for friendship. *Child Development,* 48:495–506, 1977.

Piaget, J.: *The Moral Judgment of the Child.* New York: Free Press, 1965.

The American family: Bent but not broken. *U.S. News and World Report*, June 16, 1980, pp. 60–66.

Wallerstein, J. S., Kelly, J. B.: The effects of parental divorce: Experiences of the child in late latency. *American Journal of Orthopsychiatry*, 46:256–265, 1976.

Wallerstein, J. S., Kelly, J. B.: *Surviving the Breakup. How Children and Parents Cope with Divorce*. New York: Basic Books, 1980a.

Wallerstein, J. S., Kelly, J. B.: California's children of divorce. *Psychology Today*, 13(8):66–76, 1980b.

Zimbardo, P. G.: *Shyness: What It Is. What to Do About It*. Reading, Mass.: Addison-Wesley, 1977.

HEALTH CONCERNS IN SCHOOL-AGE CHILDREN

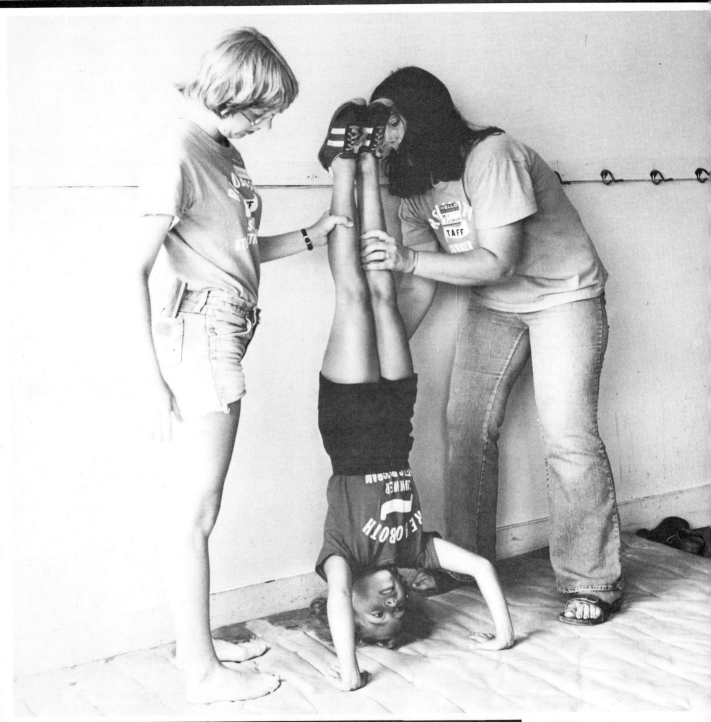

CHAPTER 9

School-age children, from 5 to 12 years old, are generally healthy. The constant "runny-nose" has passed, the chickenpox has come and gone, and the endless trips to the pediatrician have ceased. Unless there is an underlying chronic or congenital problem, the ages between 5 and 12 are probably the most uncomplicated, when viewed in the context of what has gone before and what is on the horizon. Although growth spurts vary and secondary sexual characteristics may become evident in some children, the real roller coaster ride of adolescence is still a few years away. As Chinn (1974) indicates, these are the years when children fight off infection easily, recover quickly from injury or illness, have increased motor coordination, and experience high energy levels.

What, then, are the health issues of concern in this basically healthy population? Children at this age are beginning to establish the habits that will determine health for a lifetime. They are "sponges"—alert to every television commercial and ready to consume all the junk food available in the supermarket—unless guided by parents or educators to learn healthy food habits. If given the chance, most children are eager to discover how their bodies work, and they can develop a healthy attitude toward nutrition, hygiene, sleep, and behavior. By age 11, for example, the average American child has decay in three permanent teeth. Yet we know that dental decay can be greatly reduced or eliminated by alterations in diet (chiefly by elimination of sugar) and preventive measures such as fluoridation of water and regular professional attention.

In this chapter we discuss:

1. Physiological and sexual development of the school-age child.

2. The major health issues pertaining to this age group—sex education, nutrition, safety, and accident prevention.

3. The prevention and identification of sexual assault in children.

4. The special role of the school in the health of the child and the contribution of the school nurse.

PHYSIOLOGICAL DEVELOPMENT

Children change and develop according to their individual timetables. The 6-foot tall 11-year-old boy may be no more or less able to accept his growth than his 4½ foot classmate who would give the world to have a few of those inches. Models can be created to show children how their body organs work and how the whole system is neatly and remarkably put together to keep everything humming along without a hitch. When children have the opportunity to use a microscope (preferably one of their own) to see what a cell looks like, they will be likely to listen and absorb much more readily everything a teacher or parent has to say.

Body Systems

The Brain

By 6 years of age, the brain has achieved most of its ultimate size, and by puberty it has reached adult proportions. In terms of internal brain structure, cortex development proceeds as intellectual function expands. Neurological development occurs from the head down, with large muscles gaining control first and those muscles responsible for fine motor coordination developing secondarily. The process takes a long time and is evident in the mastery of voluntary movement. Both gross and fine motor coordination appear more exact. This increased capability is also due to increase in both the size and strength of the large and small muscles. By the time children reach school age, they have also achieved the capacity to make associations between auditory, visual, and verbal cues and to integrate them.

The Eyes

By age 6 or 7, the eyes are fully developed. Both side *(peripheral)* vision and accuracy *(acuity)* are at their maximum levels. By the time a child enters school, his or her vision should be tested, in order to detect any problems. This may be done in school. If the school system does not do vision testing, parents should have a child's eyes tested at an eye clinic or physician's office. Children should be made aware that good eyesight is the key to both motor and intellectual functioning, and should learn basic safety measures to protect their eyes. Eyes should be retested every few years.

The Ears

If an infant is born with fluid-filled ears, the fluid is gradually absorbed. The resulting transient hearing loss in the young child will not usually affect future hearing. By the time the child enters school, however, a hearing test using specially designed equipment is recommended. The test, utilizing gradually diminishing sounds, can detect auditory problems.

The Gastrointestinal and Respiratory Systems

By late childhood, the gastrointestinal and respiratory systems are mature. Lung capacity continues to increase as the lungs grow in size, but functionally the lungs are mature. This is a good time for the child to be introduced to the issue of cigarette smoking and to the effect it has on the lungs. Hearing a description of the important job that lungs must do every day, even in the absence of nicotine, may help the child make a decision not to smoke.

The gastrointestinal system is capable of dealing with all adult foods by the time a child enters school, and children will have established well-entrenched food likes and dislikes by this time. Later in this chapter, the nutritional requirements for school-age children are discussed.

The Circulatory System

Circulatory functions are influenced by physical size. Because of the thinness of the chest wall and the changing relationship between chest structure and the inner organs that occurs as the child grows, as many as 50 per cent of all children may have soft, or functional, heart murmurs (Holm, 1978), These murmurs are generally of no consequence.

The Endocrine System

During this age period, control of *homeostasis* (body equilibrium) and the ability to respond to stress increase. By *puberty*, only the reproductive system has yet to reach adult capacity.

The Musculoskeletal System

Perhaps the most spectacular changes occur in the musculoskeletal system. Although there are fewer growth spurts during this age, the ability of the muscles to respond is dramatic. From tying shoes to jumping rope and riding a bike, hardly a week goes by without some accomplishment in learning a new skill. This also means skinned knees, perhaps broken bones, and, occasionally, broken front teeth. Parents who may be concerned about letting their children engage in activities that carry the risk of injury need to be reassured that torn pants and black-and-blue marks are the signs of an active, happy child. The child who is overprotected and constantly nagged to be careful will soon stop trying out new skills and can become a worried, fearful stay-at-home person.

The Skin

Although the skin has become structurally mature by this time, the sweat glands and sebaceous glands remain immature. Skin eruptions and excessive sweating, which are associated with puberty and adolescence, have not yet started.

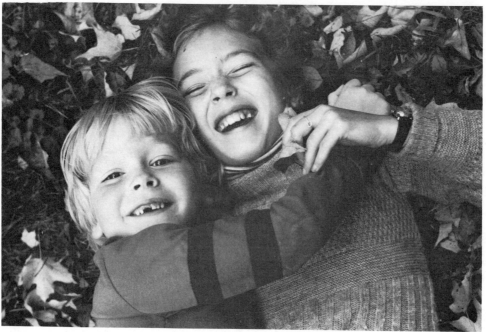

Judith Kruger Michalik

Children from the ages of 5 to 9 seem generally happier and healthier than at any other time.

The Teeth

Just looking at a grinning 7-year-old tells you what is going on in that mouth. Those big front teeth look very out of place beside the little baby ones, but in a few years, most children will have lost all their *deciduous* (first) teeth. It is not unusual, however, for even a 12- or 13-year-old to have several primary teeth removed as part of the business of getting braces. Although it is small comfort to children who have to have teeth removed, it might help for them to learn that they are fortunate to have kept their first teeth for so long because they have less chance of developing decay in the permanent teeth.

Sexual Development

As children reach what we call late childhood—10 to 11 years of age—physical changes, particularly among girls, become noticeable. Bodies that were blocky, straight up and down, and waistless begin to round out, and a vision emerges of how the adult woman may look. Table 9–1 presents some characteristic changes that occur at this time.

All of these changes are in response to the female hormones, estrogen and progesterone, which are now being produced in preparation for the childbearing years ahead. Because the hormones are produced at an uneven rate, mood changes can occur. A mother may begin to wonder if the child she sees before her is the same one who lived in the house last year! An ebullient "butterfly" one moment and sensitive to the point of tears the next, negativistic one minute and wonderfully accommodating the next, girls of this age can be a riddle to their parents. It's also hard for a young girl to understand what is going on inside her body. If she is developing faster than her peers, she may feel isolated and strangely out of joint because peer acceptance and imitation are the essence of existence at this age.

Although the average age of menarche (beginning of menstruation) has decreased in the United States, probably as a result of improved nutrition, most girls start menstruating around 11½ to 13 years of age. There are always a few fifth or sixth graders who start developing very early. As their bodies assume more adult outlines, they become the

TABLE 9–1 PHYSICAL CHANGES IN GIRLS

Breasts
 Nipples become larger.
 Area around nipples becomes larger.
 Breasts begin to develop, generally reaching adult size by 14 years of age.

Hair
 Pubic hair starts to appear, usually curly and lighter than other hair.
 Axillary (underarm) hair begins to emerge.
 Hair on head may become coarser and seem more "greasy."

Body Fat
 Hips begin to round out and a waist appears.

Skin
 Pimples may appear.
 Hair may become oily and need washing frequently.
 Skin on face may become oily as glands develop.
 Body odor develops as axillary hair traps bacteria produced by active sweat glands.

centers of curiosity and speculation among other girls. Elementary school personnel should be aware of these children and become sensitive to the issues surrounding such early development. In addition to stocking necessary sanitary supplies, schools must be prepared to offer understanding support to these youngsters in the person of the school nurse.

Sexual development in boys is generally 2 years behind that of girls, but it must not be assumed that 10-year-old undeveloped boys are any more comfortable with their bodies than their precocious female friends. The physical changes in boys are summarized in Table 9–2.

HEALTH ISSUES

The Medical Examination

Assessment of a child's current health status should review past history, family history, and the mother's labor and delivery. An attempt should be made to gain an understanding

TABLE 9–2 PHYSICAL CHANGES IN BOYS

Voice
 Starts to change; sometimes is squeaky and cracks. Change in voice is due to thickening of
  vocal chords, influenced by increase in testosterone (male hormone).

Hair
 Hair begins to develop in pubic and axillary area.
 Facial hair develops later.

Skin
 Pimples may appear.
 Sebaceous glands become more active.

Muscles
 Biceps, triceps, and pectoral muscles begin to enlarge

Genitals
 Penis begins to enlarge.
 Scrotum enlarges.
 Nocturnal emissions may begin as early as 11, but more generally around 12 or 13 years.

of the lifestyle of the family, cultural habits, whether one or both parents are working, what hours, and any other information that has a bearing on the events that shape the child's life. A medical examination should check all body systems and may include certain tests.

The Neuromuscular System

The neuromuscular check tests the strength and agility of the muscles. Sometimes the child may be asked to draw, cut out a picture, or walk on a straight line. A sensory functioning test might check whether the child can identify an object without seeing it, using only the sense of touch.

The Musculoskeletal System

A musculoskeletal examination includes a check for *scoliosis* (a sideways curvature of the spine). This examination is particularly important for prepubescent girls, who are the most prone to developing scoliosis. Approximately 10 per cent of children have this condition. If scoliosis is detected early, many children can be helped by treatment, which includes wearing a special brace. Severe abnormal curvatures of the spine can be helped by surgery.

The examination also checks the joints for tenderness or swelling. Boys may be examined for tenderness in the area just below the kneecap. Pain and tenderness in this area may be a sign of *Osgood-Schlatter disease*, a condition brought on by the uneven growth of muscles and tendons in the knee. It is most common among rapidly growing boys between 12 to 14 years of age.

The Circulatory and Respiratory Systems

The heart, lungs, pulse, and blood pressure are checked. The *upper respiratory tract examination* includes the ears, nose, and throat, as well as palpation of the neck to determine if there are any swollen glands.

The Reproductive System

In addition to a general checkup, boys need to be examined for any sign of undescended testicles. This is done by gently manipulating the scrotum to make sure that the testicles are in the scrotum. The examination is important because testicles that remain unde-scended may prohibit normal development of sperm, since sperm cannot be produced at the higher internal temperature, but only at cooler temperatures.

Sex Education

The establishment of any course called "sex education" usually causes controversy in the community. Some school systems avoid the whole subject; others offer a few sessions with the physical education teacher or school nurse on "personal hygiene," using films on menstruation produced by the manufacturers of sanitary products. This, of course, is *not* sex education. In thinking about a truly informative sex education program, we should note that the ages of unwed mothers are decreasing at an alarming rate in the United States, as more and more young people become sexually active. Although it is true that ovulation and the ability to reproduce occur months after the onset of menstruation, few young teen-aged girls understand how their bodies work and the consequences of unprotected sexual activity. It is distressing for health workers to counsel 12-year-olds at an abortion clinic, and to realize the potential for child abuse of babies born to such young mothers.

If the public does not allow school systems to present programs on sex education or human reproduction, health personnel working in clinic settings can make pamphlets and books on sexual development available for parents and children to read in the waiting room. Some clinics also have anatomical models available and include the mother in any discussions on sexual development; sometimes this can be the beginning of good communication between mother and daughter.

Some syndicated newspaper columns for teens contain straightforward answers to questions sent in concerning growth, behavior, and sexual development. A reading list of popular books written for this age group can be found in most libraries. Many focus on issues that are of vital importance to both boys and girls during these ages.

Since many girls between 9 and 12 years of age are very sensitive about their changing bodies, they may prefer to receive routine care from a female pediatrician, or, if available, a female nurse practitioner. Boys may not be any more comfortable being examined than girls, particularly if their mother is around. Boys should have the opportunity to choose whether a parent is present during medical examinations. Boys are also very curious about what is going on with their bodies. Many books, pictures, models, and articles are available to help dispel a lot of anxiety as well as to put to rest some myths, particularly those surrounding such topics as masturbation and nocturnal emissions. Both boys and girls need to be able to obtain information on sexual growth and sexual feelings from their parents or another adult in an open, matter-of-fact manner.

Nutrition

School-age children need fewer calories than younger children, but their daily caloric needs remain somewhat greater than those for adults. Young school-age children require about 35 calories per pound of body weight. By the age of 12, this is down to approximately 30 calories per pound. The total caloric intake should be between 1600 and 2200 calories per day. Protein requirement is 50 to 80 grams a day. Vitamin and mineral requirements are similar to those of a preschooler. Because of rapid large bone development, more vitamin D (400 units) and calcium (1.5 to 2 grams) are needed daily (Murray et al., 1979).

An adequate daily diet for a school-age child will include the following: milk, 3 cups; fruits and vegetables, 4 servings; meat and eggs, 2 servings; and breads and cereals, 4 servings. Substitutions can be made for animal proteins by using beans, whole wheat, and other complex carbohydrates. Milk can be either whole or skim, and powdered milk can also be used.

Parents need to view food as nourishment for developing bodies and not as a reward or punishment. Establishing good eating habits at this age will go a long way in preventing one of the most prevalent findings among young people—obesity. Obesity is rarely the result of hormonal or metabolic disturbance. Children who are obese are frequently underactive in relation to the amount of calories consumed.

Safety and Accident Prevention

Accidents are the leading cause of death in children from ages 1 to 14. In 1977, almost 10,000 children in the United States died from accidents, more than three times as many from the next leading cause, cancer.

Among the most common accidents are those involving cars (20 per cent), drownings (8 per cent), and fires (6 per cent). These accidents are the result of a combination of factors, including the same types of environmental factors that affect adults (poor highway or car design), poor parental supervision or judgment, and the lack of recognition of safety risks by children because of their level of development. Children follow the example of their parents in regard to using seat belts and in developing basic attitudes toward pedestrian and bicycle safety. Children need to be taught to wear seat belts when riding in cars and to swim only in supervised areas.

Because children are very active, they will have a higher proportion of broken limbs, most often arms, as they try to break falls by putting out their arms. Although these kinds of injuries are almost unavoidable, the injuries associated with too-rigorous organized sports activity can be avoided. Murray (1979) states: "Youngsters who play in Little League baseball are likely to develop chronic throwing injuries, especially of the elbow and shoulder, if the ball is repeatedly thrown with the arm too high." Knee trauma is common in children who play football, with the chance of permanent injury to the ligaments of the knee.

Organized sports may put undue pressure on a child to perform as a way of receiving approval from a parent. When children feel unable to keep up the level of performance expected by a parent, they will feel tense and may be more injury prone. Parents need to monitor such organized activities, as well as to realize that there are physical hazards in structured, competitive sports.

By the time children are in school, they should know basic safety rules concerning cooking, the use of knives and household tools, and the use of the stove. School-age children should know what to do in an emergency at home. They should be taught basic fire safety rules at home, and every family should plan and practice how to get out of the house or apartment in case of fire. School-age children should also know how to use the telephone to call the police or other community emergency agency.

Outside the house, the parent's job is more difficult. Responding to peer group pressure, a child who is generally sensible and cautious may well become a daredevil when it comes to bike riding, tree climbing, and other activities. Some school systems

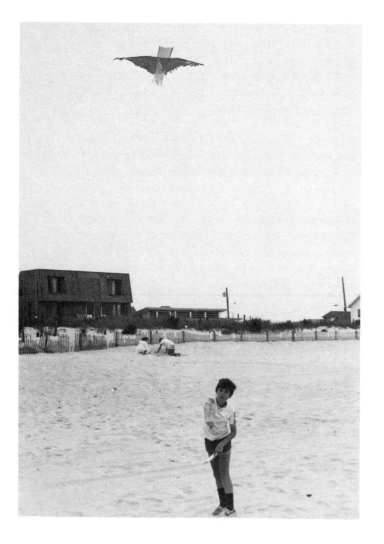

As a school-age child's interests and activities grow, simple safety rules must be taught by responsible adults. Even when it comes to such enjoyments as flying a kite, children should be shown how to avoid wires, other people, and other possible hazards.

promote a bike safety program, teaching safety rules and allowing only those children who pass a safety test to ride their bikes to school. Sometimes parents volunteer to take groups of children on bike trips along the most used routes, demonstrating signals and correct biking behavior. It is an activity that brings parents in contact with the school and enables children to feel part of a group.

SEXUAL ASSAULT OF CHILDREN

There is one problem about which every nurse, health aide, social worker, teacher, guidance counselor, or any other person involved with some aspect of a child's life should be acutely aware. This problem is *child sexual assault*. Sexual assault of children has become more apparent, with more and more cases being reported each year. Recent estimates have put the number of American children involved annually at more than 100,000 (Henderson, 1975). With only one in ten cases being reported, some investigators have estimate the figure to be as high as 750,000 cases per year (Cohen et al., 1979).

Child sexual assault is defined as any sexual contact with a child, in which a child is coerced into sexual activity by means of treats, threats, or force. It does not have to involve actual intercourse but can include fondling, oral-genital contact, digital manipulation of sexual organs, child pornography, or child prostitution.

Sexual assault of children is generally hidden. Because most children do not display obvious signs of external injury, it is the responsibility of caregivers to be alert to the signs and symptoms of assault, to acknowledge the possibility of its occurrence, and to act on behalf of the child involved, ensuring that proper measures are instituted to help prevent further victimization and exploitation.

The ages of children involved may range from preschoolers to adolescents. Although approximately a third of all reported cases are actually incestuous (the perpetrator being the child's father), 80 per cent of all child victims know their assailant as a family friend, baby sitter, mother's boyfriend, foster father, or person who is perceived by the child to be an authority figure (Burgess, 1978). Schechter and Roberge (1976) concur that 90 per cent of all victims are females assaulted by males. However, cases involving male children are being reported more frequently, with the most commonly identified offender being baby sitter, neighborhood boy, or older man who may have been involved with many children over a long period of time. We rarely identify children who have been assaulted by their mothers. There is some speculation that these figures are higher than reported, however, since many of the victims of this sexual activity are boys, who have a tendency to report abuse less often than girls.

The fact that there is rarely any severe or violent physical trauma associated with child sexual assault does not imply cooperation by the child in the activity. Children respond to authority figures in their lives by compliance and obedience. When confronted by a father who gives orders or states "all daddies do this," or "I'm going to teach you something," most children accept what they are told without question. In some instances, children are even rewarded for engaging in the sexual activity. Special trips, treats, or new toys are all enticements used by perpetrators to gain access to the child. The stakes are high. Children are told that the activity is secret and that it is a special time for them. They are warned that if they tell anyone, they will be punished and sent away, or that the father (or other assailant) will have to go to jail.

On the average, sexual assault begins around the age of 6 or 7 and may continue into adolescence, when the child, more skillful at making decisions and more able to function independently, will disclose the activity to a teacher, nurse, or guidance counselor.

Children who have been molested are frequently labeled "seductive" by family members and even by professionals. These children have learned at an early age only one way of gaining affection from men. Again, in our society, we tend to socialize little girls to be pretty, affectionate, cuddly, and compliant. We teach them to beware of strangers; but we do not make it clear that their bodies are their own to control. Frequently what is termed "seductive behavior" is what a little girl perceives of as acceptable behavior for females. Seductive behavior is learned in response to a desperate need to be accepted and loved and to bolster pervasive low self-esteem. Sometimes, in a distorted way, it is an attempt to keep the family intact. Many of these children are the oldest daughters in the family, who often have had to assume heavy adult house-keeping and child-care responsibilities and seem to be trying to fill the role of an inadequate mother.

Identification of Sexual Assault Victims

Reliance on a single behavioral sign is of little value in identifying sexually abused children. Although something may arouse suspicions, it is usually a pattern of the characteristics of the family, the child, and the whole family system that may signal the possibility of abuse. Table 9–3 identifies the family patterns associated with child sexual assault (James, 1975; Spector, 1979).

Examination of the Child

Sexual abuse of children is usually ongoing and long term. As such, evidence of recent activity is not needed. However, a physical examination is absolutely essential. There are two primary reasons for performing a medical examination on a child who is *suspected* of being an assault victim. The first is to diagnose and treat any injury, possible venereal disease, or pregnancy (11-year-olds can and do become pregnant). The second is to gather evidence that might be pertinent if the case is going to go to court.

Sgroi (1976) has formulated some guidelines for an appropriate examination as follows:

1. A complete history is taken and a physical examination is done to identify any signs of physical abuse or neglect. Many sexually abused children are also physically abused.

2. A skeletal roentgenogram is taken if physical abuse is suspected. This can show classic twisting fractures of the upper arm or other healed fractures of the long bones, skull, and other structures.

3. The examiner should check all parts of the body for trauma, particularly the genital and rectal areas and should look for foreign objects placed in the vagina or rectum.

4. The examiner should note the condition (or absence) of the hymen including the hymenal ring, and size of the vaginal and rectal openings.

5. A blood test for syphilis and cultures for gonorrhea of the throat, genitals and rectum should be done.

6. The child should be retested for syphilis in 3 months and for gonorrhea in 2 to 3 weeks if the assault has been recent.

It must be remembered that boys, as well as girls, are assaulted, and although sexual assaults are usually nonviolent, any diagnosis of gonorrhea in a young child is nearly always an indication of molestation. The examiner should be a licensed physician who can testify in court if necessary. Sometimes it is beneficial to do an examination to reassure the child that nothing is wrong physiologically.

Interviewing the Child

Because they are generally reluctant to talk, the child should be interviewed privately, without the mother present if possible. The interview should be conducted in a private, relaxed atmosphere without interruptions and in a comfortable setting. The interviewer should establish a relationship with the child by explaining what will happen and what the child can expect as a result of the conversation.

TABLE 9–3 IDENTIFICATION OF SEXUAL ASSAULT VICTIMS

Family Characteristics
1. Family tends to keep secrets about many things
2. Anti-social behavior on the part of family members
3. Poor impulse control on the part of the father
4. Signs of some violence toward children
5. History of physical or sexual abuse of parents
6. Isolation of family in community (few friends)
7. Denial of any trouble to the outside world; boundaries are rigid to outsiders but virtually nonexistent within the family

Characteristics of Mother
1. Passive, easily manipulated
2. Dependent on daughter to assume maternal or marital role
3. Inability to contemplate severing relationship with man involved in the abuse for fear of losing the relationship, financial support, or sexual contact
4. Poor self-image

Characteristics of Father or Other Authoritative Person
1. Dominant and overpowering
2. Poor impulse control
3. Alcohol abuse
4. Abused as a child
5. Denial that anything has happened
6. Tendency to blame child or mother for what is happening

Behavioral Signs in Young Children
1. Fecal soiling
2. Regression in developmental milestones
3. Explicit knowledge of sexual acts
4. Excessive masturbation
5. Anxiety about being left alone with a particular person or about visiting a particular person
6. Open sexual behavior after the age of 6 or 7

Medical Identification
1. Extreme distrust and fear of physicians or examinations
2. Somatic complaints (headache, stomachache)
3. Persistent sore throat resulting from gonorrhea
4. Sudden onset of bed wetting day or night
5. Vaginal, rectal, or any genital discharge or irritation
6. Preoccupation with anatomy and an explicit knowledge of sexual behavior

School-Associated Identification
1. Depression or withdrawal
2. Hyperactivity and an inability to pay attention to school tasks; frequently labeled as "learning disabled"
3. Arrival at school very early
4. Afraid to go home, staying at school after everyone has gone
5. Poor self-image
6. Poor performance in school
7. Inability to get involved in any school activities because of inappropriate, heavy responsibilities at home

The interviewer should use the child's terminology for sexual organs and activities. It is important not to show distaste or humor at a child's vocabulary. To do so makes the child feel unaccepted. The interviewer can use drawings, puppets, and dolls to help the child relate what has happened. Children find it easier to speak through a "third" person. The child should not be present when the interviewer is speaking to either the mother or the perpetrator.

The interviewer should use familiar events to elicit information and not ask direct questions. Children should be asked what they want to have happen as a result of disclosure.

The interviewer should not show anger or repulsion toward the offender. Many children have warm feelings toward the assailant and may feel that the only affectionate person in their life was that assailant.

The child should be made to feel blameless for anything that happened. It is also helpful for the child to be told that sometimes adults get confused in the ways they behave toward children.

Arrangements should be made to interview other children in the family. Often more than one child in the family has been assaulted by the same person. The interviewer should report all cases of intrafamilial sexual assault to the child protective service responsible for the monitoring of such cases. Child sexual assault is considered child abuse (Burgess, 1978).

Children do not lie about such events. The details are too graphic, the behavioral indicators are too evident, and the trauma is too profound for any health professional to question the occurrence. It is always important to believe the story until and unless it is proved unfounded.

Effects of Sexual Assault

The effects of sexual abuse can be distinctly varied, depending on who the offender was, his or her relationship to the victim, and how long the abuse went on. If the assault was recent and sudden—as in the cases of children who are assaulted by strangers—the trauma may be of limited duration. Although it is indeed a crisis, the event is easier to talk about because the child does not perceive that he or she had anything to do with it. If the family is supportive, believes the story, and acts in a protective manner, the child may feel reassured that the parents will prevent molestation from happening again and the long-term effects may be negligible. Unfortunately, some parents feel that if the child does not talk about the assault, it must have been forgotten or that the child was not concerned about what happened. Children should be allowed to talk as much as necessary about the assault. A silent child may be one who is mulling over what went on and is unable to integrate the experience.

Children who have been assaulted over a long period of time are traumatized even more. Feeling helpless and pressured, unable to tell anyone who will believe them, confused as to their role in the family and afraid of disclosure, they remain silent. Their victimization continues and may have profound lifelong consequences. These are the victims, most often girls, who as adults become depressed, run away from home, become sexually promiscuous, become dependent on alcohol or drugs, show suicidal tendencies and fantasies, and have major difficulties experiencing a mature, satisfying relationship with a man. Many later experience marital and sexual dysfunctions. They become angry at their fathers for exploiting them and angry at their mothers for their lack of protection. They show up as in-patients in psychiatric facilities in great numbers (Herman, 1980).

Handling Cases of Sexual Assault

Child sexual assault is a complex problem that no one agency or professional can handle individually. Coordination of resources and cooperation between agencies are essential. The work is frustrating and anxiety provoking. Professionals, including physicians, may be loath to report their suspicions or findings. Sometimes they are family friends. Others may be reluctant to get involved for fear of the time that may have to be committed or because they might have to testify publicly in court. For these reasons, the team approach is the only viable one for handling assault cases.

Medical personnel may be called upon to act quickly if they feel that the child is in potential or actual imminent life-threatening danger, if the family is unprepared to acknowledge the assault or to stop the activity, or if the mother is unable or unwilling to protect the child from further abuse. Procedures should be well in place to handle cases, with liaisons firmly established, and the responsibilities of all involved clearly defined and acknowledged.

Difficult as it may be to imagine any man or woman sexually abusing a young child, child abuse is a known and tragic fact. These children must be helped, as must their families. The consequences of inaction on the part of professionals—owing to disbelief, fear of reprisal, or recrimination—are morally unacceptable. In many states, failure to report abuse is a punishable offense and may involve a fine or imprisonment, just as in cases of child battering. Acting sensitively and quickly may, in the long run, enable a sexually abused child to work through the trauma and continue to develop in a healthy, normal fashion.

THE ROLE OF THE SCHOOL NURSE IN HEALTH PROMOTION

Many children receive only episodic health care in response to an active illness. The recognition of the importance of early detection and prevention of diseases has led to a more thorough exploration of the roles of the school and the school nurse as agents in promoting the child's total well-being. The school nurse thus assumes the role of educator, screener, and detective. Allanson (1978) states; "No school can choose to either maintain or not maintain a school health program. The only question is how adequate it will be."

Keeve (1966) expressed concern over the state of the school health program:

"For too long we have been much too concerned with the mere problems of quantity—the number of children examined each year, their height, weight, immunity, etc. The question now facing us all is: Height and weight for what purpose? Greater life expectancy for what?"

The traditional responsibilities of the school nurse to weigh and measure pupils, test their ears and eyes, and dispense occasional first aid constitute the misuse of a professional. (There is even some question concerning the appropriateness of weighing-in sessions. For many children, getting weighed in front of their friends represents an invasion of privacy that is painfully embarrassing whether they are chunky or skinny.)

Allanson (1978) believes that adequate school nursing services should include health programs, health counseling for parents and children, and follow-up of identified problems. When this is not done, there tends to be an excessive use of community health resources with increased costs to parents and the community.

The major health problems of school-age children have changed over the years. The incidence of communicable diseases such as measles, mumps, and German measles, as well as physical handicaps, has decreased in largely middle-class school populations. Yet these illnesses remain distressingly high among low-income populations who live in areas where preventive health programs are either rudimentary, nonexistent, or malproportioned in terms of monies distributed.

It is enlightening to see how school health programs have fared in various locations. In Sweden, for example, children are checked every 3 years after entrance to school in an effort to prevent, detect, and respond early to health problems. A study by Kornfält (1978) done in 1975 in the Dalby area in southern Sweden, involved 223 children (110 boys and 113 girls) born in 1965. All the children had been examined previously as part of the regular school health program. After a health questionnaire was returned by the parents to the school, the children were examined by a pediatrician and nurse.

Only 4.4 per cent of the children had newly discovered health problems, with visual defects being the major finding, and 13.5 per cent had allergy problems. (Approximately 33 per cent of children of the same age in the United States have allergy problems. It was concluded that the general health of Swedish children had improved mainly as a result of the better socioeconomic level of the families involved.

Although the Swedish investigators questioned the validity of conducting such comprehensive examinations on a healthy population, the study does point out some important considerations for school-age children in the United States. Because higher socioeconomic standards could be considered to be a salient factor in the decrease of health problems, the support of adequate school breakfast and lunch programs, low-cost health maintenance programs, and adequate housing programs appears to be cost-efficient when compared with the cost to society in caring for ill, deprived people.

Another approach to detecting current and potential problems was used by Holt (1979). In this study, two school nurses initiated home visits with the families of elementary school children to determine the role of the family in the child's overall development and health. The nurses were able to learn a great deal about a child by watching family interactions. Based on their questionnaire findings concerning the developmental and health history of each child, the nurses were then able to recommend procedures that were specifically designed for the individual child.

In an effort to measure the effectiveness of a school health progaram, Gilman (1979) conducted a study of 742 randomly selected elementary school children from tri-ethnic backgrounds in Galveston, Texas. The children matched those of the total elementary school population in the following ways: 76 per cent lived in households where the head of the household either was unemployed or was an unskilled or semiskilled laborer, and 40 per cent of these homes were headed by someone with less than a high school education. Of the total study, 29 per cent of the children were from single-parent families; 18 per cent lived in a variety of situations ranging from orphanages to extended families. Of the families interviewed, 64 per cent indicated that they took their sick children to many places for medical assistance. Many used the emergency rooms and clinics in local hospitals but did not use the same one consistently.

The tendency to take a child from one institution to another makes it impossible for a health worker to develop a total picture of the true health status of that child. Only a small proportion of the families indicated that they considered the school nurse as a resource and almost never reported any history of illness to the nurse. Their perception of the nurse was a person whose services were used for single-contact episodes, such as trauma, stomachaches, and so forth. This is a common perception, unfortunately based often in reality, for in many states, school nurses are prevented from doing more. If the nurse is visible only occasionally at school, is seen and instructed to administer only first aid, is not part of the educational process, and has little interaction with most children, the children will not see the nurse as a person who can do much for them. This perception is carried home, and parents may rightly assume that the nurse has no role in monitoring the health of their child.

In an effort to change the image and accessibility of school nurses, Lewis (1980) designed a project in the elementary school associated with the University of California in Los Angeles. The pupils were allowed access to the school nurse when they desired at any time during the day. Initially a data base was established for each child involved. The child was then asked to participate in any decisions about handling health problems. The results showed that approximately 15 to 20 per cent of the children never came to see the nurse. The majority of those who did come were boys. Many children used the service to seek solutions to nonmedical issues. The pattern of use was well established by the age of 6. The investigators concluded that those children who were taken regularly to a pediatrician for check-ups even when healthy used the system more frequently. In addition, the perceived health status of the child's mother had a bearing on the perception by the child of his own health. Thus, most children learned to use the system offered and overuse was not viewed as a problem. It thus seems reasonable that if children are able to incorporate the school nurse as part of their school routine, they might also incorporate the nurse as part of their educational program as health educator.

The school nurse is also involved in health education. Health education goes beyond pinning up glossy pictures of people sitting at an immaculately set table, eating a well-balanced meal. Health education involves a comprehensive in-depth approach. As indicated in the Berkeley School Health Curriculum Project (1976), the overall goals of a health education program are as follows:

1. Self-enhancement for every child.
2. Appreciation of the human body.

3. An understanding of how the body integrates with the environment and the daily practices of the individual.

4. Knowledge of the body systems and functions in order to understand health maintenance and disease and to better equip students to make their own decisions.

5. Pupil interaction for peer teaching and stimulation of critical thinking.

6. Contemporary community health problems.

7. Interaction with people in the community who are also concerned with health.

The Berkeley Project describes a program that differs from more traditional ones in several respects. For example, everyone who is involved in the program receives special training. This includes nurses, teachers, and school administrators. Teaching methods involve much student participation. The emphasis is on the individual, how the body works, health and well-being, options, and responsibilities. Few lectures are given; instead, active tools are used, trips are taken, and visual aids are employed.

In 1975, a similar project had been launched in Seattle, Washington, involving kindergarten through the third grade (Andrews, 1976). The kindergarten unit focused on teaching children about themselves, their five senses, awareness and appreciation of their teeth, good foods and nutrition, germs and disease, and safety. Each of the subsequent grades focused on the same topics but concepts and teaching tools became progressively more sophisticated.

In all the studies described in this chapter, the school nurse was in some way an active participant, sometimes visible in the classroom or working with children to develop healthful habits and concepts. Without a doubt as Tackett (1981) suggests, the school nurse is in a position to help children and their families evaluate all medical options available and to assist them in carrying out the option that makes the most sense. The role of the school nurse remains vital.

References

Allanson, J.: School nursing services: Some current justifications and cost-benefit implications. *Journal of School Health*, 48:603–607, 1978.

Andrew, R.: Evaluation Report: The Seattle School Health Project, 1976. Atlanta: Community Program Development, Center for Disease Control, 1976.

Berkeley Project. School Health Curriculum, 1976. *Focal Points*. Atlanta: Community Program Development, Center for Disease Control, 1976.

Burgess, A., et al.: *Sexual Assault of Children and Adolescents*. Lexington, Mass.: Lexington Books, 1978.

Chinn, P.: *Child Health Maintenance: Concepts in Family-Centered Care*. St. Louis: C. V. Mosby Company, 1974.

Cohen, M., et al.: *The Sexual Offender Against Children*. Speech given at Bridgewater Correctional Institution, Bridgewater, Mass., 1979.

Gilman, S., et al.: Measuring effectiveness of school health program. *Journal of School Health*, 49:10–14, 1979.

Henderson, J.: Incest. In Freedman, A., Kaplan, H., Sadock, B. (eds.): *Comprehensive Textbook of Psychiatry*, Vol 2. Baltimore: Williams & Wilkins, 1975.

Herman, J.: Father-daughter incest: Families at risk. Paper presented at the 133rd annual meeting, American Psychiatric Association, San Francisco, May 1980.

Holm, V.: Childhood. In Smith, W., Bierman, E., Robinson, N. (eds.): *The Biologic Ages of Man*. Philadelphia: W. B. Saunders Company, 1978.

Holt, S. J., et al.: The school nurse's family assessment tool. *American Journal of Nursing*, 79:950–953, 1979.

James, M.: *Little Victims*. New York: David McKay 1975.

Keeve, J.: Overcoming obstacles to a creative school health program. *School Health Education*, 26–32, 1967.

Kornfält, R., et al.: Physical health of 10-year-old children: An epidemiological study of school children. *Acta Paediatrica Scandia*, 67:481–489, 1978.

Leonard, B., Murray, R., et al.: Assessment and health promotion for the school child. In Murray, R., Zentner, J. (eds.): *Nursing Assessment and Health Promotion Through the Life Span*. Englewood Cliffs, N.J.: Prentice-Hall, 1979.

Lewis, C.: Child-initiated health care. *Journal of School Health* 50:144–165, 1980.

Murray, R., Zentner, J. (eds.): *Nursing Assessment and Health Promotion Through the Life Span*. Englewood Cliffs, N.J.: Prentice-Hall, 1979.

Schechter, M., and Roberge L.: Sexual exploitation of children. In Helfer, R. Kempe, C. (eds.): *Child Abuse and Neglect*. Cambridge, Mass.: Harper & Row, Ballinger Publications, 1976.

Sgroi, S.: *Comprehensive Examination for Child Sexual Assault. Sexual Assault of Children and Adolescents*. Lexington, Mass.: Lexington Books, 1978.

Spector, P.: Incest: Confronting the silent crime. Minnesota program for victims of sexual assault. St. Paul, Minn.: Department of Corrections, 1979.

Tackett, J.: Managing health. In *Family Centered Care of Children and Adolescents*. Philadelphia: W. B. Saunders Company, 1981.

THE ADOLESCENT:
Identity

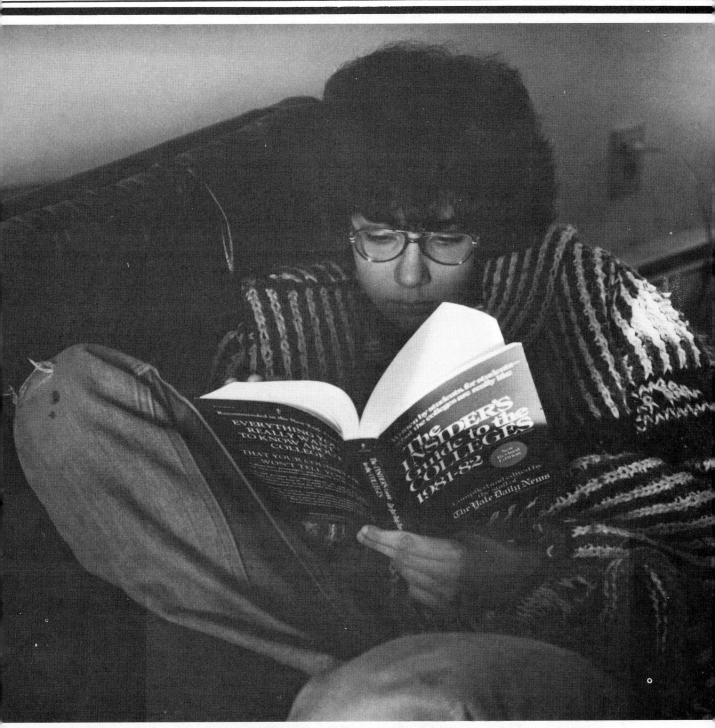

CHAPTER 10

Adolescence. Growing up. Time of upheaval and turbulence. Time of the generation gap, with parents trying frantically to maintain some control over the young person's behavior. The face of scorn and taunts that "we don't trust anyone over 30." These are widespread pictures of adolescence, given even broader currency since the youth rebellions and riots of the late 1960s and early 1970s.

So, it is interesting to inquire why this time of life should be marked by conflict and turmoil. Even more interesting is the question of whether this is, indeed, an accurate description.

The characterization of adolescence as a time of "sturm und drang" (storm and stress) was given broad reach as a "scientific" idea by G. Stanley Hall (1904), former president of Clark University and the man who invited Sigmund Freud to the United States to give a series of lectures. Hall pioneered some advanced (for the day) methods of studying children and his works were published extensively; thus, his thinking and theorizing were accorded considerable respect. The time was an exciting one, with new ideas bubbling everywhere. One of these was Charles Darwin's *Origin of Species*, which offered the notion of evolutionary development. Hall incorporated some of Darwin's thinking into his suggestions that human beings re-create their evolutionary history in the development from embryo to adult; he pointed to the aquatic fetus "recapitulating" the supposed aquatic origin of life, the creeping child mirroring ancestors who traveled on all fours, and the adolescent who, according to Hall, was passing through the stage of human existence when primitive emotions and violence were typical of the race. Hall also saw the stage as one of transition (in an evolutionary mode) from uncontrolled, impulse-driven passions to civilized restraint with profound accompanying psychological changes.

Psychoanalytic theory of the day offered support for the idea of a particularly stormy period after the "calm" of latency. Freud saw adolescence as the time when the sexual urges of the Oedipal situation, having been dampened down during latency, suddenly resurge because of the physiological maturation. Furthermore, for psychoanalytic theory, these impulses are powerful and imperative, producing high anxiety and a variety of frantic defenses. A great struggle to free the self from parents was seen as part of the effort to resolve the Oedipal attachments with sound and fury in proportion to the strength of the conflict.

Margaret Mead, representing a more contemporary view, was one of the first to question the idea of the inevitability of adolescent tension, pointing to her studies of Samoa (1950), where the young people were essentially unrestricted with regard to sexual behavior and did not need to fight or rebel, so that "coming of age" was serene and tranquil. Mead's lasting contribution was to place a brake on our own cultural ethnocentrism—the tendency to presume that "our ways" hold everywhere. She assisted in bringing about the understanding of the influence of cultural institutions and values in producing widely different behaviors and personalities.

There is present-day research, too, that should help to temper the picture of adolescents as out to overthrow all semblance of parental authority. Offer and Offer (1975) found relatively little parent-adolescent conflict in their systematic, well-designed study of middle-class adolescent boys. Adelson (1979) suggests that the number of rebellious adolescents has been greatly overestimated because psychologists and psychiatrists are primarily involved with disturbed youths and tend to generalize these troubles to the group as a whole. Like the Offers, Adelson believes that adolescents, taken as a whole, are coping with their problems calmly and responsibly.

The fact is that each age has its own parent-child conflicts, and these are determined by the cultural expectations for that age. Ask a group of parents from any part of the world to list their problems of child rearing. It is possible to predict the problems if something is known about the parents' society.

In our own society, in the day when it was considered vital to toilet train an infant by the age of 1 year, toilet training was a huge problem in every parent's mind. Few parents would list this as a problem now. These days, children tend to be toilet trained "when ready," much closer to the age of 2, and it usually takes place without fuss or frustration.

We would never expect an American mother to list as a problem the rearing of a son so courageous that he could endure a circumcision rite at age 13 without flinching. Yet, this could be a problem cited by another mother in another culture. We would probably expect a middle-class American parent to be concerned about achievement in high school and chances for college acceptance. A traditional Iranian parent is likely to describe the difficulty of rearing a marriageable daughter.

In every instance, a "problem" exists in a parent's mind because it touches upon what the child is expected to do or become. All child-rearing problems, the world over, *are* problems because of the necessity for imposing on the child the cultural expectations of the society to which she or he will belong. Insofar as these dovetail with the child's own inclinations or capabilities, or insofar as the child is able and willing to modify impulses and desires to fit, the process tends to go smoothly. However, there are instances in which the impositions are untimely (such as the insistence on too-early toilet training) or they make enormous demands that sometimes cannot be fulfilled (to endure frightful pain stoically); or there may be cases in which the child simply refuses to match the expectations (the present-day Islamic girl who will not don the veil). When there is a mismatch between expectation of the parent and the child of whom it is being required, the stage is set for a parent-child "problem."

It might very well be that the relationships between adults and adolescents flounder on the matter of expectations. We are about to take a closer look at the age period, taking note of its special features and distinctions. Perhaps this will permit a better judgment with regard to the commonly held expectations for adolescent youth in our society.

PHYSIOLOGICAL CHANGES

During no other period, except in the transformation from the stage of infancy to that of upright locomotion, are the changes as extensive and complete as in adolescence. In the course of several years, the child will acquire, literally, an entire new body—considerably larger, with muscles and fat distributed differently, growth of hair on formerly smooth areas, voice differences, larger internal organs and expanded lung capacity, a new center of gravity, changed genitalia, the addition of breasts (for girls) and last, but by no means least, new cognitive powers and emotional inclinations.

First, some terminology:

Pubescence is a period of some 2 to 2½ years during which all of the biological and physiological changes that lead to sexual maturation take place. This time is sometimes referred to as "preadolescence" because it may actually include the last several years of middle childhood, the period described in Chapter 8. For some girls, pubescence could begin as young as 8, whereas for some boys, it might begin at 10.

Puberty is the term used for the period in which the pubescent changes result in an individual who is capable of reproduction. Whether that time arrives with the first menstrual flow, *menarche*, for girls and ejaculation for boys (these events are usually cited as the hallmarks of puberty) is conjectural. There are some indications that ovulation and sperm production may be delayed for several months to a year. First menstrual periods tend to be scanty and irregular, and a full sperm count is not achieved immediately (Dusek, 1977). However, the possibility of an "adolescent sterility," a period of relative infertility during early puberty, has not been confirmed. Certainly, the increase in incidence of pregnancy among very young teenage girls casts some doubt.

Adolescence is a term that comes from the Latin verb meaning "to grow up." It, too, is an imprecise designation in both its sociological and psychological expressions. Sociologically, it is used to describe the period of transition from dependent child to self-sufficient adult. This may be clear in the instance of the individual who, at the end of high school, moves out of the parents' home, takes a job, and becomes self-supporting. But what of college students and those in graduate school whose financial needs may be supplied by the family for many years? Psychologically, adolescence is the bridge from childhood to adulthood, encompassing all of the adjustments as behavior is transformed from the "childish" into that typical of an adult. With full acknowledgment of the problematic characteristics of the term, we are going to refer to adolescence to include the years from ages 13 to 20.

Ordinarily, pubescence is heralded by a sudden increase in growth, beginning a year or two before the actual onset of puberty. Until this time, the child (whether male or female) has been progressing steadily and moderately in height and weight at a rate of some 4 to 6 pounds and approximately 1½ inches per year. This period brings about a dramatic increase of about 25 per cent in height and 50 per cent in weight, taking place over a time span of about 4 years for girls and 6 years for boys.

Body proportions also change radically. Boys undergo a broadening of the shoulders, a redistribution and enlargement of muscles, and a loss of a considerable portion of subcutaneous fat. Girls acquire wider hips, reflecting the new pelvic measurements, and retain much of the fat—with consequent softening and rounding of contours of the body. The growth process is uneven so that parts of the body grow faster than other parts, accounting for the leggy, coltish look of early adolescence. Hands and feet enlarge before the arms and legs lengthen, and, unaccustomed to the new size, adolescents literally trip over their own "clodhoppers." Nose and ears—and sometimes the lower jaw—may seem disproportionate to the rest of the face for a while.

The gargantuan appetites of teenagers support the accelerated growth, requiring more calories now than they will ever need again unless there are conditions of extraordinary physical activity. One of the results, for girls, is a preoccupation with

The appetite of the teen-ager must support the accelerated growth spurt. The teen-age boy can astound his parents by what he can "put away."

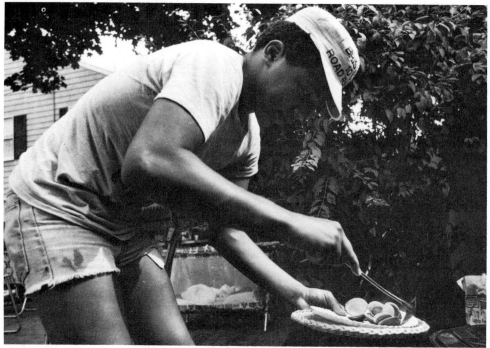

staying slender. In our society, thin is beautiful, and even the slimmest of maidens is likely to consider herself "too fat." Denying the compelling appetite is no mean feat and can result in a condition known as *anorexia nervosa* (Bruch, 1979). This is a state of extreme emaciation—the result of dieting, but maintained by abnormal and disordered psychological perceptions. Because the condition is one that can proceed to death, it is important to obtain both medical and psychological treatment.

The "growth spurt" is only a prologue to the main physiological events, however. Sexual maturation and all of the associated developments are the conspicuous outcomes of this period. First, a complex pattern of hormonal activity stimulates appearance of the secondary sex characteristics—nongenital development such as breasts, voice changes, and growth of hair. It can be a bewildering time, especially since the beginning frequently occurs while the youngster is chronologically still a child. One 10-year-old, looking down on the unmistakable protuberances on her chest, protested, "My body has gone on without me!"

It is not only the budding breasts; it is all of the agonizing questions. About a brassiere, when do you buy it? What size? Will the sales clerk laugh? The first pubic hair is thin, straight, and light-colored: is it normal and whom could you ever ask? How do you tell your mother you need your own razor for underarms?

The burgeoning hormones cause greatly increased activity for oil and sweat glands. Perspiration takes on its characteristic odor, causing crushing self-doubt among youngsters who are convinced that they are the most odorous and repugnant ones around, despite almost hourly showers. The active glands on the face and back also cause acne, a problem for two thirds of all boys between the ages of 14 and 19 and about 50 per cent of girls. Damaged self-confidence and poise from the psychological burden of acne can last well into adult life.

The primary sex organs, those directly concerned with reproduction, also develop remarkably during this period, although neither ovaries nor testes will reach full adult size until about age 20. The great majority of American girls have their first menstruation between the ages of 11 and 15, though there is an interesting "new" phenomenon that suggests the onset can be considerably delayed if the young woman is engaged in extremely strenuous exercise. A recent survey of ballet schools found many dancers who had not had a first menstrual period even in the late teen years (Frisch, 1980). This is a "new" observation only in the sense that more women are participating in arduous athletics, and there are more frequent reports concerning the effects of competitive sports on menstrual functioning. The training that goes into maintaining top form in gymnastics, marathon running, skating, tennis, and swimming is often related to cessation of menstruation. Periods resume when the training is relaxed (Feicht et al., 1978).

It is our impression that girls, currently, are better prepared for menarche and its questions than in former years. Even tampon use is not the mystery it once was. These days, hardly anyone would ask seriously whether it was all right to wash hair or bathe or go swimming during a period. Girls still check each other for a possible telltale stain on the back of jeans or skirt, but even this seems to be less an occasion for harrowing embarrassment. The one thing a generation of wholesome educative efforts has not erased is the term "curse" for the monthly period. But the onset of menstruation is no longer a shock or the subject of fearful myths for most young women.

Not so for the pubescence of the young male, who is left almost entirely to the not-so-tender mercies of his peers in dealing with the perplexities of erections, erotic dreams, ejaculation, and penis size. Grown men write, recollecting their torturing self-doubts when the entire world seems to have taken on a libidinal aura (Lester, 1973). Few adults seem able to provide the pubescent boy with credible assurance that the size of his penis, his erotic dreams, and his ejaculations are all O.K. and that the incomprehensible erectibility will simmer down. It is one of the large gaps existing in the jigsaw puzzle that teen-agers must piece together to picture their sexuality and its meaning in their own lives. We will be discussing this further later in this chapter.

Whether a teen-ager matures early or late makes a difference. The classic studies were done more than a generation ago, but there is still a message in the results. We need to be aware that there are possible long-term effects of beginning pubescence "late," say at age 14 when friends have all shot ahead in size and maturity. According to the Mussen and Jones study (1957), the late-maturing boy is at a competitive disadvantage in athletic activities and this spills over into unfortunate negative feelings about the self, feelings of being rejected by others, rebellious attitudes toward parents, and prolonged dependency. The last quality, perhaps, could be a function of being regarded as immature by others. In contrast, the early-maturing boy achieves pre-eminence because of his superior size, strength, and endurance. In a society that stresses male dominance and authority, the value of being physically able to overpower contemporaries is clear. Early-maturing boys were reported by Mussen and Jones to be significantly more self-confident and less dependent, to feel more accepted by parents, and to perceive themselves as more mature and capable of fulfilling an adult role in interpersonal relationships.

All of this would be moot if there were no long-term effects. However, a follow-up study of these same boys (Jones, 1965) revealed that the feelings of inferiority, generated by delayed development, carried over into adulthood. Late maturers were less successful in careers, with few holding positions of heavy responsibility or leadership. The Mussen and Jones studies should serve as a reminder of the need for maximum reassurance when an adolescent male is slow to develop. His plight is easy to overlook because the adult knows that all will catch up in time. But the suffering young person does not have this perspective. Even if the lad seems to angrily reject the words, he needs the promise that he will not be "runty" for much longer. The best prescription for a late-maturing boy's self-concept is assistance in gaining some kind of special skills that might bring him admiration and high regard from age-mates. Size is not requisite for earning a black belt in karate, but perseverance and discipline are. A late maturer would have as good a chance at such an endeavor (and many others) as anyone and should be encouraged to seek his own areas of excellence.

The report on early-versus-late-maturing girls did not show differences that were as great as those of the boys (Jones and Mussen, 1958). The prediction of these investigators that early-maturing girls would be disadvantaged by being "out of step" was not upheld. The outlook of both early-maturing girls and their less mature friends seems to depend much more on their own perceptions of themselves as attractive or unattractive and the circumstances that support the perception. The early-maturing girl, for example, may be able to date older boys until her age group catches up, enhancing her self-esteem and making her the envy of her friends. Furthermore, the time gap between early- and late-maturing girls is not as great as that between individual boys. When Mussen and Jones were investigating, the young subjects were all 17 years old. Whereas some of the late-maturing boys in the study were still undergoing changes and still experiencing the reactions of the world to their incomplete maturity, the 17-year-old girls, whether early or late maturing, were no longer unlike their peers.

The close relationship between one's physical self and the psychological attitudes toward the self and the world is reflected in these findings. An interesting approach to a better self-concept through physical fitness was demonstrated at Brigham Young University with a group of self-rejecting seventh graders (McGowan et al., 1974). The youngsters were enrolled in an 18-week success-oriented endurance training program that featured running on 4 days a week and competitive sports on the remaining days. The boys were reinforced by their own improving records, by approval, and by regularly experiencing the joy of winning a competition. The winning was ensured, without detection, by the experimenters. At the end of the training period, significant increases were found both for cardiovascular fitness and in self-concept. Neither change was evident for the control group.

The extensive bodily and physiological functioning changes that take place during adolescence are accompanied by psychological upheavals—joy, excitement, despair, and gloom. Even the possibility of such free-ranging mood changes is new to the adolescent. Younger children's emotional states are not experienced subjectively as being this profound. New capacities for feeling and thinking are another facet of adolescence.

COGNITIVE DEVELOPMENT

For each of the periods studied, we have noted the distinct differences between the children at the entrance to the period, some of whom retain the characteristics and behavior patterns of what went just before, and others who begin to merge with those just ahead. The fact that it is impossible to capture the child at a point in time and say "this is it!" with reference to a particular growth period pays tribute to the concept of development as a continuing process of change.

Adolescents, too, exhibit great differences between those just entering the period and those who are about to leave. One of the real tension points between adolescent and parent is the lack of clearly defined points at which privileges (and responsibilities) can be conferred. The bar mitzvah of the Jewish boy takes place when he is 13 and admits him to the ritual life of adult males. Confirmation is supposed to be a conscious decision of the Christian young person to join the church at age 14, "confirming" the baptism of infancy into the faith. "Sweet 16" parties and debuts introduced young women as "of an age" in yesteryear, to be courted. But the rites of passage are no longer as meaningful as they once were.

The occasions and celebrations point up a difficult contradiction in modern life. The young person involved in bar mitzvah, confirmation, or a coming-of-age party will not be accorded adult status for a number of years. The body is beginning to take on adult contours; the young man is probably able to arm-wrestle his father at least to a stand-off, but the family still controls the adolescent's time, furnishes board and room and clothes, monitors his or her spending, and provides a certain amount of guidance, counsel, and emotional support.

There is a limbo quality to the period, which is felt keenly by all participants.

New capacities for feeling, thinking, and expressing oneself are another facet of adolescence.

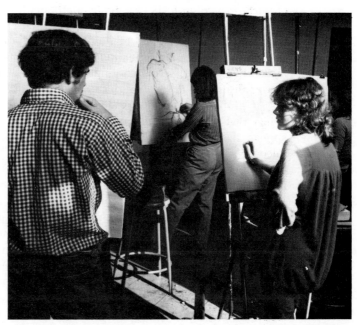

Judith Kruger Michalik

Patrick, age 13, complains at Christmas time, "I'm too old for toys and too young for anything else." The long preparation for assuming the tasks of a technological and industrialized world contrasts vividly with another time when a 15-year-old boy could be supporting himself and might soon be supporting a family. The early mills at Lowell, Massachusetts employed many 15-year-old girls and some who were younger. Shakespeare's Juliet was not yet 14 and Joan of Arc was 17 when she led the armies of France. It is the marginal state of today's adolescents that makes "status symbols" so important to them. The car or motorcycle, cigarettes, alcohol and other drugs, having a girlfriend or boyfriend are all eagerly sought-after badges that proclaim a measure of independence.

It is true that independence does not arrive with either car or cigarette. But to even consider it, to yearn for it, necessitates a capacity for a kind of thinking that is very different from that of the middle-years child whose thinking was closely tied to concrete operations. Adolescents acquire an entire new ability to think in terms that are abstract and propositional. They begin to think with the intellectual forms that will be practiced in adulthood.

Piaget terms the period *formal operations*. It is a time during which tools of thinking that are applicable to larger reaches of the world, including construction of hypotheses and reflections upon one's own thinking, can be developed. This brings about a subtle self-consciousness and range of expression for the adolescent—a time of wonder and sensitivity. The long hours of looking at oneself in the mirror not only serve the search for identity (about which we will have more to say) but also create a vibrant self-awareness and sense of discovery. Ideas become important. The adolescent wonders seriously why the whole world isn't excited about the insights of the *Communist Manifesto* of Marx and Engels or the writings of Sigmund Freud. The new cognitive abilities also lead to idealism—and wrath toward injustice, greed, corruption, and other sins of mankind.

Such a description of these cognitive changes is, of course, a generalization. Piaget's observations of formal operations (abstract, symbolic, and logical reasoning) were gleaned from young people who had pursued a classical European education. More recently it has been reported that youngsters in nonliterate societies do not manifest this type of thinking (Berry and Dasen, 1974). Niemark's survey (1975) of the research on formal operations indicates that the capabilities are far from universal and that many American adults cannot reason logically or think in mathematical terms. Furthermore, the quality of performance on tests of logic or mathematics varies widely according to the nature of the task. Piaget himself (1973) recognized that experience and, especially, education that stresses science, logic, and mathematics may be necessary to promote the ability to think in the formal operations mode. The maturation of body and brain during adolescence makes higher intellectual attainments possible, but relinquishing the egocentrism, phenomenalism, and other qualities of earlier thinking does not occur for everyone.

It probably is not necessary for all adolescents to reach the high peaks of cognitive ability that enable an understanding of symbolic logic and finite mathematics, but it does appear that for many, this period between childhood and adulthood constitutes an unconscionable waste of brain power and energy. Adolescence as an unproductive period occurs because industrialized societies have not yet figured out peacetime uses for large numbers of youths who are untrained and unschooled for most of the available jobs.

However, assigning this period to schooling leads in too many instances to boredom and dropping out. The present school system especially fails minority youths, including uncounted numbers of offspring of recent immigrants, most of whom are poor and nonwhite. A recent Ford Foundation report (Schrank, 1980) points not only to continued discrimination against black and Hispanic young people and a continuing shortage of entry-level jobs on all counts, but also to the tragic fact that so many youngsters leave school unable to read or to do simple arithmetic. The report points to a New York City bank that, attempting to obtain 300 viable entry-level job candidates, had to interview

4000, half of whom could not fill out the application form and a quarter of whom could not do elementary 3-digit arithmetic.

Without opportunity to learn the conventional skills or, in many instances lacking motivation and encouragement to do so, groups of young people all over the world seem to be feeling a deep sense of having nowhere to go. It is not a mere coincidence that rioting in Florida, South Korea, Iran, South Africa, and elsewhere has been notable for the major presence of teen-agers. They are a volatile mass and can constitute a "powder keg" in any society that fails to recognize and deal with them. The prime need is for jobs that can both serve for training and give the adolescent some sense of the self as a useful person.

The question of one's future—"what am I going to do?"—becomes possible at this age because of the advances in cognition that enable a more mature notion of time. This includes the ability to conceptualize both past and future and to contemplate different alternatives. Because of an awareness of many possible paths to the future, questions and possible plans and goals are formed.

Though the discussion separates these aspects of the adolescent experience, the interlocking effects of maturing organ systems, physical growth, and the new cognitive capacity should be plainly clear. The combination of a maturing physical self and cognitive powers, in turn, enables consideration of the task of becoming a productive worker. What kind of a worker one should become is, in its own turn, part of the search for identity.

IDENTITY
The Independent Self

Identity is, according to Erikson (1968), the critical task for this period—the necessity of acquiring a clear sense of self, apart from family and the family patterns. Identity will include elements of the changing body, one's own sex role, relationships with the opposite sex, emotional independence, economic independence, new intellectual skills, and socially acceptable values. It does not, of course, occur in a vacuum. The identity of a minister's son is likely to take shape along different lines from that of the son of a day laborer. The daughter of a suburban career-couple family will have identity options that might seem wholly alien to the daughter of an Appalachian rural-poor family.

Nor does the process of identity formation go forth without connections to previous periods. The measure of basic trust, autonomy, initiative, and industry and accomplishment will have been contributed to the personality and character. The fundamental view of the world, the quality of inner confidence, the comfort taken in being male or female, and the learning base for future effort will all be in place, according to Erikson's view of the sequential nature of these developmental tasks. However, the quest for identity is also on a different scale from those that went on before. The previous acquisitions were controlled mainly by other people and were limited and circumscribed by immaturity. Now the task will be primarily accomplished alone, not wholly without input from the world, but the basic shaping and processing of inner and outer convictions can be done only by the self.

"Who am I?" is the identity question. The changing body offers ample evidence that you are not the person you were yesterday. You spend hours getting used to some of the changes, studying different facial expressions—smiling, surprise, anger, disdain. Change the hair, look at the profile, decide which is the best side for photography, head up, head down, look over the shoulder, as if in regret. And the body! It is mourned or approved partly in terms of who is being idolized on television or at rock music concerts.

"Who am I if I am not the person I was yesterday?" necessitates a new look at parents. The reassessment includes examining parents' beliefs and values, often question-

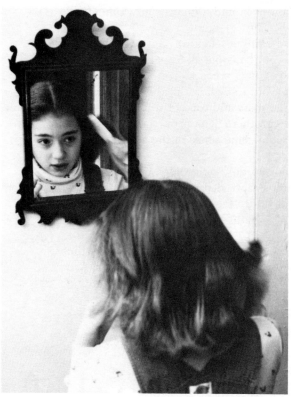

The adolescent can spend hours at the mirror studying facial expressions and trying to become familiar with the strange new person she is becoming.

Judith Kruger Michalik

ing and sometimes disparaging them. It is a time for parents to stay "cool," though this may be difficult on several counts.

1. Though the relationship between parent and child continues, marked by its previous qualities, the new factor is that parents are no longer seen as all-powerful and all-wise. Whether the parent descends gracefully or reluctantly from the pedestal contributes an important ingredient to the situation.

2. The fact that the child is indubitably growing up means that parents are growing older. Many parents find themselves more than a little ambivalent about this clear signal that middle age looms on the horizon.

3. Parents are acutely aware of the dangers "out there" and are likely to have real fears for their adolescent's well-being and safety, especially with regard to drug use and sex.

Parent-offspring relationships are complicated by the fact that parents themselves are now uncertain about the world in which their children will live. When they were growing up, the American dream seemed an attainable goal and the roles men and women played as adults were relatively clear. Now the world seems overwhelmed with unsolved problems—overpopulation, limited natural resources, environmental pollution, failing economy, violence, lawlessness, and terrorism. The feminist movement, affirmative action, and the statistic that one in every three marriages is ended by divorce contribute further to the unsettling notion that there are no models for what children should be. Lacking a secure sense of direction, even for themselves, parents are not easy in the role of guide. Counsel, cautions, requests, and orders may be issued with some lack of confidence, quickly sensed and quickly challenged by the young person. The parent bristles and the joust begins. These kinds of confrontations can be decreased if parents are able to decide in advance which issues are critical and which are extraneous. Keeping the number of critical issues to a minimum, but making it clear that these count, will help to define the absolute limits and make it easier for everyone involved.

The search for an answer to the question of "Who am I?" finds a considerable portion of the answer in the fact of being female or male. The extreme conservatism of teen-agers with regard to sex-role behavior provides ony a limited range of possibilities for that behavior. Both boys and girls tend to settle into the stereotyped roles, almost with a sigh of relief, and any questioning of the premises under which the role is carried out will have to wait until later (Conger, 1973). It is almost impossible to interest young high school girls in the philosophical base for women's liberation or to convince high school boys that they should be expressive and feel free to cry. It is very difficult to consider changing something you aren't wholly comfortable with for yourself at this stage.

The Sexual Self

So boys will be boys and girls will be girls, at least through the high school years. A generous portion of the time and energy of the adolescent is occupied with being a boy or girl in relation to a person of the opposite sex. Ideally, the eventual result would offer one of the answers to the identity question: "I am a responsible sexual being."

That answer would be hard to claim for most adolescents in American society; such an answer is made more difficult because of ambiguous and hypocritical guidelines from adults. Protection of girls so that they remain virgins is still the parental ideal, whereas the adolescent male is given tacit permission for sexual expression because "boys will be boys." Though his sexual experiences will have to involve someone's daughter or sister, parents do not challenge the double standard.

This system of restricted sexual behavior for girls and relatively unrestricted behavior for boys is grafted on the social necessity for adolescent girls to win male approval. It is called the "popularity neurosis" by Stone and Church (1975), referring to the intensity of the need to be admired and desired as verification of one's worth. A multitude of commercial interests, guaranteeing instant beauty, capitalize on the adolescent insecurity.

A good deal of the time of the adolescent is occupied in being a boy or girl in relation to a person of the opposite sex.

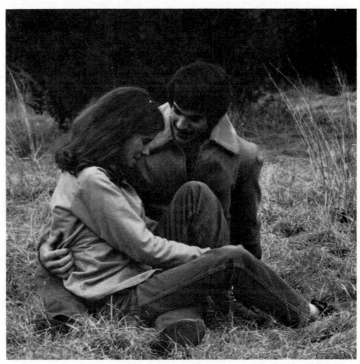

Judith Kruger Michalik

Sexual stimuli in American society are everywhere and explicit. Erotic invitations are used to sell everything from cars to sink cleaners. Movies and television provide a backdrop of blatant sexual fantasy, both glorifying and making it essentially valueless. Yet, there is a general societal pretense that adolescents are oblivious to the messages. It is remarkable that adolescents have played this game so gallantly: no wonder their sexual relationships are often furtive and guilty, having little to do with good feelings, pleasure, and delight.

Has there been a sexual revolution? The answer is that what revolt exists has been directed against the double standard. The change in the number of single women experiencing intercourse before the age of 20 is startling. Kinsey, publishing in 1953, reported 21 per cent of his sample of unmarried women had sexual experience. Twenty years later, Sorenson (1973) found that 45 per cent of the 13- to 19-year-old girls had had premarital intercourse. Three years later a national survey of unmarried women found the number of 19-year-olds reporting premarital intercourse had risen to 55 per cent, an increase of 10 per cent over Sorenson's figure (Zelnick and Kantner, 1977).

The compelling need of the adolescent age period is for authoritative information from individuals who can be trusted and respected by young people. There is continuing dissatisfaction among youths with regard to the "sex education" that they have received (Diamond, 1976), in the main because parents and teachers concentrate on safe, nonsensitive details of reproduction. We have already noted the virtual blackout of any helpful communication for the young maturing male with regard to his special problems of growing up. The same deafening silence surrounds other issues that are of vital interest to adolescents. They need straightforward facts about *being* sexual, including the act of intercourse, male and female genitalia, contraception, venereal disease, and sexual functioning. They need opportunities to explore, in a nonjudgmental atmosphere, their own and others' sexual attitudes. They need assistance in figuring out what is myth and what is authentic in the rumors, stories, and testimony they've heard. They need help and reinforcement for making their own decisions without bowing to peer pressure and without pressuring each other.

Parents tend to be almost violently opposed to school-sponsored programs that promise realistic information. The fear seems to be that, once the details are revealed, their teenagers will begin an unbridled orgy of sexual experimentation. However, there is absolutely no evidence or indication that adequately informed adolescents behave more promiscuously than those who are unknowing.

On the contrary, the epidemic of teen-age pregnancies suggests that failure to equip adolescents to deal with sexuality has not succeeded in maintaining innocence. Teen-age pregnancies account for one in every five births in the United States—some 617,000 in 1974. In addition an estimated one out of every three abortions is performed on a teen-ager (Green and Lowe, 1975). Even more frightening is the fact that 13,000 babies were born to girls age 10 to 14 years in 1975 (Ventura, 1977). A national survey taken that same year (Zelnick and Kantner, 1977) found that only about half of the sexually active adolescents had used a contraceptive during their last intercourse and only about 20 per cent of the entire sample used contraceptives with any consistency. This game of "Russian roulette" played out by young people seems to have several features.

First is the general disinclination of the adolescent male to seriously associate the possibility of pregnancy with his own sexual activity. He tends to dismiss any concern by presuming that contraception is *her* responsibility. *She*, however, is most likely to be operating with an assumption that runs directly counter: "Good girls do not engage in sexual activity unless they are carried away by the passion of the moment." To be prepared with contraceptives indicates a beforehand decision, something with which few adolescent girls could be comfortable.

There are also several premises common to both sexes: That a pregnancy can't happen when participants are so young; or that it can't happen unless intercourse is regular and frequent, as in marriage; or that pregnancy only happens if you really want a baby. It may well be that good instruction would not ensure sexual responsibility for all young people, but it could focus their attention on the issues ahead of time and perhaps encourage conscious deliberation rather than impulsivity, for some.

Adolescents also need honest information about venereal disease (V.D., or S.T.D.—sexually transmitted disease), now the second most common infection (exceeded in incidence only by the ordinary head cold), with half the reported cases occurring in persons under age 25 (Katchadourian, 1977). There is a general mythology that persuades youth that knowing your partner is adequate protection and that "nice people don't get V.D." Even in this day and age, adolescents know almost nothing about sexually transmitted disease, its causes, symptoms, and treatment. They are quite unaware of the consequences of failure to obtain medical attention, and many are not even clear that disease can be transmitted by sexual activity (Gordon, 1973).

What would be desirable by way of getting in touch with one's own sexual identity? The experience of a husband and wife team, Leona and Philip Sarrel (1979), who served Yale University as the student enrollment turned coeducational, led them to suggest that, optimally, coming into sexual being is a gradual process, involving many quiet awakenings . . . a kind of gentle "unfolding." It should lead to an evolving sense of the sexual self and would include:

1. A developing sense of the body and body image, without distortion and without disclaiming any aspects, especially with regard to the genitals.
2. A lessening and moderating of the guilt and shame associated with things sexual (which almost none of us escape in the course of growing up).
3. A loosening of sexual ties to parents and siblings.
4. A recognition of what is erotically pleasing and displeasing, along with an increasingly satisfying and enriching sex life, with acceptance, for most individuals, of a healthy autoeroticism.
(ADAPTED FROM SARREL AND SARREL, 1979).

The listing of a healthy autoeroticism (masturbation) as one worthwhile result of wholesome sexuality is an important point. Adolescents still believe that "you shouldn't do it too much"—and agonize in wondering how much is too much. They are fearful that "too much" might indicate or cause homosexuality. They learn (if fortunate) with overwhelming relief that masturbation is not harmful and does not interfere with heterosexual pleasure but may, in fact, enhance it, especially for women (Kelly, 1980).

The search for sexual identity during adolescence should result in awareness of the self as a sexual person, with a good feeling for the value and place of sex in one's life. It can best be assisted by adults who are comfortable with their own sexuality or who can admit that their background does not permit real easiness, but they earnestly wish for something better for the young people they contact. The outcome of an "unfolding" like that described by the Sarrels would be an individual who can establish intimate bonds with another, joyously, freely, and honestly. This will be a major topic in a forthcoming chapter.

The Occupational Self

"Who am I?" demands an answer in terms of our productive life. One of the necessities of the period of youth is the process of vocational choice. Ideally, this would involve several years of "trying on" different occupations, probably with peripheral participation but with some firsthand observations of what the work entails. The adolescent needs to be a part of the world of work. Employers' claims that the high minimum wage prevents them from hiring teen-agers suggest the need of some possible readjustment of the minimum wage law. This is not to suggest that adolescents as unskilled, untrained workers should be exploited, but ways need to be found so that the young person can

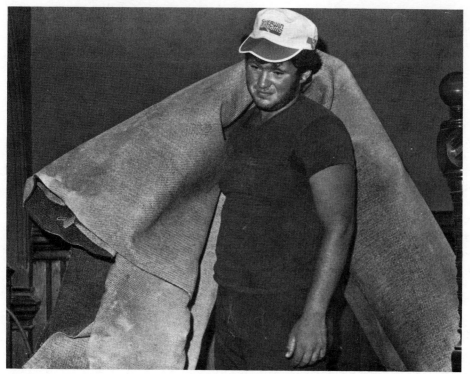

J. V. Barry

It is better for an adolescent to have a low-paying job and a chance to learn than no job at all.

obtain experience at a rate of pay that makes reasonable economic sense. It is better to have a low-paying job, especially if it offers a chance to learn, than none at all.

Deciding what you want to be, however, involves much more than after-school and summertime employment. Career choice reflects motivation, knowledge, personality, and ability (Holland, 1973). The world of work is so extensive (there were more than 20,000 job descriptions in the fourth edition of the Dictionary of Occupational Titles) that contemplation of the possibilities is dizzying and, inevitably, a vast number of possibilities will be unknown and overlooked.

Furthermore, because occupational choice is very central to American life, young people feel the pressure to decide and there is considerable danger of becoming locked into a premature decision. Parents, counselors, and adolescents themselves all need to be cautioned to guard against foreclosing alternatives, and all need to be encouraged to see choices as tentative. Parents have to be encouraged to restrain the anxiety when their adolescent has not declared a preference. It would be a relief to liberal-arts majors not to have to fight off the inevitable question, "But what are you going to *do* with it?"

As a matter of fact, a moratorium on this issue, lasting several years during late adolescence before career choice becomes imperative, is often a splendid notion. Traditionally, adolescents from well-to-do families spent a year in traveling, seeing the great cities, museums, and theaters of Europe. For some young people military service has always been a way to "see the world." The Peace Corps, also, frequently serves as a career-decision postponement device, productively occupying the young person and permitting deferment of vocational commitment for a while longer. A possibility for the future would be some type of universal national service, with all adolescents required to enroll for 2 years. Many kinds of useful endeavors could fulfill the obligation. Such a program could provide skill training and broadening of career options, in addition to mixing young people from all socioeconomic levels and different backgrounds, while furnishing young energy and strengths to many tasks that currently lie undone.

An important consideration in the area of occupational identity is career choice for young women. Girls have not been expected to stake out careers for themselves, except secondarily. First wife and mother; second, teacher or nurse or whatever, but clearly subordinate to the first. The encouragement to think of herself as being supported by a husband for most of her life creates a heavy psychological disadvantage for every woman. She does not, then, focus seriously on discovering a vocation that will capture her enthusiasm and to which she can commit herself. Her training becomes more casual, and her jobs are regarded as temporary, a "fall-back" position.

However, most women can no longer afford to be less than in total earnest about becoming financially independent. The number of families with children supported solely by the mother doubled between 1970 and 1979. The average family income for these families headed by females plunged nearly 50 per cent in the transition from two-parent to single-parent household! Any adolescent woman who believes that she does not need to worry about vocation or career is deluding herself and needs to be dissuaded by parents, teachers, and vocational counselors, armed with the facts of contemporary life.

A related issue is that of male perceptions of what women do. Enwisle and Greenberger (1972) asked ninth grade boys and girls a series of questions regarding their views on what women should be like, what women should do, and how they thought women saw the world. Both sexes suggested that women are curious and exploratory, but the girls were significantly more positive with regard to the possibility of women succeeding in careers. On the contrary, almost all the boys felt that women would be most successful staying home and caring for children. The authors conclude that girls' aspirations and achievement will suffer because of the expectations of male peers.

There is, also, need for a plea that the young adolescent girl not receive the message that she is "no good" in math and science or that she "doesn't need it." Too many girls accept the news gratefully, avoid further pursuit, and succeed in cutting themselves off from a good portion of the technical world's best jobs.

This section, it must be acknowledged, is influenced by a middle-class perspective—as if all adolescents were able to choose and, having chosen, could pursue the career or vocation without hindrance. Actually, *choice* of most kinds depends upon socioeconomic status. The ghetto dweller, the child of recent immigrants, and many minority group children, including American Indians, are not likely to be able to pick and choose among careers with confidence or facility. Not only does the world of work seem to be alien territory because of lack of access to role models, but the skills and training necessary will neither be as discernible nor as available. Good techniques have not yet been invented to help jobless and hopeless youths break out of the poverty cycle. It remains one of the most pressing problems of our time. Rich or poor, the answers to one's own question "What can I do in the world of work?" determine a large portion of the feelings about self. In work-oriented American society we tend to *be*, in good measure, what we do for a living.

The Self of Values, Moral Judgments, and Conscience

The "I" of the question "Who am I?" is also the possessor of beliefs, evaluator of issues, and holder of attitudes. The beliefs, values, and attitudes are claimed as belonging to the self. As we have seen, the developing cognitive powers especially permit thinking about problems of conduct, considering whether events are good or bad according to abstract principles, and ruling on one's own behavior in relation to a set of inner standards. Kohlberg's (1963) account of evolving moral judgments through an individual's lifetime described four levels of coping with "right" or "wrong" for the young child (see Chapter 8), with a possibility of reaching stage 4—the unquestioning respect-for-law-and-order level—during the late middle years or preadolescence.

Two higher levels are yet to be discussed (see Table 8–1, p. 138). These are considered the most mature levels, attainable only by someone who is capable of advanced cognitive processes; therefore, the last two stages are not reached by all adolescents or even by all adults. Stage 5 demands an ability to conceive of an abstract "social contract," whereby the rights of the individual are seen as important but must be balanced and weighed in light of the overall well-being of society. It includes the idea of laws formulated on the basis of mutual "good" and that these can be changed. The notion of democratic procedures, in theory and practice, is also a feature of this stage.

Stage 6 is, for Kohlberg, the highest form of moral judgment, based on abstract principles of absolute, ethical standards. Now there is capacity to envision universal "good" in the form of justice, equality, and human rights for all. The golden rule as a perfect prescription for all human affairs becomes conceivable. The ultimate decision residing in the individual conscience is also recognized, as is the fact that one might "morally" defy an edict on the basis of a personally perceived universal principle. The conscientious objector who goes to jail rather than kill in a war is seen as behaving according to such principles by those whose development has reached stage 6. Stages 5 and 6, if they occur at all, cannot occur before adolescence because of the necessity for the highest level of cognition. Studies by Kohlberg and Elfenbein (1975) found a certain amount of stage 5 thinking at age 16 but infrequent use of stage 6 concepts.

Idealism and a pledge to change the world for the better are a vital part of the existence of many adolescents, however. It all seems so easy if only the jaded adults would give it a chance. "Make love, not war." "What if they gave a war and nobody came?" These are typical slogans, almost undebatable, because they are so *right* in spirit. The person over 30 can hardly bear to ask what is intended for all those individuals who simply can't or don't or won't love.

The idealism makes youth especially vulnerable to movements that offer solidarity with a group and conviction of having found "the answer." The young people selling flowers in airports and the ever-smiling "Moonies" are examples. Although it might seem that traditional religions could fulfill this deep need, this does not seem to be the case. Church attendance by adolescents has suffered a dramatic decline in the last 15 years (Johnson, 1974), and the number of adolescents who felt that religion was becoming less important to their lives increased from 62 per cent in 1965 to 78 per cent in 1969 (Graham, 1972). Churches will need to heed youthful charges of hypocrisy and irrelevance if they wish to counter the trend.

Choosing whether to use drugs or not is still another value-laden decision, partaking of the young person's attitudes toward law and society and turning somewhat on allegiance to a particular peer group (Kandel, 1978). Adolescents are using more drugs at earlier ages than ever before (Johnson and Bachman, 1975). The drug most commonly used at all levels is alcohol, with about half of all junior high school students and three quarters of all high school students reporting that they have used it (Holden, 1975). Tobacco is next, with about 1 million adolescents beginning to smoke every year (Rice, 1975). Third in incidence of use is marijuana, though statistics are difficult to gather because marijuana is illegal. A 1972 Gallup poll indicated that a majority of college students have used marijuana at least once. It would be difficult to be part of a college community today (in the early 1980s) without observing both the casual acceptance and casual use of this drug.

However, increasing drug use is a problem not only of adolescents. Blackwell (1973) reported that physicians were writing an estimated 50 million prescriptions each year for tranquilizers such as Valium and Librium. Mass advertising encourages widespread use of drugs for every minor disequilibrium—headache, backache, arthritic pains, sleepless-ness, or difficulty in waking up. The use of alcohol and cigarettes is encouraged by association with glamorous models in exciting settings. Young people, with some justifi-cation, can point to nay-saying elders and suggest that though the drugs may be different, the use of drugs is similar.

Several investigators (Kandel, 1974; Maddox, 1970; Prendergast and Schaefer, 1974) indicate a relationship between parental practices with regard to drugs—ranging from parental use of alcohol and tobacco to reliance on prescription and nonprescription medications during the adolescent's childhood and the adolescent's present behavior with regard to drugs. As one young college student put it, "Don't tell me about the evils of marijuana with a martini in your hand!"

A quick backward look along the route that we have followed with our adolescent youth will recall that the overall theme of this period is "change." Hall (1904) perceived it early, describing the transformation of child into adult. Erikson (1963) carried the idea further, suggesting that the transformation takes place during the course of intensive search for answers to the question, "Who am I?"—the seeking of identity for the self. If successfully undertaken, the search will lead to answers that give a degree of independence from family, make peace with sexuality, obtain direction for productive economic future, and discover purposes, values, attitudes, and inner regulations of one's own. Like the other "developmental tasks," Erikson suggests that this one, too, can be short-circuited. If the young person is unable to attain a relatively secure sense of personal identity because of failures at a previous level or unyielding social circumstances, the result is *role confusion*. A sure sense of self will be deficient, lacking focus and without belonging. The youthful capacity for fidelity will be impaired (Erikson, 1968). Rather than self-confidence in ability to deal with life's events, there will be resignation to feelings that life's events are the determiners.

However, failure to establish a firm sense of personal identity does not doom one to perpetual failure. Indeed, even the young person who attains a good working sense of the independent self will continually have to defend against threats and invent solutions to new problems throughout life. Erikson stresses a view of life as never-ending change. Accomplishing a developmental task at one period does not finish it for all time, but only facilitates coping with the next challenge.

While we are talking, our adolescents are off, changing, hurrying on to encounter the next life tasks of the young adult.

GLOSSARY

ADOLESCENCE   An imprecise term used to describe the period of transition from dependent child to self-sufficient adult.

ANOREXIA NERVOSA   A state of severe emaciation, the result of dieting, but maintained by disordered psychological perceptions.

FORMAL OPERATIONS   The fourth and last period, and highest order, of cognitive development, according to Piaget. It enables an objective view of the world, along with the ability to assess reality, to perform inductive and deductive reasoning, to engage in abstract thinking, to formulate and test hypotheses, to use formal logic in reasoning, and to understand higher mathematics.

IDENTITY   The critical task for adolescence, according to Erikson. It entails acquiring a clear sense of self, apart from family and childhood patterns.

MENARCHE   First menstrual flow.

PUBERTY   The point in time at which the pubescent changes result in an individual who is capable of reproduction.

PUBESCENCE   Period of about 2 years during which all of the biological and physiological changes that lead to sexual maturation take place.

ROLE CONFUSION A result of the failure to achieve a sense of identity, bringing about an impaired capacity for focus and fidelity.

REFERENCES

Adelson, J.: Adolesence and the generation gap. *Psychology Today*, 12(9):33–37, 1979.

Berry, J. W., Dasen, P. (eds.): *Culture and Cognition: Readings in Cross-Cultural Psychology*. London: Metheen, 1974.

Blackwell, B. Psychotropic drugs in use today. *Journal of the American Medical Association*, 225:1637–1641, 1973.

Bruch, H.: *The Golden Cage*. The Enigma of Anorexia Nervosa. New York: Vintage Books, 1979.

Conger, J. J.: *Adolescence and Youth: Psychological Development in a Changing World*. New York: Harper & Row, 1973.

Diamond, M.: Human sexuality: Mass sex education—Student and community reaction. *Journal of Sex Education and Therapy*, Fall–Winter, 1976, p. 1–11.

Diamond, M., Karlen, A.: *Sexual Decisions*. Boston: Little, Brown, 1980.

Dictionary of Occupational Titles, 4th ed. Washington, D.C.: U.S. Department of Labor, U.S. Government Printing Office, 1965.

Dusek, J. B.: *Adolescent Development and Behavior*. Palo Alto, Cal.: Science Research Associates, 1977.

Enwisle, D., Greenberger, E.: Adolescents' views of women's work role. *American Journal of Orthopsychiatry*, 42:648–656, 1972.

Erikson, E.: *Childhood and Society* (2nd ed.). New York: W. W. Norton & Company, 1963.

Erikson, E.: *Identity: Youth and Crisis*. New York: W. W. Norton & Company, 1968.

Feicht, C. B., Johnson, T. S., Martin, B. J.: Secondary amenorrhoea in athletes. *Lancet*, 1:1145–1146, 1978.

Feldman, B. H., Rosenkrantz, A. L.: Drug use by college students and their parents. *Addictive Diseases, an International Journal*, 3:235–241, 1977.

Frisch, R. E.: Delayed menarche and amenorrhea in ballet dancers. *New England Journal of Medicine*, 303:17–19, 1980.

Gordon, S.: *Facts about V.D. for Today's Youth*. New York: John Day, 1973.

Graham, D.: *Moral Learning and Development: Theory and Research*. New York: Wiley Interscience, 1972.

Green, C., Lowe, S. J.: Teenage pregnancy: A major problem of minors. *Zero Population Growth National Reporter*,7(6):4–5, 1975.

Hall, G. S.: *Adolescence* (two vols.). New York: Appleton, 1904.

Holden, C.: Drug abuse 1975: The "war" is past, the problem is as big as ever. *Science*, 190:638–641, 1975.

Holland, J. L.: *Making Vocational Choices: A Theory of Careers*. Englewood Cliffs, N.J.: Prentice-Hall, 1973.

Johnson, A. L.: Age differences and dimensions of religious behavior. *Journal of Social Issues*, 30:43–67, 1974.

Johnston, L., Bachman, J.: *Monitoring the Future: A Continuing Study of Lifestyles and Values of Youth*. Ann Arbor, Mich.: Institute for Social Research, 1975.

Jones, M., Mussen, P. H.: Self-conceptions, motivations and interpersonal attitudes of early and late maturing girls. *Child Development*, 29:491–501, 1958.

Jones, M. C.: Psychological correlates of somatic development. *Child Development*, 36:899–911, 1965.

Kandel, D.: Inter- and intragenerational influences on adolescent marijuana use. *Journal of Social Issues*, 30(2):107–135, 1974.

Katchadourian, H. A.: *The Biology of Adolescence*. San Francisco: W. H. Freeman & Company, 1977.

Kelly, G. E.: *Sexuality: The Human Perspective*. Woodbury, N.Y.: Barron's, 1980.

Kinsey, A. C., Pomeroy, W. B., Martin, C. E.: *Sexual Behavior in the Human Female*. Philadelphia: W. B. Saunders Company, 1953.

Kohlberg, L.: The development of children's orientations toward a moral order. *Vita Humana*, 6:11–33, 1963.

Kohlberg, L., Elfenbein, D.: The development of moral judgements concerning capital punishment. *American Journal of Orthopsychiatry*, 45:614–640, 1975.

Lester, J.: Being a boy. In Pleck, J. H., Sawyer, J. (eds.): *Men and Masculinity*. Englewood Cliffs, N.J.: Prentice-Hall, 1974.

Maddox, G. L.: Drinking prior to college. In G. L. Maddox (ed.): *The Domesticated Drug: Drinking Among College Students*. New Haven: College and University Press, 1970.

McGowan, R. W., Jarman, B. O., Pedersen, D. M.: Effects of a competitive endurance training program on self-concept and peer approval. *The Journal of Psychology*, 86:57–60, 1974.

Mead, M.: *Coming of Age in Samoa*. New York: Morrow, 1950.

Mead, M.: *Culture and Commitment: A Study of the Generation Gap*. New York: Doubleday, 1970.

Mussen, P. H., Jones, M. C.: Self-conceptions, motivations and interpersonal attitudes of late and early maturing boys. *Child Development*, 28:243–256, 1957.

Niemark, E.: Intellectual development during adolescence. In Horowitz, F. D. (ed.): *Review of Child Development Research*. Chicago: University of Chicago Press, 1975.

Offer, D., Offer, J.: *From Teenage to Young Manhood*. New York: Basic Books, 1975.

Piaget, J., Inhelder, B.: *Memory and Intelligence*. New York: Basic Books, 1973.

Prendergast, T. J., Schaefer, E. S.: Correlates of drinking and drunkenness among high school students. *Quarterly Journal Studies on Alcohol*, 35:232–242, 1974.

Rice, F. P.: *The Adolescent: Development, Relationships and Culture* (2nd ed.). Boston: Allyn and Bacon, 1975.

Robinson, I. E., King, K., Balswick, J. O.: The premarital revolution among college females. *Family Coordinator*, 21:189–194, 1972.

Sarrel, L. J., Sarrel, P. M.: *Sexual Unfolding: Sexual Development and Sex Therapies in Late Adolescence*. Boston: Little, Brown, 1979.

Schrank, R.: Poor data on unemployed youths. *New York Times*, editorial page. July 13, 1980.

Shah, F., Zelnick, M., Kantner, J. F.: Unprotected intercourse among unwed teenagers. *Family Planning Perspectives,* 7:39–44, 1975.

Sorenson, R. C.: *Adolescent Sexuality in Contemporary America.* New York: World Publications, 1973.

Stone, J., Church, J.: *Childhood and Adolescence* (4th ed.). New York: Random House, 1979, pp. 488–489.

Tanner, J. M.: Physical growth. In Mussen, P. H. (ed.): *Carmichael's Manual of Child Psychology* (3rd ed., vol. I). New York: John Wiley & Sons, 1970.

Thornburg, N. A.: Comparative study of sex information sources. *Journal of School Health,* 52(2):88–91, 1971.

Tillman, K.: Relationship between physical fitness and selected personality traits. *Research Quarterly,* 36:485–489, 1965.

Ventura, S. J.: Teen-age child bearing in the United States. *Monthly Vital Statistics Reports.* National Center for Health Statistics, Vol. 26, No. 5, 1977.

Zelnick, M., Kantner, J. F.: Sexual and contraceptive experience of young unmarried women in the United States, 1971, 1976. *Family Planning Perspectives,* 9:55–71, 1977.

HEALTH CONCERNS IN ADOLESCENCE

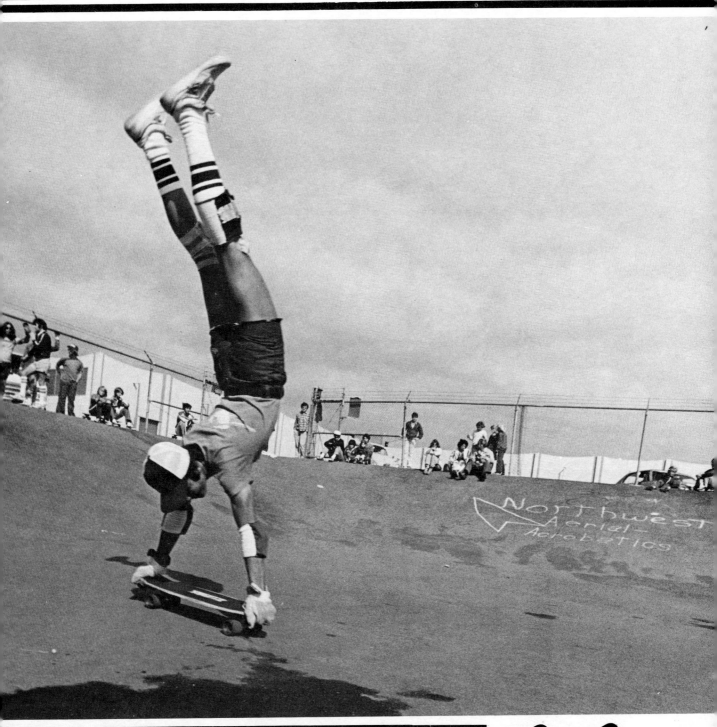

CHAPTER 11

*In adolescence is the astonishment of the Universe
and the triumph of God.
For when the child is young, the mother and father
are chewed on
That the child may be nourished into a likeness
of themselves.
But when the child is almost grown it chews on itself
that it may be transformed
Into shapes and spirits that will surprise the angels.
Therefore, as you welcome the rending which frees
the shimmering butterfly from its dull cocoon,
Welcome also the frenzy which seizes your child
in its rough and passionate grip
Releasing, at last, not your child but someone else,
a familiar stranger
Whom you can still love but never again possess.*

LEONARD HASSOL

Welcoming, applauding, and tolerating the changing "cocoon" as it turns into a shimmering butterfly is not easy. Nor is it dull. It is, however, vital; for perhaps at no other time is there a greater need for a young person to have access to and acceptance from peers and adults. Adolescence may be turbulent for some, smooth for others, and a roller coaster of ups and downs for many more. What is consistent is that changes are taking place, physically, emotionally, and intellectually.

Varying widely, perfectly normal healthy adolescents differ from one another in the timing, rate, and extent of their growth. For some, physical growth speeds up and maturation is complete in 2 years. For others, the mechanisms of growth and development are slower and less perceptible. For these reasons, chronological age can be deceptive as a consideration in the evaluation and management of health care of adolescents.

This chapter will emphasize the following:

1. Delivery of services to adolescents.
2. Assessment of health status.
3. Physical change.
4. Relevant health issues.

DELIVERY OF SERVICES

Adolescents tend not to be in regular contact with the health care system. In the absence of chronic disease or disability, adolescent health care concerns are of the short-term or crisis type—pregnancy tests, testing for sexually transmitted disease, sports injuries, birth control information, and injuries resulting from accidents.

Adolescents are old enough to have their own physician, to tell their own story, to ask questions, to listen to explanations, and to take advice. In short, adolescents should begin to be responsible for their own care (Gallagher, 1976). The goal in providing medical assistance is to avoid perpetuating immaturity and to foster effective adult behavior.

Services for Adolescents

In 1951, the first general clinic for adolescents was established by Dr. J. Roswell Gallagher in recognition of the need for adolescents to have their own physicians and some input concerning their own health care. During the decade of the 1950s, 35 such clinics were opened within the United States, located mainly in large teaching institutions.

In the 1960s, these specialized outpatient units were joined by adolescent inpatient units. In the mid-1960s free clinics, crisis centers, hot lines and shelters for runaways opened in substantial numbers in an attempt to deliver medical and other services to the thousands of adolescents who, adopting alternative lifestyles, took to the highways. By 1973, patient visits by teen-agers totaled more than 2 million (Garell, 1976). As more adolescents began to visit these clinics, they became more knowledgeable and demanding consumers of health care. Some of the demands focused on the kinds of services available, whereas others emphasized the relationship with the caregiver, either professional or voluntary. What has evolved is a subspecialty in medicine with some basic criteria, which are described next.

Prerequisites for Clinics

Trust

The primary patient is the adolescent, not the young person's parent. Focusing on the parent as a conduit to the patient will inhibit the development of a trusting relationship.

Treatment of the Whole Person

Many areas of adolescent existence impinge on health. Job, homelife, finances, peer relationships, and self-image are all determinants for well-being. Service must be available to deal with these issues as well as with medical problems.

Education and Involvement

Frequently, the success of any medical intervention with teen-agers depends on their understanding of what is wrong. When adolescents have an actual perceived need, they will seek care. When the need for care is prescribed by family members, many adolescents will either select inappropriate services or neglect to seek help at all. If an experience with a medical facility has been positive and supportive, the adolescent is much more likely to return (Garell, 1976).

Remembering their own adolescence, without ruffles or flourishes, will have a significant impact on how health workers respond to the teen-ager who seeks assistance. As Garell (1976) states:

Each adolescent has a personal impact upon the health worker. Unresolved issues acquired during the health professional's own adolescence, the presence of adolescents in his or her own family, and the capacity to deal with change . . . all have a significant influence on that health professional's ability to care for the adolescent.

Although staff attitudes may be more important than the physical setting, the location, attractiveness, and degree of privacy, as well as the hours of operation, will influence the adolescent's acceptance of the facility. A free-standing or separate facility that cooperates with local medical institutions is frequently seen by teen-agers as less bureaucratic, more flexible, and less inhibiting. Multiservice centers offering professional and social services, as well as peer counseling, may be one example of an appropriate adolescent resource.

One such center, known to the authors, is centrally located, accessible by public transportation, and housed in an older Victorian building. The services offered include general medical, gynecological, and sexually transmitted disease clinics. Professional and well-trained lay staff members are available for group and individual counseling. In addition, peer counseling can be used for a variety of issues. The center is furnished comfortably and informally. Uniforms are not worn by the staff, and the atmosphere is supportive, nonjudgmental, and professional. The hours are structured to avoid conflict with school and work schedules, and many of the services are offered during the evening.

Fees are set on a sliding-scale basis with additional monies provided by communities adjacent to the center. Professional staff members are drawn from local community hospitals and mental health clinics. Referrals are possible for acute or serious long-term problems. After several years of operation, the center has come to be seen as a vital link in providing the best possible care to a population often ignored by more traditional institutions.

To sum up, the ideal system for the care of adolescents should include comprehensive, continuously available services, staffed by an appropriate mix of professional and allied health workers with linkage to external resources. Such services should maintain a close relationship with the young people who are served by being responsive to their changing needs. Such a system eliminates red tape and legal restrictions that would limit usage and provides subsidized and, therefore, low-cost service, which increases the utilization by adolescents. Most important, perhaps, such a system regards health services as a universal right and not a privilege or a luxury. Such a system functions primarily for the individual client asking for assistance (Garell, 1976).

ASSESSMENT OF HEALTH

Sometimes, assessing the health of an adolescent requires more listening with the "third ear" than with the stethoscope. Listening is the key, allowing the adolescent to describe in personalized terms, without interjections from parents, what is perceived to be the problem. Because contact with adolescents is of such a sporadic nature, a thorough physical examination and history are essential. How often a checkup is needed may be a controversial issue. Factors include the type of health insurance coverage held, the relatively insignificant yield in terms of detection of disease that the annual examination produces, and the patient's mobility. In early adolescence, children may be covered by family health plans, but when they reach 19 or 20 years of age, or are not in school and not covered by employee group insurance, medical coverage typically ceases.

PHYSICAL CHANGES

Adolescence is the second greatest growing period in a person's life. After infancy, there is no other time when the rapidity, extent, and variety of growth are as pronounced.

Many of the accelerated changes can be attributed to the gradual but considerable increases in the various hormone levels in both boys and girls. For girls reaching puberty (typically from ages 10 to 12), *estrogen* levels are as much as 20 times higher than in childhood (Gallagher, 1976). In boys, pubertal changes generally occur 2 years later than for girls, and the increase in male hormones is about four times what it was before puberty. This increase in estrogen in girls and *testosterone* in boys triggers a sequence of growth changes in many of the body systems (see Table 11–1).

Although many teen-agers take all these changes in stride, there are others whose negative feelings about their size and shape will be reflected in physical symptoms, poor posture, aches and pains, and other signs of a troubled self-image. Girls may develop slouched posture and may appear hunched over as a way of hiding new breast development. Poor posture may also be an indication of *scoliosis*. Because scoliosis is most common among girls in the 13- to 15-year age range, any persistent slumped position should be evaluated.

For both boys and girls, the rapid skeletal growth, offset by lagging muscle development, may produce the familiar "all hands and feet" syndrome. Parents who develop a good sense of humor and a tolerance for spilled milk, dropped dishes, and stumbles go a long way toward helping an adolescent feel less self-conscious about being so clumsy. Buying a full-length mirror to help an adolescent daughter monitor her own posture is a more supportive and positive approach than nagging.

TABLE 11–1   PHYSICAL CHANGES IN ADOLESCENCE

Girls	Boys
Growth (height)	
2 to 4 inches in 1 year	2 to 5 inches in 1 year
Cardiovascular System	
Pulse Slows to 60–68	Slower rate
Blood Pressure 100/50–120/70	Higher systolic pressure
Respiratory System	
Rate 16–20/minute	Greater volume, greater vital capacity, increased respirations
Gastrointestinal System	
Stomach capacity increases Stomach becomes longer Intestines grow in length Stomach and intestinal muscles become stronger Liver attains adult size	Similar changes
Urinary System	
Bladder capacity increases	May void up to 1500 ml (1½ quarts) daily
Fluid and Electrolyte Balance	
Percentage of body fluids decreases (50% of female body is fluid) Sodium and chloride levels decline Potassium levels rise	60% of body is fluid Similar changes 15% higher potassium level
Musculoskeletal System	
Increased estrogen levels, causing earlier unity of the epiphyses and shafts of the long bones and shorter stature Fat distribution over thighs, breasts, and buttocks because of estrogen production	Greater length in arms and legs; later ossification of bones Muscle growth continues for a longer time because of androgen production

When given the opportunity in a setting that is noncoercive, many adolescents will help themselves to available information. In any clinic, materials should be available for teen-agers to take with them to read and to share with their friends. Topics might include nutritional needs, contraception, obesity, sports injuries, venereal disease, and normal development. Included in these handouts should be a listing of "hot lines," free clinics, sexual assault units, and other community agencies that can be contacted independently.

HEALTH ISSUES

Nutrition

Daily Requirements

Adolescents, growing rapidly, are always hungry! Any parent shopping for a family that includes teen-agers knows that the recently purchased food seems to vanish as soon as it is brought into the house. It is sometimes hard for parents to believe that the midnight snacks of quarts of milk, the newly baked cake, and jars of peanut butter are essential. They *are* essential, for at no other time in their development do boys, in particular, have such high nutritional needs. The adolescent girl's nutritional needs are surpassed only during pregnancy and lactation. Failure to eat an adequate diet at this time can retard growth and delay sexual maturity.

Caloric Needs.   Caloric intake differs significantly for boys and girls. The difference is most often attributed to the lesser degree of physical activity for many girls. Whereas girls usually consume the most calories between the ages of 12 and 13 (2550 calories daily), the caloric intake of boys rises steadily until the age of 16 (3470 calories daily) and then decreases approximately 500 daily calories over the next 3 years (Marino and King, 1980).

Protein Needs.   Protein supplies about 12 to 14 per cent of the energy intake throughout childhood and adolescence (Marino and King, 1980). Although there is little evidence to show that most American adolescents are deficient in protein, those who limit their protein consumption because of economic problems or in an attempt to lose weight will not have the necessary protein available for the synthesis of new tissue. The result could be slower growth and delayed sexual maturity.

Mineral Needs.   The three minerals most likely to be inadequate in the diets of adolescents are calcium, iron, and zinc. During the rapid growth of adolescence, there is an increased need for all three: Calcium for the increase in skeletal growth; iron for the increase in muscle mass and blood volume; and zinc for the development of both skeleton and muscle mass. Both boys and girls need about 1200 mg of calcium daily. Boys need 42 mg of iron daily and girls 31 mg. Both boys and girls need about 15 mg of zinc every day (Marino and King, 1980). Table 11–2 lists sources of these important minerals and foods rich in the three most important vitamins, A, B$_6$, and C.

Many adolescent girls limit intake of these important dietary nutrients in an attempt to lose weight. Marino and King observed that as many as 50 per cent of all girls eat less than two thirds of the recommended calcium intake, have lower levels of iron, and

TABLE 11–2   SOURCES OF ESSENTIAL MINERALS AND VITAMINS

Nutrients	Food Source
Minerals	
Calcium	Dairy products, such as cheeses, milk, yogurt, ice cream
Iron	Red meat, dried beans, green vegetables, fortified cereals, peanuts, dried fruits
Zinc	Seafood, meat, eggs, milk
Vitamins	
A	Dark yellow and dark green vegetables, such as squash, carrots, sweet potatoes, broccoli, spinach, kale, Swiss chard
B$_6$	Whole-grain cereals and seeds, such as sunflower seeds, sesame seeds, wheat seeds, nuts, beans, potatoes
C	All citrus fruits, mangoes, tomatoes, rose hips (the seed pod of a rose)

consume less than two thirds of the recommended intake of zinc. The reasons for this alarmingly deficient diet among adolescent girls can almost always be attributed to the desire to look like women portrayed in fashion magazines. Often, adolescents attempt to lose weight rapidly on a "quick weight-loss" diet, limiting not only foods high in carbohydrates, but also important proteins and fats.

Nutritional Counseling

In order for a counselor to evaluate the quality of an adolescent's daily diet, it is best to know what was eaten the day before, without indicating how "bad" or "good" that intake was. It should be remembered that most teen-agers are snackers, fast-food consumers, and meal skippers. Pilliteri (1977) suggests an interview with the adolescent alone, without the parent present, to prevent a "padding" of the menu to meet familial criteria. Although meal skipping should not be encouraged, between-meal snacks can provide significant contributions to the total nutrient intake and provide a fairly adequate balance of nutrients. Pilliteri suggests that a pizza made with cheese, tomato sauce, and sausage, accompanied by ice cream, contains all the essential elements from the four food groups. Pointing out nutritional concepts in this manner may make good nutrition more acceptable to the adolescent rather than trigger an automatic negative response. Some good snack foods include whole-grain crackers, nuts, seeds, fruit, yogurt, cheese, and raw vegetables.

When teen-agers and their parents are being helped to appreciate dietary needs and nutritional requirements, the stage may sometimes be set for another child–parent confrontation. A light touch of humor on the part of the counselor and encouragement of the young person to assume more responsibility for good food habits may be more rewarding for all involved. Allowing or encouraging a teen-ager to shop for the family's weekly groceries is one way for a youngster to learn not only what food costs, but also what foods are important for the whole family. Families can plan menus a week in advance, allowing each child to pick a night to be responsible for cooking supper, selecting the food, and helping to shop. For this plan to be successful, the parents must stay out of the kitchen when the person in charge is cooking. Even if the kitchen has always been the mother's domain, the experience of planning, buying, and preparing meals is one of the best ways to establish patterns for adolescents that will have long-term benefits.

Obesity

There are several nutritional problems associated with adolescence. One of these is the problem of body image and obesity. For the teen-age girl, obesity can be very harmful to social and psychological development. Taunted by images of thin women in fashion magazines, the overweight girl is likely to feel rejected by her peers, self-conscious, and depressed. These feelings of rejection, isolation, and depression can cause more overeating, making the problem worse.

Heald (1976) defines obesity as "an excessive disposition and storage of fat and thus should be distinguished from overweight, which does not explicitly express fatness." The use of height and weight guidelines may be misleading. Many adolescents who appear to be overweight are not; they may have a large frame or greater muscle mass. It is therefore important that physical activity, food habits, and rate of physical growth be considered when determining if obesity is a problem.

Predisposition to Obesity. The tendency toward adult obesity is laid down between birth and 5 years of age (Heald, 1976). Obese children tend to have either a greater number of fat cells (hyperplastic obesity) or fat cells that are larger than those of normal-weight children (hypertrophic obesity) (Murray, 1979). There seem to be three vulnerable times for the onset of this predisposition—during the first 3 or 4 years of life, adolescence, and the last trimester of pregnancy.

Obese children are often more advanced than normal-weight youths in some physical growth characteristics and sexual maturation, and they are somewhat taller when entering adolescence. Often, obese female adolescents do not eat as much as their thinner peers. They may eat more rapidly and sometimes have little sensation of hunger. There is also some indication of a genetic predisposition to obesity. In early-onset obesity, 60 per cent of the parents of obese children and 40 per cent of their siblings also have been obese (Smith, 1978).

Weight Control.   In an attempt to become slim or remain slim, many adolescents adopt restrictive diets. A diet of fewer than 1600 calories daily cannot be tolerated by an adolescent, and such a diet provides insufficient protein as well as vitamins. Adolescents also tend to adopt "fad diets." A boy who wants to make the football team may eat nothing but carbohydrates, whereas another, wanting to fulfill requirements for the wrestling team, may literally starve himself. Diets that eliminate breads and cereals also eliminate essential riboflavin and thiamine, whereas the macrobiotic diet or other such diets are deficient in important nutrients.

Curing obesity is difficult. Prevention is more appropriate. Teaching good nutrition, not using food as a reward or punishment, and accepting the teen-ager "as is," with a de-emphasis on physical appearance, may help to take the pressure off and to be more effective in a program of weight reduction.

Establishing realistic goals is also important. It might be helpful for the adolescent to join an organization (such as Weight Watchers) in which everyone is struggling with the same issue. For some girls, a particularly glamorous mother who spends a great deal of time involved with her "image" may present an impossible role model. Counseling for both mother and daughter might be appropriate to discuss the issues of body image, acceptance, and nurturance. The goal is to take the conflict out of eating and to bring about a permanent change in eating habits.

Anorexia Nervosa

"Self-inflicted starvation, in the absence of recognizable organic disease" is called anorexia nervosa (Bruch, 1976). Preoccupied with a mania to be thin, some patients are involved with their body image, others with the relentless pursuit of diminished body size, and others with a phobic fear of being fat. Adolescence is the characteristic time for this disorder to become evident. Anorexia nervosa appears to be a bitter struggle to gain a sense of control and identity. Many anorectic adolescents come from affluent families who describe their home life as "happy," but who expect a great deal from their children with stress on success and conformity to family rules.

Anorexia nervosa may be manifested in several ways. Bruch (1976) indicates that the syndrome is likely to have the following components:
1. A disturbance in body image and body concept.
2. An inaccurate, confused perception and interpretation of hunger stimuli.
3. A paralyzing sense of personal ineffectiveness.

Some victims are unaware of hunger but are preoccupied with food; they may develop bizarre food habits, places to eat, and ritualistic eating routines. Some starve for long periods of time and then go on uncontrollable eating binges, followed by self-induced vomiting, and may lose 40 per cent of their body weight.

Many anorectic teen-agers do not see their body as their own; they see the condition as "just happening" without any reason. They are unable to recognize that this behavior is a desperate attempt to extricate themselves from their families. They hurt their parents by not eating and get satisfaction from doing so.

Health care professionals working with anorectic patients need to be supportive and understanding. Any indication of rejection will intensify the feelings of loss of control that is already evident in these girls. Anorectic adolescents need help in understanding how emotional stress can affect their bodies and how these emotional needs are being met by their eating behavior. Referrals should be made for psychological counseling, which may include family therapy, behavior therapy, or biofeedback therapy. Family therapy focuses on identifying how family members are triggering these responses in the adolescent, with the goal to develop more healthy ways of interacting (Luckman, 1980).

Nutrition and Sports

There are many misconceptions about nutrition and athletics. Many believe that vitamin and protein supplements are necessary for good performance, but there is little indication that these supplements are necessary with the exception of a small increase in iron supplements for young female adolescents in active training (Marino and King, 1980). During heavy physical activity, there are losses of sodium and potassium. These losses can be made up by drinking electrolyte-rich beverages (rich in sodium and potassium) and by including oranges and bananas in the diet. School nurses could assist athletic coaches in developing a list of appropriate foods for distribution to team members.

One of the most serious consequences of continuous physical activity is the loss of body water by sweating, urination, and evaporation from the respiratory tract. With increased temperature and intensity of activity, water requirements are dramatically increased. Fluid balance should be met by frequent small drinks of water. Limiting water intake during training or conditioning may lead to fatigue, elevated body temperature, and possible heat stroke and death (Marino and King, 1980).

Vegetarian Diets

In some cases, adolescents have adopted a vegetarian diet because of health, ecological, or moral beliefs. For some, vegetarianism becomes a lifelong practice; for others, it is a short-lived fad, adopted as an experiment, a gesture of independence, or something to try because friends are doing it. For those who eat dairy products, careful planning will eliminate the need for supplementary vitamins and minerals. For those who refuse to eat any animal products and wish to fulfill their dietary needs with fruits, grains, and vegetables alone, very careful counseling will be needed to provide information on which foods are rich in the necessary nutrients and how these must be combined to meet daily nutritional needs. If a teen-ager does not like to eat those soybean products that are high in vitamin B_{12} (such as tempeh and tofu), supplemental vitamins are recommended.

Smoking

Teen-agers smoke to relax, to be part of the group, to appear sophisticated, and to escape boredom . . . just like adults. The elimination of cigarette advertising from television had been intended to reduce the seductive influence on young people. However, advertisements continue unabated in the printed media, depicting "virile" men lighting up after stopping a cattle stampede or a handsome mountaineering couple sharing a cigarette on a snowy peak. It is not hard to understand why the repeated warnings of health professionals on the dangers of smoking, the pictures of diseased lungs, and the published results of lung capacity tests all seem to have failed to convince boys and girls of the present and future consequences of smoking. Smoking a cigarette proclaims that one is "old enough" during a period in which it is hard to gain that kind of assurance in other definitive ways.

Helping adolescents build self-confidence and pride in the capability of the body may deter some would-be smokers. During the past few years, a campaign against smoking that was carried on through the media had a positive impact, and similar efforts ought to be mounted again. Role models are of greatest importance; the health professional who smokes in the presence of young people is abdicating a critical responsibility. By the same token, the adolescent who lights up a cigarette in the clinic office or waiting room needs to be informed whether smoking is permitted.

Alcohol and Drug Abuse

Drug and alcohol usage among adolescents has risen dramatically in the last decade. In a society in which advertising encourages anyone with an actual or imagined ache, anxiety, or sleepless night to relieve the symptoms with a pill; when strenuous physical activity must be rewarded with a beer, it is no wonder that alcoholism and drug abuse are major national problems.

Alcohol

Alcohol abuse is being observed in an ever-younger teen-aged population. Drinking that starts at an early age is often part of a familial pattern linked to families in which drinking is common and frequently excessive.

Robinson (1978) gives an idea of the prevalence of adolescent alcohol consumption. In suburban high schools 82 per cent of all students reported using alcohol in the early 1970s; among middle-school children, the figure was 50 per cent. Alcohol is responsible for almost 50 per cent of all automobile fatalities in the United States each year. In 1977 49,000 people died in automobile accidents; about one-third of these were between the ages of 15 and 24. These figures mean about *7000* young people die every year because of the combination of driving and drinking.

Counseling and teaching adolescents about alcohol consumption is an important responsibility of the home, school, and health care facility. Instruction should focus on how to drink sensibly, how much alcohol is in each drink, how the body metabolizes liquor, as well as the physiological and psychological consequences of alcohol abuse. Parents and chaperones can make sure that parties provide nonalcoholic beverages for those who do not want to drink but who want to feel included.

Drug Use

It is estimated that at least 50 million people in the United States have tried marijuana at least once. A report of the National Academy of Sciences Institute of Medicine indicates that "More high school seniors smoke pot daily than drink alcohol." However, it also notes that marijuana use among teen-agers has leveled off. The proportion of high school seniors who smoke marijuana every day dropped from 11 per cent in 1978 to 7 per cent in 1981. The report detected a link between teen-agers who smoke pot and a lower level of achievement in school. However, it is not clear whether the use of marijuana causes the apathy and lack of interest in school or whether adolescents who lack interest in school for other reasons also tend to begin regular use of marijuana (*Newsweek*, March 8, 1982).

Although little long-term research has been done on the physical effects of marijuana, its use can contribute to the same types of respiratory problems that cigarette smoking causes. There have been some reports that marijuana use can decrease fertility or affect future children of users, but no conclusive evidence supports these claims.

Nurses and other health care workers should be alert to signs of substance (drug) abuse and should know the characteristics of specific drugs, the antidotes for overdose, and the community agencies that are available for counseling. Adolescents need to know the consequences of drug or alcohol abuse, such as loss of job, loss of friends, alienation from family, potential for criminal records with all the legal ramifications, poor health, and the inability to function competently. Murray (1979) states, "Every person with whom you work is a potential drug abuser or addict. All drugs and chemical substances have a potential for harm from allergy, side-effects, toxicity or overdose." It is therefore important that young people be aware of the dangers of self-medication; they should know how dangerous unsterile, unknown drugs may be. Parents also need help in understanding how their own drug use affects children; how their alcohol consumption becomes a not-so-subtle message, and how they can help decrease their teen-ager's dependency on substances that make the teen-ager feel adequate, relaxed, and accepted.

We live in a stressful society. Adolescents are aware of the problems they face in the world. They need help in order to develop a positive sense of self, satisfying activities, and supportive, constructive relationships with parents and peers. As members of the community in which we work and live, all of us have the ability to affect the lives of teen-agers by advocating habits for promoting vibrant good health.

Mortality

Violence (suicides, homicides, and accidents) is the leading cause of death for those ages 1 to 39. For young people age 15 to 24, the violent death rate is currently the highest ever recorded. Over the 15-year period from 1961 to 1975, the suicide and homicide rates for 10- to 24-year-olds more than doubled (Holigen, 1980). In 1965, the mortality rate from violent deaths in the 15- to 19-year-old group was 76.5 per 100,000. This figure escalates dramatically for the next 10 years of age before leveling off.

According to Holigen, for every death in this age group, there is a loss of expected years of life. It is painfully clear that the American population is being robbed of its greatest regenerative potential—its young people.

Adolescent Suicide

Adolescent death by suicide ranks second only to all other kinds of accidental deaths. Some experts even feel that many so-called accidents are probably suicides. Some of the factors leading to suicide are:

1. Increased stress.
2. Isolation and depression.
3. Drug and alcohol abuse.

Figure 11–1 Major causes of death for ages 15–24 years in the United States, 1976. (From *Healthy People: The Surgeon General's Report on Health Promotion and Disease Prevention, 1979.* Washington, D.C., Department of Health, Education, and Welfare, Pub. No. 79-55071, p. 45.)

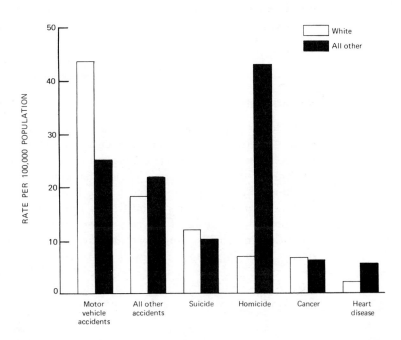

Greuling (1980) has concluded that although many of the teen-agers who commit suicide are substance abusers, the abuse is not necessarily the cause of the suicide. A more valid explanation seems to be that teen-agers who abuse drugs are often depressed and isolated and are the same ones who would attempt suicide in any case.

Professionals working in a school or clinic may be the first to identify potential suicide victims. Whereas adults may exhibit depressive symptoms such as withdrawal, the suicidal adolescent is more likely to show the following:

1. An inability to concentrate.
2. Restlessness.
3. Declining school grades.
4. Somatic complaints, such as persistent headaches, gastrointestinal complaints, and nonspecific aches and pains.
5. Obvious drug or alcohol dependency.

Services for depressed adolescents who are contemplating suicide should be available 24 hours a day, 7 days a week, as part of outpatient units, clinics, and drop-in centers. In many cities, 24-hour suicide-prevention "hot lines" have sprung up, offering crisis counseling, referrals, and a ready ear. Crisis counseling attempts to help the person react in an adaptive and creative way to the immediate crisis. After the crisis has been diffused, more intensive psychotherapy is indicated and referrals should be made. At all times, anyone working with an adolescent who expresses the intent to commit suicide must take such expressions seriously. Because the teen-ager contemplating suicide feels isolated and cut off from those who can be nurturing and supportive, nurses and counselors must never give an indication that they are condemning the behavior of the adolescent. Nor should the suicidal adolescent be addressed in a casual manner. This might give the teen-ager the impression that the situation is not serious and that it can be handled lightly.

School personnel are frequently the first to detect changes in mood, behavior, and achievement. Although intensive counseling is not within the province of every teacher or school counselor or nurse, school personnel can play an important and active role in suicide prevention. Workshops might be offered to acquaint teachers and parents with adolescent suicide. Adults need to learn something of the myths, symptoms, and causes of suicide, as well as the community agencies that are appropriate for referral. McKenry and associates (1980) also suggest that concerned adults might be interested in participating in a crisis "hot line" operation; all who are involved with adolescents need to be aware of the life stresses with which the student is dealing and that any indication of trouble is important.

Sexuality

Sex Education

As children enter adolescence and shed the "cocoon" of childhood, they have to begin making decisions about many conflict-laden behaviors— driving, drinking, drugs, smoking, relationships with their peers, and sexuality. All are issues that consume inordinate amounts of time and energy. Though families may become involved in the driving and drinking issues, the one subject that brings irate and frightened parents to school committee meetings and administrators' offices is sex education in the school curriculum.

Indeed, in the last few years there has been a rising tide of opposition to any sex education in schools. Some parents have always raised reasonable questions about the quality of the programs, how well the teachers involved are trained, what topics should be covered, and at what age certain sensitive subjects should be addressed. When these parents are involved in the design of the courses to be taught, much of the opposition dies away. For the opponents of any sex education, the issue has become one of parental rights, patriotism, and perversion. Scales (1981) states: "To the attacker of . . . sex education and other assorted targets, analysis, inquiry, skepticism, judgment, and dissent are all evils." Providing information about or even discussing human sexuality in the school appears to engender fear of sexual promiscuity; that adolescents will hasten to try out what they have learned.

A desire to return to an idealized concept of a cohesive nuclear family and a time when children were less tempted by assorted worldly evils has produced a groundswell of highly charged thought and rhetoric. But adolescents are living in a complex world that is undergoing exponential change. Lack of knowledge will not make it a simpler place. Professionals working in the health field have a responsibility to teen-agers to provide a forum in which all opinions are valued, information is accurate and uncolored by personal preference, and guidance and counseling are structured to help clients make decisions about their own behavior and lives.

Contraception in Adolescence

Sexual Activity. The sexually active teen-ager is no longer a rarity. Zelnik and co-workers (1979) reported that one in ten girls will have one pregnancy before their 19th birthday; 25 per cent of all those who are sexually active are likely to have a premarital conception by age 17; 33 per cent of all sexually active adolescents can be expected to conceive by age 19.

Studies done by the Guttmacher Institute indicate that the numbers of sexually active teen-agers increased by two thirds in the 1970s. Of the 29 million people ages 13 to 19 in the United States, 7 million boys and 5 million girls have had sexual intercourse. Teen-agers constitute only 18 per cent of the sexually active women in the United States considered capable of becoming pregnant, but they account for 46 per cent of the out-of-wedlock births and 31 per cent of all abortions. In 1978, 554,000 American teen-age women became pregnant; only 17 per cent of the births were conceived after marriage; 38 per cent were terminated, 22 per cent resulted in live births, and the rest miscarried. These statistics are sobering in light of what we know about the potential for babies born to teen-age girls to be abused, the problematic ability of teen-agers to mother, and the economic and social implications of this tragedy.

Contraceptive Information. Teen-agers learn about contraception and pregnancy risk in a variety of ways. Zelnik (1979) investigated the number of adolescents who had had sex education courses, the adequacy of such courses, and how much the students learned. His survey, done in 1976, demonstrated that 69.3 per cent of the students interviewed indicated that they had had a sex education course, and 67 per cent said that they had the course in school. Ninety-two per cent of the courses included information on sexually transmitted disease and the menstrual cycle, and 72 per cent included information on modern contraceptive techniques. Although more than 60 per cent claimed that they knew "when during the monthly cycle pregnancy is most likely to occur," only 57 per cent (36 per cent of those having had a course) correctly identified the period of greatest risk. This information is important, for many sexually active teen-agers indicate that a major reason for non-use of contraceptives is that intercourse took place at a time of the month when they thought they could not become pregnant.

Providing Contraceptive Services. It can be assumed that health care professionals who work in clinics for teen-agers or who are involved in counseling them will be called upon to advise their clients about sexual activity and sexually transmitted disease, contraception, and pregnancy. In an attempt to provide multidisciplinary health care to adolescents, living in St. Paul, Minnesota, a health clinic was opened in a local junior-senior high school in 1973. The project took 2 years to implement because of the objection of school administrators, plus the concern, on the part of the students, that their parents would be notified if they came to the clinic, and the fear, on the part of the parents, that services would be provided without their consent. Because parents objected to the dispensing of contraceptive devices in the school, the school clinic staff set up a special evening adolescent clinic at a local hospital for students requesting such devices (Edwards et al., 1980).

Initially, the services offered were prenatal and postpartum care, venereal disease testing and treatment, pregnancy testing, Pap smears, and contraceptive counseling. The clinic was housed in a small room in the basement, and few students utilized it. When the clinic was moved to a more visible and accessible space, expanded to include athletic, job, and college physicals, immunizations, and weight control programs, sexually active students became more relaxed about their anonymity and the use of the clinic grew rapidly. The program was subsequently offered in three high schools and has been scheduled to be expanded to include the junior high school population.

Although initial use of the original school clinic was low, Edwards and colleagues (1980) report that by the end of the third year, 50 per cent of the total school population has visited the clinic at least once and that 92 per cent of the pregnant students had obtained prenatal services. Those students who gave birth tended to return to school, and the dropout rate due to pregnancy decreased from 45 to 10 per cent. There were no repeat pregnancies among students who delivered and then returned to school. Fewer premature infants were born; there were fewer complications and the infant mortality rate dropped. Teen-age girls requesting contraceptive services rose from 7 per cent in 1976 to 30 per cent in 1979. The pregnancy rate declined 40 per cent between 1976 and 1979.

Edwards and co-workers (1980) concludes that well-trained, committed professionals, available on a daily basis, providing quality care and consistent follow-up in a setting that guarantees anonymity and confidentiality, have a great impact on the health consciousness of many sexually active adolescents.

Basic Methods of Contraception. Contraceptive methods are frequently described in two ways:

1. Use effectiveness (how the contraceptive method was used).
2. Theoretical effectiveness (potential effectiveness under ideal conditions, without errors or omissions in application).

When adolescents are counseled about various methods of contraception, the difference between the two kinds of effectiveness and the client's role in determining effectiveness of any form of birth control should be pointed out. Care should also be taken not to give the theoretical usefulness statistics for those methods preferred by the health care worker and use effectiveness for those that seem personally less acceptable. Clients deserve to hear statistics for each category of effectiveness. The best method of birth control is the one that makes the couple most comfortable and is most likely to be consistently used. Hatcher and co-workers (1979) list questions that a teen-age girl might ask herself in deciding which method is best for her:

1. Am I afraid of using this method?
2. Will I have trouble remembering to use this method?
3. Has anyone in my family strongly discouraged me from using this method?
4. Will I be embarrassed using it?
5. Is my partner opposed to my using this method?
6. Do I feel uncomfortable asking my partner to use this method?

Every "yes" response to these questions indicates some possible difficulty using that method consistently and effectively.

Birth Control Pills. Birth control pills containing both estrogen and progesterone approach 100 per cent effectiveness (Hatcher et al., 1979). In actual practice, however, many women run into difficulty, stop taking the pill, and do not substitute an alternative method. It is recommended that any woman going on the pill should be provided with an alternative method of birth control before she leaves the physician's office for the first time and should know how to use the second method (Hatcher et al., 1979). Then if for any reason she decides that she does not want to continue taking the pill, she will have a back-up method. Only 45 to 75 per cent of all women who start on the pill continue to use it for at least 1 year. Some of their reasons for discontinuance are the following:

1. Desire for pregnancy.
2. Anxiety about side effects.
3. Side effects.
4. Termination of the sexual relationship.
5. Ethical or religious reasons.
6. Inadvertent pregnancy.
7. Permanent sterilization.

HOW THE PILL WORKS. Estrogens and progesterone work in several ways to prevent pregnancy. Estrogens inhibit ovulation by their effect on the hormonal secretions necessary to produce ovulation. Progesterone prevents pregnancy by changing the mucus in the vagina, slowing down the rate at which sperm move, inhibiting inplantation of an ovum in the uterus, and possibly subtly altering the hormones secreted by the *pituitary* or master gland.

CONTRAINDICATIONS. Table 11–3 lists some conditions that make use of birth control pills ill advised. The decision as to which pill is appropriate is left to the physician, who needs to be aware of any possible contraindications. Health care professionals referring patients for a possible pill prescription should therefore take a careful history, asking about any family history of disease as well as current health status. Clients ought to be informed about current research regarding smoking and effects of the medication. The physician prescribes the pill, but it might be the responsibility of a nurse or other health care worker to explain its use.

TAKING THE PILL. Pills come in two forms, either a 21-day or a 28-day pack. With the 21-day pack, the woman takes the pills for 21 days, stops for 1 week, and starts a new pack. The 28-day pack comes with seven "sugar" pills at the end. The woman takes one pill every day; when the pack is empty, she starts another one, without a break.

TABLE 11–3 CONTRAINDICATIONS FOR BIRTH CONTROL PILLS

1. Evidence or history of circulatory problems
2. Impaired liver function
3. Breast malignancy
4. Pregnancy (known or suspected)
5. Severe migraine headaches
6. High blood pressure
7. Diabetes
8. Gallbladder disease, including removal
9. Mononucleosis (acute phase)
10. Sickle cell disease
11. Abnormal vaginal bleeding
12. Elective surgery planned in next 4 weeks
13. Long leg casts or major surgery to lower leg
14. Cystic breast disease
15. Failure to establish normal menstrual cycles
16. Heart or kidney disease
17. Being a young teen-ager or being judged as potentially unreliable
18. Onset of lactation (production of breast milk)
19. Over 35–40 years of age, particularly if the woman is obese, has high blood pressure, is a heavy smoker, has a family history of diabetes or has a high cholesterol level.

All women should be advised to use another form of birth control for the first month because the effects of the pill might not be fully potent for that month. The pill is taken at the same time every day. Some women find that they tend to be less nauseated (a common side effect for the first few weeks) if they take the pill just before going to sleep.

The patient should make sure that a pill was taken the day before. If one pill is missed, it should be taken when the omission is discovered and the regular pill should be taken at the regular time. If two pills are missed, two are taken when the omission is discovered and two are taken the next day. Another means of contraception should be used until the pack is empty. If three or more pills have been forgotten the client should ask herself whether she ought not change to another form of birth control unless such flagrant omission is an isolated instance. If one or more pills have been missed and the woman skips a period, she should arrange for a pregnancy test (Hatcher et al., 1979).

All patients using birth control pills should have a physical examination once a year, including a Pap smear, a test for sexually transmitted disease, and a breast examination. Some physicians believe that teen-agers who are using the pill should be examined every six months (Garfinkel, 1978).

Garfinkel finds little evidence to indicate that there is any benefit from taking a rest period from the pill or changing pills. In addition, the patient runs the risk of becoming pregnant. All patients should mention to their physician that they are on the pill when they are seen for other reasons, particularly if they are going into the hospital.

The Diaphragm. The diaphragm is a dome-shaped latex cup surrounded by a flexible ring. It must be inserted before having intercourse, left in place for 6 to 8 hours after intercourse, and used with a spermicidal jelly or cream. Diaphragms must be fitted to the individual patient's vaginal size and can be purchased only with a prescription or through a family planning clinic.

Although some adolescents are motivated enough to use the diaphragm consistently, it is not as reliable a method for them as other methods. Adolescents who do believe they will feel comfortable using a diaphragm need explicit instructions for its use and should be allowed to practice putting it in and taking it out several times during the office visit. The patient should be advised to return for another fitting if she loses or gains more than 10 to 20 pounds or if the diaphragm causes pain or discomfort. In addition, teen-agers should use a back-up method the first few weeks until they are very comfortable using the diaphragm.

After use, the diaphragm should be removed and washed with warm soapy water and dried. It can be dusted with cornstarch; talcum powder is not suitable because it has a perfume additive that can cause the latex to deteriorate. Diaphragms should be checked for defects after each use; the edges around the rim, especially, should be searched for pinholes. Petroleum jelly can also cause the diaphragm to deteriorate and should never be used as a lubricant or instead of a spermicidal cream. A good rule of thumb is for the patient to be refitted for a new diaphragm once a year at the time of the annual Pap smear.

The Condom. The oldest known method of birth control, the condom, also offers protection against sexually transmitted disease. There are several advantages for using condoms, particularly among teen-agers. They are cheap, can be bought without prescription, and promote participation of males in birth control responsibility.

The user should buy a good brand and store the condom away from heat. Keeping condoms in a wallet hastens deterioration of the rubber.

Condoms *must* be put on when the penis is erect, before any penetration into the vagina. Because the male secretes a small amount of seminal fluid that may contain sperm when he is aroused, he should apply the condom before foreplay. Vaseline should not be used as a lubricant because it will cause the condom rubber to deteriorate.

The condom should be put on so that there is a reservoir, or empty space, at the end. Some condoms are made with this "nipple" built in. The space holds the semen. The condom should be removed before the penis loses its erection. If the condom is left on and the penis is not withdrawn, the condom might fall off in the vagina, spilling the semen.

The effectiveness of condoms is greatly increased with the added use of foam. It is never a good idea to use a condom more than once.

Foam.   Spermicidal foam is an agent containing a medium to hold sperm-killing ingredients close to the cervix. Foam is placed deep inside the vagina, preventing the sperm from entering the cervix. The spermicidal agent immobilizes and kills the sperm. Foam can be purchased without a prescription, is inexpensive, and, when used in conjunction with a condom, is about as effective as the pill. The high failure rates that seem correlated with foam generally are caused by the carelessness of the user; thus only highly motivated adolescents should be encouraged in this method.

Some brands of foam can be bought with premeasured or preloaded applicators, ready for use. If the foam comes in a separate container, the container should be shaken 20 times to activate the bubbles and to ensure good adhesion to the cervix. The applicator, full of foam, should be inserted no earlier than 10 to 20 minutes before intercourse; although this may require interruption of foreplay, some couples use the insertion of the foam as part of lovemaking. A separate applicator of foam should be inserted for each intercourse.

Because it is difficult to tell when the foam in the container will be all used up, it is a good idea to have another one available at all times. At least 6 hours should elapse before douching. Some people practicing oral-genital sex find the taste of foam objectionable, but there is no other contraindication for use of foam.

The effectiveness of foam is greatly increased when used with a condom. This is the method that should be encouraged. Some newer foam-type contraceptives come in the form of small oval suppositories that create foam when correctly inserted in the vagina. Most family planning clinics suggest using a condom in conjunction with the oval suppository. Couples who use the oval suppository must wait 10 minutes before having intercourse and should not have intercourse later than 2 hours after insertion (Hatcher et al., 1979).

Intrauterine Device.   The intrauterine device (IUD) is sometimes suggested as the contraceptive measure of choice in instances when the adolescent requesting birth control has had a poor history of adhering to any other method consistently. IUDs have stringent contraindications for use. These are as follows:
1. Any previous history of pelvic infection.
2. Acute inflammation of the cervix.
3. Disease of the heart valves.
4. Abnormal Pap smear.
5. Prolonged or heavy menstrual bleeding.
6. Anemia.

During the last few years, there has been increasing concern over the use of the IUD because of the complications that have been reported. One type of IUD, the Dalkon Shield, has been taken off the market because of an association with pelvic inflammatory disease. The risk of infection is noted by Garfinkel (1978): "It is for this potential threat to fertility that [I] prefer other methods of birth control unless there is an overriding reason for an IUD." A pelvic inflammatory infection can cause scarring of the fallopian tubes, thus resulting in sterility.

Adolescents having an IUD inserted should report any fever, abdominal pain, foul-smelling discharge, painful urination, or bleeding between periods. Garfinkel also indicates that women using IUDs have a three times greater chance of contracting a pelvic infection than those who use a different kind of birth control. If the patient has never had a baby, as is the case with most adolescents, the risk is even higher.

In addition, the insertion of an IUD requires experience and skill. In most cases, it should be inserted at the time of a menstrual period. This practice thus rules out an existing pregnancy and tends to minimize pain because the cervix is opened a bit wider.

Rhythm Method. There are three types of rhythm methods: One uses a calendar; another observes basal body temperature, and the third notes the mucus secreted by the vagina. Because the menstrual cycle of a young teen-ager is often irregular, all three methods should be used simultaneously to increase effectiveness.

The calendar method requires the patient to keep track of her menstrual periods for about 8 months. She can then calculate the "safe" periods in her cycle. Only the most conscientious adolescent could be expected to remember to do this month after month.

The basal temperature method requires taking the temperature every morning before getting out of bed. There tends to be a slight dip in the basal temperature rate just before ovulation and a slight rise in temperature for the 3 days following ovulation. Because some women ovulate as early as the seventh day of their cycle, the woman using this method should have protected intercourse from day 3 of the cycle until after 3 consecutive days of temperature elevation.

The third "natural" method of birth control involves observing changes in the mucus secreted from the vagina. Women interested in this method should be aware of the thinning of the vaginal secretions around the time of ovulation. Changes need to be recorded for several months before an ovulatory phase can be considered to be reliably discerned.

All the rhythm methods are useful for adolescents who are in touch with their bodies, are not self-conscious about touching themselves, and are not reluctant to discuss these issues with their partner. They are not acceptable methods for most teen-agers.

Abortion

Historically, abortion has been described in folk medicine since about 2700 B.C., and mention is made of it in the writings of ancient Greeks, Romans, and Hebrews. The controversy surrounding abortion continues to swirl through Congress and the Supreme Court, state legislatures, and local communities. For those opposed to abortion under any circumstances, the issue is when life begins. Opponents of abortion believe that life begins at the moment of conception and that abortion is murder. For those who favor abortion, the issue is the right of any woman to decide for herself when and if she should have a child.

Court decisions in the early 1970s supported the view that abortion is a private matter between a woman and her physician. Various state and federal actions have been taken to limit abortions. Many people feel that abortions should be prohibited even for women who become pregnant as a result of rape or incest. A strong movement continues to promote the passage either of a constitutional amendment to prohibit all abortions or some form of legal definition of conception as the beginning of life.

The first restrictive abortion law was passed in the United States in 1830 to protect women against the high mortality rate associated with abortions done under unsanitary conditions by unskilled operators. Designed to save the life of the patient, the primary consideration was medical, not moral.

Abortions are usually requested because of contraceptive failure or lack of knowledge of contraception (Nadelson, 1979). In 1977, 28 per cent of all pregnant women chose to terminate their pregnancies, and in 1978 more than 1.2 million abortions were performed in the United States. Of these abortions, 90 per cent were performed during the first 3 months of pregnancy, with about 50 per cent of that total done within the first 8 weeks. The shift to earlier abortions with safer methods has had much to do with the dramatic decrease in complications (Witters, 1980).

Adolescents and Abortion. Adolescents make up the majority of women requesting abortions. Statistically, two thirds of all women asking for abortions are between 14 and 24 years of age, the highest rate being among the 17- to 19-year-olds. Approximately 75 per cent of all abortions are performed for unmarried women, and more than 1 million abortions are done each year in the United States (Robinson, 1978).

Methods of Abortion. There are several ways to terminate a pregnancy, but the three most common are as follows:

Vacuum Aspiration. This method is used during the first 3 months of pregnancy. The contents of the uterus are evacuated by means of a machine that suctions out the fetus after the cervix has been dilated. Generally accomplished under local anesthesia, the procedure can be done on an outpatient basis, takes approximately 10 minutes, and requires that the woman stay in the office for several hours of observation in case there is excessive bleeding.

Suction and Curettage. After the 12th week, vacuum aspiration can no longer be used because the uterus has become spongy and soft and there is risk of perforation of the uterus or excessive bleeding. Abortions done at this time usually require general anesthesia, involve both suction and curettage (scraping) of the lining of the uterus, and, according to many state laws, must be performed in a hospital setting.

Induction of Labor. In the 16th to 24th weeks of pregnancy, abortion can be performed by inducing labor and a subsequent miscarriage. Until recently, the most common procedure involved withdrawal of about 200 ml of amniotic fluid and the introduction of an equivalent amount of *saline solution*. Labor generally begins within 8 to 24 hours, with the expulsion of the fetus within 8 to 15 hours. The use of saline solution has been generally replaced by the use of *prostaglandins*, hormone-like substances that cause the uterus to contract. Normally occurring in the body, they are responsible for menstrual cramps and contractions of other smooth muscles. In an abortion, prostaglandins are injected into the amniotic sac. Labor and the ensuing delivery of the fetus occur more quickly than with saline. Saline or prostaglandin abortions must be done in a hospital setting and in a unit specifically organized for this kind of operation.

Adolescents requiring second-trimester termination of pregnancy need extensive counseling as well as supportive, nonjudgmental care. Although no abortion is an easy, anxiety-free experience, a late abortion is considerably more traumatic, a frightening and lonely experience.

Sexually Transmitted Diseases

The term "sexually transmitted disease" is generally applied to a series of conditions that are most often transmitted through sexual activity. As our society becomes more open about sexual activity and as sexual activity becomes less restricted, the risks of contracting a sexually transmitted disease will increase. One of the most important considerations is the number of sexual partners in an individual's experience. It appears that there is a correlation between the number of partners and such conditions as cervical cancer. In addition, Garfinkel (1978) and others have investigated the relationship between common sexually transmitted diseases and cervical cancer. For these reasons, it is very important that adolescents understand the hazards of early intercourse and multiple partners.

The diseases most common among teen-age populations and young adults are herpes simplex virus 2, gonorrhea, trichomoniasis, and syphilis. Syphilis has become a lesser danger because of routine screening. However, herpes and gonorrhea are not similarly controlled. Because gonorrhea frequently presents no symptoms in some 60 to 70 per cent of all female patients, routine testing for it should be a part of every physical examination. Gonorrhea may also cause long-term adverse consequences. Sterility can occur in those women who are not diagnosed and treated before the organism has spread to the fallopian tubes, producing scar tissue that prevents passage of the fertilized ovum into the uterus.

Herpes simplex virus 2 presents an urgent danger for the babies of women who are actively infectious at the time of delivery. Many infants who contract the disease die during the birth process, others suffer serious intestinal ailments. There has been added concern over herpes and the later development of cancer of the cervix. In several studies reported by King and colleagues (1980), there is indication of an increase in the antibody to type 2 herpes simplex virus in a significantly higher percentage of women diagnosed as having cancer of the cervix than among a control group who did not have the antibodies

TABLE 11–4 SEXUALLY TRANSMITTED DISEASES

Disease	Symptoms	Prevention
Gonorrhea		
Females	Vaginal discharge, painful urination, lower abdominal pain, fever; no symptoms in 60–70%	Urinate before and after intercourse. Use foam and condom. Know your sexual partner well.
Males	Penile discharge, painful urination, testicular pain, fever	Use condom during intercourse. Urinate before and after intercourse. Wash penis after intercourse. Know your sexual partner well.
Syphilis		
Primary	Small painless lesion on vagina, mouth, anus, or cervix	Know your sexual partner well.
Secondary	Rash on body, particularly palms of hands and soles of feet 6 weeks after first lesion; fever; sore throat; headache	Limit numbers of sexual partners. Use condoms.
Third stage	Blindness, heart disease, and brain damage as much as 20 years later	Get attention for any lesions that appear on the genitals, or ones that are painless and go away leaving a crater.
Herpes simplex virus 2	Multiple blisters on vulva or penis; discharge; painful urination	Know your sexual partner. Limit number of partners. Use condoms.
Trichomoniasis		
Females	Frothy, greenish-white discharge, vulvar itching, pain on urination, frequent urination.	Know your sexual partner. Avoid multiple partners. If infected, both partners must be treated.
Males	Frequently asymptomatic; occasional painful urination, penile discharge	Use condoms.

present. For this reason, it is vital that adolescents suffering from herpes simplex understand the need for regular Pap smears.

Table 11–4 lists the most common sexually transmitted diseases, their symptoms, and the preventive measures that can be taken. A glance at the table makes clear that use of a condom could be a key to preventing infection and spread of sexually transmitted disease, as well as providing a measure of contraceptive security. Teen-agers who are sexually active should be encouraged to use this inexpensive and readily available device.

CONCLUSION

Issues of adolescent health and well-being, whether confronted in traditional settings or in less structured environments, present a challenge to parents, teachers, health care professionals, and all others involved with youth. Hazards of the age period are great but so, too, are the rewards. There are few delights as heart-warming as that of watching turbulent adolescents change into steady, responsible, goal-directed young adults.

REFERENCES

Bruch, H.: Anorexia nervosa. In Gallagher, J., Heald, F., Garell, D. (eds.): *Medical Care of the Adolescent.* New York: Appleton-Century-Crofts, 1976.

Edwards, L., Steinman, M., Arnold, K., Hakanson, E.: Adolescent pregnancy prevention services in high school clinics. *Family Planning Perspectives,* 12(1):6–14, 1980.

Gallagher, J.: Physical assessment. In Gallagher, J., Heald, F., Garell, D. (eds.): *Medical Care of the Adolescent.* New York: Appleton-Century-Crofts, 1976.

Garell, D.: Health care delivery systems. In Gallagher, J., Heald, F., Garell, D. (eds.): *Medical Care of the Adolescent.* New York: Appleton-Century-Crofts, 1976.

Garfinkel, B.: Common gynecologic problems of the adolescent. In Shenken, I. (ed.): *Topics in Adolescent Medicine.* New York: Stratton Intercontinental Books Corporation, 1978.

Greuling, J.: Adolescent suicide. *Adolescence,* 15(59):591–601, 1980.

Hatcher, R., et al.: *Contraceptive Techology, 1978–1979.* New York: Irvington Publishers, Inc., 1979.

Heald, F.: Adolescent obesity. In Gallagher, J., Heald, F., Garell, D. (eds.): *Medical Care of the Adolescent.* New York: Appleton-Century-Crofts, 1976.

Holigen, P.: Violent deaths as a leading cause of mortality: An epidemiologic study of suicide, homicide and accidents. *American Journal of Psychiatry,* 137(4):472–475, 1980.

King, A.: Herpes virus 2. In King, A., Nicol, C., Rodin, P. *Venereal Disease,* 4th ed. London: Bailliere, Tindall, 1980.

Marino, D., King, J.: Nutritional concerns during adolescence. *Pediatric Clinics of North America,* 27(1):125–138, 1980.

McHenry, P., Tishler, C., Christman, K.: Adolescent suicide and the classroom teacher. *The Journal of School Health,* 50(3):130–132, 1980.

Murray, R.: Assessment and health promotion for the adolescent. In Murray, R., Zentner, J. (eds.): *Nursing Assessment and Health Promotion in the Life Span.* Englewood Cliffs, N.J.: Prentice-Hall, Inc., 1979.

Nadelson, C.: Emotional impact of abortion. In Nadelson, C., Notman, M. (eds.): *The Woman Patient.* New York: Plenum Press, 1979.

Pilliteri, A.: Nutritional needs of the adolescent. In *Nursing Care of the Growing Family.* Boston: Little, Brown & Company, 1977.

Reich, P.: A historical understanding of contraception. In Notman, M., Nadelson C. (eds.): *The Woman Patient.* New York: Plenum Press, 1979.

Robinson, N.: Adolescence. In Smith, D., Bierman, E., Robinson, N. (eds.): *The Biologic Ages of Man,* 2nd ed. Philadelphia: W. B. Saunders Company, 1978.

Scales, P.: The new opposition to sex education. *The Journal of School Health,* April 1981, pp. 300–303.

Smith, D.: Growth. In Smith, D., Bierman, E., Robinson, N. (eds.): *The Biologic Ages of Man,* 2nd ed. Philadelphia: W. B. Saunders Company, 1978.

The Hazards of Marijuana. *Newsweek,* March 8, 1982, p. 89.

Witters, W., Jones-Witters, P.: Fertility control: Contraception, sterilization and abortion. In *Human Sexuality: A Biological Perspective.* New York: D. Van Nostrand, 1980.

Zelnik, M.: Sex education and knowledge of pregnancy risk among teenage women. *Family Planning Perspectives,* 11(6):355–358, 1979.

Zelnik, M., Kim, Y., Kantner, J.: Probabilities of intercourse and conception among U.S. teenage women, 1971–1976. *Family Planning Perspectives,* 11(3):177–183; 1979.

Zelnik, M., Kantner, J.: Sexual activity, contraceptive use and pregnancy among metropolitan-area teenagers. *Family Planning Perspectives,* 12(5):230–237, 1980.

THE YOUNG ADULT:
Intimacy

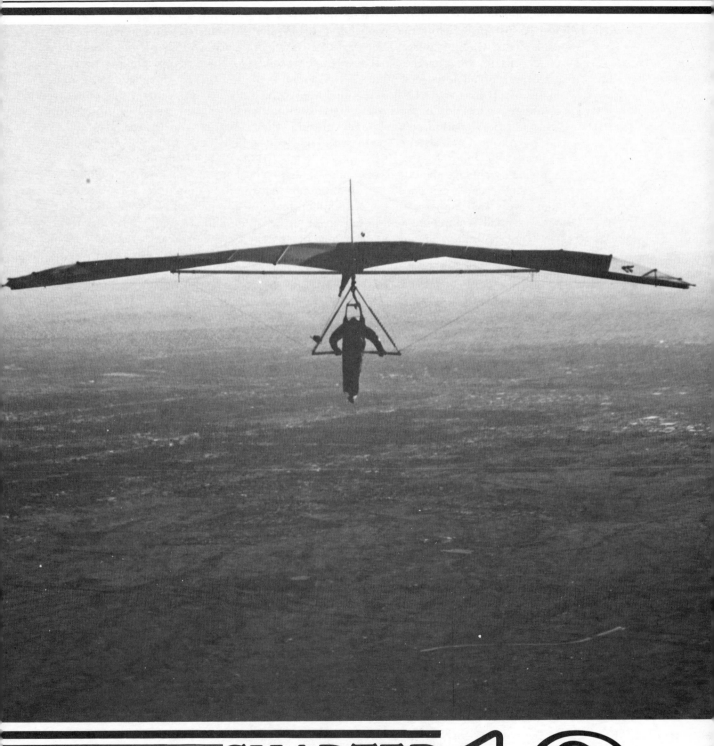

CHAPTER 12

Developmental psychology has come only lately to the study of adulthood. There are several historical factors that contributed to the almost exclusive focus on children and adolescents. One, of course, is the fact that Freudian theory, with its profound influence on all considerations of emotional development, concludes the description of psychosexual maturing with adolescence (Table 12–1). Another is the fact that psychology in the United States, flourishing since 1900, responded to perceived needs of the country that intended to educate all children. Such an ambitious educational program would cope with the large numbers of immigrants, "Americanizing" their offspring and indirectly providing the new, robust industrial economy with knowledgeable and energetic workers. William James (1890), John Dewey (1916), and G. Stanley Hall (1911) all emphasized the idea of applying psychological methods of inquiry to the practical purposes of improving education and using research evidence to create programs that would be suited to children's needs. Along with this emphasis went an assumption that the "product" of education, the adult, was essentially completed and did not need further attention.

The possibility of significant development after age 20 was not given serious attention. When intelligence testing became widespread in the 1920s and 1930s, there was an almost taken-for-granted presumption that intelligence declines with advancing age. The tests, contrived for children, yielded relatively poor adult performances, and it seemed that the idea of failing adult cognitive powers had received confirmation, as expected.

Erik Erikson's "eight stages of man" (1963) provided for the concept of continuing growth

TABLE 12–1   FREUD'S STAGES OF PSYCHOSEXUAL DEVELOPMENT

Period	Approximate Age	Characteristics of Period	Results of Fixation (Problems)
Oral	Birth to 18 months	Mouth is center of comfort: Sucking Biting	Overeating, overdrinking, oversmoking, overdependency, argumentativeness, polemics.
Anal	1 to 4 years	Holding on versus letting go, interest in feces, toilet-training conflict.	Messiness, rigidity, overscheduling, overneatness, hoarding, negativism, stubbornness.
Phallic	3 to 6 years	Oedipal conflict for boys: Desire to have mother is resolved through castration fear and identification with father. Comparable conflict for girls: Electra complex. Basic tenets now largely rejected because they were based on Victorian view of women.	Sexual identity problems, inability to give up mother or father as sex object: Guilt Aggression.
Latency	6 to 12 years	Previous conflicts go underground temporarily while child preoccupies self with school and sports.	Presumably no fixations at this stage.
Genital	12 to 18 years	Remnants of old conflicts (Oedipal and Electra) must be resolved. Homosexuality is a transitory phase. Sexual experimentation and masturbation.	Failure to resolve old conflicts will prevent full maturity. Goal is full, genitally focused heterosexuality.

and change during adulthood, but occasioned hardly more than a cursory nod. Research with adults as subjects was actually focused on children, attempting to discover the effects of parental practices and attitudes, the absent father, the working mother, family conflict, and divorce. The only adults who began to come into view were the aged, primarily because of interest in elderly adults on the part of the federal government, with much of the research turning to health and social problems of that population. The "no-man's land" between adolescence and old age did not begin to attract sustained concern until the 1960s, and it has taken two decades to begin to build the research.

In this chapter, we will be looking at the young adult emerging from late adolescence at age 18, 19, or 20 through the decade of the 20's. If the adolescent years have passed favorably, the matter of identity—a good sense of one's own strengths and direction— ' will have been formed. Acceptable independence from family will have been settled to offer a certain security in making decisions. It is this capacity for self-determination that characterizes the young adult and sets the period apart from adolescence. It is time not only of setting future courses but of being able to take the steps for implementation.

PHYSICAL ATTRIBUTES

Both men and women reach a peak of physical form during this period. Never again will stamina, strength, endurance, agility, grace, coordination, and balance be so readily accessible for strenuous or controlled body performance. As a matter of fact, certain organ systems will already have begun a slow decline, to be gradually joined by other

Both men and women reach a peak of physical form in young adulthood. Stamina, strength, endurance, agility, grace, and coordination combine to allow superb physical performance.

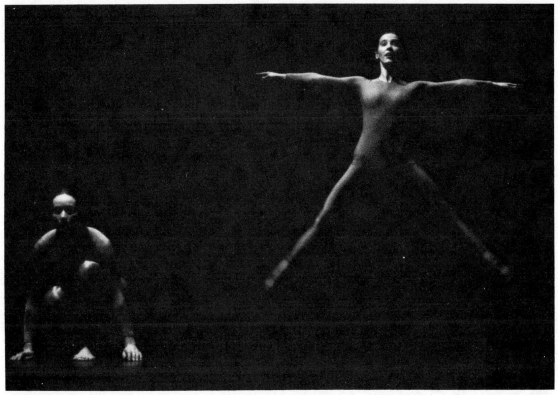

Richard M. Grabbert

systems so that general body functioning continues to decrease at a rate of about 1 per cent per year in adult life (Shock, 1962). However, the traditional signs of aging—the notion of infirmity and loss of vigor—will seem as far off as the moon for most young adults. Many will continue some of the excessive practices of their adolescence: driving too fast, getting little sleep, eating an excess of "junk" food, taking hair-raising risks, and testing powers of sensory and judgmental acuity. There is often a sense of personal indestructibility that can, of course, lead to tragedy. However, all society admires and exalts the prowess of youthful jumpers, runners, swimmers, dancers, rock climbers, football players, and other examples of heavy calls upon mind and muscle. Youthful appearance is also highly prized, granting tidy profits to any industries that promise shiny hair, flashing teeth, a smooth tan, and a trim body.

So—young adulthood might seem to be a golden age. However, it is interesting to note, in this regard, a study of how individuals at different stages of life think about "prime time" for themselves (Daniel and Lachmann, 1975). The subjects, ages 13 to 85, were asked what they considered to be the prime time of their lives. Most of the adolescents felt their prime was still ahead of them, whereas most of the subjects older than age 70 felt that it had passed. Beginning at age 20, a steadily increasing number said that their prime time was "right now," with the 40- to 50-year-old age group having the highest percentage of "in the present" responses. It appears that good feelings about one's life can extend through and beyond the period of young adulthood. Though decline in some functions has already started, its progression tends to be unnoticed except in the case of extraordinary body demands. Furthermore, the observation that "youth is wasted on the young" (the complaint of jealous oldsters) fails to reflect the fact that young people themselves may not consider their age to be so ideal, having little with which to compare it. Indeed, the age contains a number of uncertainties that make it less than serene. Among these is the necessity of finding and assuming one's place in adult society.

For this task, says Daniel Levinson (1978a), who has done some of the original "passages" research on adults, the young adult male needs a Dream, a mentor, and a special woman. (This "Dream" is capitalized to set off its specific significance and unique quality.) Because Levinson's subjects were all men and because no comparable work has been forthcoming on the young adult female, the prescription for today's woman is less clear. It is additionally uncharted because the young women of today, in unprecedented numbers, are leaving the traditional roads, and what lies along the new routes is not known. Nevertheless, we propose to use the "Dream, mentor, and special other" framework for discussion of the young adulthood of both sexes, looking at the relationship between fantasy and cognition during this period, discussing the role of a mentor in certain kinds of career progressions, and examining the critical developmental task (according to Erikson) of forming intimate relationships. Levinson coined a descriptive term for this stage that connotes the young individual's foothold in adulthood. It is thought of as the period of the *novice*, which effectively demarcates its quality of "beginning," and is seen to last about 15 years, from age 17 or 18 to age 32 or 33.

COGNITIVE DEVELOPMENT

A Dream

Levinson (1978a) proposes that the most successful men at midlife, those whose work and adulthoods have been suffused with a sense of excitement and self-fulfillment, were creators of a Dream during their novice phase. The function of the Dream was to offer those able to build a life around it, despite setbacks and struggle, a focus for commitment.

Subjects whose Dream was vague and unconnected to life had difficulty sustaining a sense of purpose. Those who permitted their Dream to be eclipsed by parental opposition or various combinations of circumstances and personal factors tended to pursue a life and occupation that held no interest for them and were confronted with a point of reckoning in later life.

The place, purpose, extent, alternatives, thwartings, and enhancers of such a fantasy in young adult life need much further study. However, the particular kind of Dream described by Levinson seems to be appropriate for the powers of "formal operations," Piaget's model for cognition of adulthood. Formal operations, the last stage of developing intelligence according to Piaget, was discussed in Chapter 10, but we will recall its salient features here.

Piaget (1973) presents *formal operations* as the highest order of mental development, the most mature form of thinking. It enables the individual to look at the world objectively, assessing reality, forming hypotheses and the strategies for testing these, and understanding and dealing with abstractions. Although this final step is not universally achieved, the value of being able to process information efficiently and flexibly is obvious.

To be able to fashion a Dream would seem to represent a capacity for formal operations. To dream of one's own future, to spin out the various alternatives, trying them on mentally, sorting and discarding and retaining, calls for high-order mental accomplishment. This kind of fantasy would be quite unlike the pretend or symbolic play that Piaget described for early childhood. The very young child is *not* objective nor realistic and therefore freely distorts reality to suit egocentric needs of the moment. But the adult Dream is future-oriented and anchored in reality; it would be difficult to conceive of a young adult dreaming seriously about becoming a fairy princess.

Levinson (1978a) suggests that there is a very real difference in the Dreams of men at the various socioeconomic levels in his sample. The biologists and novelists he studied, for the most part, followed their Dreams. But the young men who were going to become workers for hourly wages tended to have Dreams (often of star athletic achievement) that they could not live out. For most of them, the Dream became lost in the pressure for survival. One of the social problems that will have to be addressed in the future is that of loss of talent and zest when individuals are sidelined into occupations that hold neither challenge nor interest. The frustration of having had to settle for so much less than one's earlier hopes may lead to depression and discontent; under some circumstances, people in their despair have fallen easy victims to the promises of demagogues (Krause, 1978).

Because corresponding research on the Dream for women has not yet been done, it is necessary to proceed with some "educated" guesses. Both men (Komarovsky, 1976) and women (Suniewick, 1971) tend to presume that women's interests should be subordinated to those of a fiancé or husband. It seems likely, therefore, that the Dream of the young woman has an "iffy" quality that does not characterize that of her male counterpart. Hers will include some contingencies: ". . . if I get married," ". . . depending on when I get married," ". . . depends on whom I marry." Each conditional proposition has a determining power over what happens next. "If" has to do with the chances of meeting an acceptable man, being considered attractive and desirable by him, and, finally, being invited to share his life. "When" involves a time span of some length during which the young woman waits to be chosen. "Who" makes the future even more problematic since the still-most-acceptable custom is that the husband's domicile becomes the wife's. If he is a local man with a position here, she stays. If his position is overseas, she goes. For centuries, the life of a woman after marriage has been determined almost entirely by the occupation, preferences, and abode of her mate. This is not likely to change overnight, despite efforts to help women become more autonomous. The sum, for many women, if not most, must be a Dream that is seen to be in the hands of fate, with a faceless man and faceless children serving as focal points. Even women who are struggling to change personal and interpersonal orientations are showing unmodified views about marriage, jobs, and income (Carruth, 1975), or have wholly unrealistic perceptions of what is involved in whole-hearted pursuit of a career and motherhood at one and the same time (Bardwick, 1971).

The young adult male is absolved from this conflict in his contemplation of the future. His Dream does not have to solve the problem of how to combine lifework and family. He can construct that bridge, or build that business, or farm that crop whether he becomes a father or not. His Dream will, in all likelihood, include options that seem to be of his own choosing and under his own control.

The difference is enormous. Whether you feel that you, yourself, guide the circumstances and manage the events in your life or whether you assume that outside forces influence the things that happen creates two very dissimilar orientations toward the future. People who see themselves as masters of their own destiny place the *locus of control* inside, coming from their own inner psychic resources. They are called *internalizers; externalizers* feel that the locus of control is outside and that there is almost nothing that can be done to change anything (Rotter, 1966). The internalizer moves to take charge, whereas the externalizer tends to react passively to events, rather than instigating them.

Women who Dream of a life of their own making (internalizers) are likely to have been reared rather differently from those who are traditional. Hennig and Jardim (1977) studied women who had achieved top rank in career-progress. These women were found to have had steady encouragement and support by their fathers all through childhood and adolescence. Fathers promoted the conviction that girls could do anything that boys could do, and especially commended the capabilities of their daughters. Relationships with mothers for these women had been warm, though most of the mothers were less than enthusiastic about the career route that the daughters selected, quite probably because the early years did not include marriage.

Internalizer or externalizer, the young adult woman's Dream will provide direction for her behavior and a beacon toward her future in a fashion similar to that of her male age-mate. Her Dream, too, might be said to gain strength from the ability to think maturely and realistically, in the mode of formal operations.

Creative Problem Solving

Not all scholars are content with the idea of formal operations as the final stage of cognitive development, however. Piaget's descriptive emphasis on rigorous analysis, mathematical precision, pure logic, and rational hypothesis testing may seem austere and even lacking in excitement for some people. Perhaps different types of individuals would thrive with different cognitive styles. Might there not be alternative modes that would qualify as mature, objective, and reality-oriented but, say, creative rather than analytical?

One of the suggestions in this regard is that of a cognition characterized by intuition and deriving its energy from conflict and crisis. Klaus Riegel (1973), whose theory this is, points out that the mature equilibrium envisioned by Piaget is not for everyone, nor is it even likely to occur for long. The normal course of life will include biological crises, such as disease and accidents; there will be catastrophes, such as earthquakes and droughts; there will be social disagreements and thwartings of entire groups. However, these "normative life crises" may actually force a new, creative adjustment of mentality. Riegel terms it a "dialectical process," noting that contradictions and problems at one level of existence force a shift to something new. Riegel's work is an optimistic model for development. He insists that frustration leads to new levels of complexity and that conflict is necessary rather than negative. Because he considers all of the aging processes to create one type of regularly recurring crisis, the possibility of continued cognitive development during all adulthood is suggested. Riegel points to Piaget—elderly, active, and productive—as a prime example.

Counselors and clinical psychologists find this dialectical interpretation of development affirming their own observations of clients who emerge from a period of great distress stronger and better than before. This is not to imply that crises are always resolved positively (Carruth, 1975), but, rather, to emphasize the potential for growth that is presented by life's troubles.

There is no need to "choose" between Piaget or Riegel. It is most likely that both will be found to contribute to our understanding and that neither will be found wholly valid. The use and value of a "model" are that it gives thinking some system and order. This raises the questions that need to be tested. Then, like good scientists, we stand ready to revise a model or try out a new one when the data are in.

The cognitive development in this period of young adulthood, whether seeking the balance of formal operations or moving with dialectical tensions, permits the formation of a special Dream for both men and women. Whether the Dream is well formed or vague, rooted in the past, or soaring toward the future partakes of the young person's total view of self and life. Whether the Dream is nurtured and brought to fruition or forgotten and allowed to die will depend significantly upon the individual's personal and environmental resources, and, in some measure, upon chance. Ideally, the Dream should lead into one of the most important tasks of this period—beginning one's life work.

CAREER DEVELOPMENT

There is a widespread belief that career and occupation ought to be well settled by the early 20s. On the contrary, Levinson (1978b) suggests that the sequence of occupational development is more complex and takes a longer time. He uses the term "forming" an occupation rather than the common "choosing" to signify the continuing effort, decisions, and experience that must contribute to the process. The initial serious interest is likely to be based on a more-or-less objective assessment of curiosity, values, and concerns. Having set one's sights, the protracted tasks of acquiring the training, skills, and credentials follow. This is not always a direct and plainly visible route; there are stations and drop-offs and sometimes detours to other places.

The value of a mentor in this regard, according to Levinson, is to keep the young adult "on track," supporting and facilitating realization of the Dream. The need for a mentor has become a standard aspect of academic industrial psychology courses and popular magazine articles on job progression, attesting to the recognition of mentoring as a prevalent practice in corporations and other institutions. Levinson's description of the mentor is invariably male. The men in his sample had almost no women friends, let alone women mentors. There simply were not enough women holding positions in which they might have served as mentors, though Levinson foresees their advent as bringing great developmental benefits to mentoring relationships.

The mentor, in a very real sense, enhances the young adult's self-identity and self-confidence by explicitly believing in him, providing a critical but supportive appraisal of efforts, sponsoring, and serving as a model of what may come. The ideal mentor offers room to grow but can point out the pitfalls along the way without robbing the young person of initiative and responsibility. It is a tricky relationship—"mixture of parent and peer," according to Levinson—and must not be too much of either. The mentor, in an optimal relationship, will enable a full transition from the insecurities of adolescence into an effective sense of one's own adult autonomy and capability for dependable, competent actions.

There are instances when the relationship is not as benign as that described, when the mentor suddenly withdraws support or becomes destructive at a critical point. The young person may break loose prematurely, unnerved by some dynamic in the situation. Of such stuff are novels fashioned!

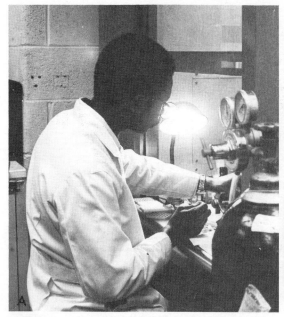

L. Newman

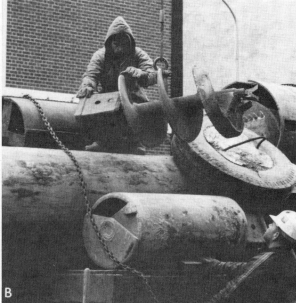

K. Pitcoff

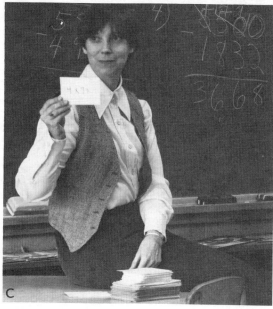

Judith Kruger Michalik

(A, B, C) The decade of the twenties is the time of choosing an occupation or career. Establishing oneself and achieving satisfaction in a career, however, extend beyond these years.

Levinson (1978b) indicates and Hennig and Jardim (1977) confirm that mentors of achieving women are somewhat different from those of men, but they essentially serve the same purpose—that of acting as guide and champion, teaching the young woman all of the intricacies of the particular organization, opening important doors, and protecting her from certain kinds of career-progression dangers. The mentors of these women were men, which may give the relationship a special erotically tinged intensity that future researchers will have to define and elaborate. The time has not yet arrived, apparently, when men and women can work together without sexual overtones. A young woman lawyer commented that it is always necessary for her to inform a new group of male colleagues that she is married. "It clears the air," she says. "We can get to work without a lot of bandying and jockeying for position." It will be interesting to watch, during the coming years, whether women co-workers as an ordinary and common phenomenon will relieve these situations.

The young women described by Hennig and Jardim (1977) did not have women mentors, in part because, as in Levinson's sample, there were no available women in executive positions. There is another question in this regard that only the future can answer. It asks whether women who attain high rank will undertake mentoring of other women. There are some unsettling indications that the generous hand up the ladder may not be offered as readily by one woman to another as it has been offered by men to other men. Tavris (1971) refers to a "Queen Bee Syndrome," a constellation of attitudes by which successful women refuse to assist those coming afterward. The Queen Bee insists, "I made it by myself. Everyone else can do the same."

The issue is somewhat more complex, however, than what is suggested as the jealous maintenance of the Queen Bee's own assuredly hard-won position. There is the further question of whether women will be capable of the kind of cooperation and "bonding" by which men have built bridges, cities, industrial empires, armies, governments, and rockets to the moon (Tiger and Fox, 1971). Tiger speaks of a special kind of male-to-male affinity that encourages cooperation and suggests that it is an evolutionary consequence of the hunting parties of tribal history. Modern feminists bristle at the implication that women are less able to join together for a major common purpose. But where can one point to a large-scale group endeavor executed wholly by women? It is necessary to look to the medieval convents to obtain an example of women working together for great projects over a sustained period of time.

Does this mean that there is good reason for doubting the ability of women to form groups for collective action? Not necessarily. A rejoinder would cite the fact that women have tended to be isolated, one from another, and preoccupied with childbearing and child rearing. There have been no opportunities to form bands and troops and maintain organizations. Women have also been restricted with regard to mobility, far less free to move around than men. Women have not been taught the building, trading, fighting or governing skills. All this argues for a social rather than a genetic explanation. There is no doubt that it has become a deeply rooted part of women's psyche. Competition with each other for the attentions of available men also colors women's relationships with hostility. There has been very little "one for all and all for one" sentiment among marriageable maidens. There may be, however, some hopeful signs. The growing emphasis on team sports for women and the increased numbers of women forming self-help organizations (such as those running crisis centers for victims of rape or battered wives) will almost certainly assist the turnaround in social attitudes whereby women can truly regard each other as "sisters."

Whether women can or cannot, will or will not, serve each other as mentors is a brand new issue, addressing an unprecedented increase in the number of women "in the marketplace." Women now make up 43 per cent of the total labor force. Although they are still segregated mainly in entry-level low-status jobs, a combination of determined women and some appropriate legal support is making small but perceptible headway toward better access and opportunities. In 1970, only 6 per cent of all bank officers were women, but in only 10 years the proportion had increased to 30 per cent (U.S. News & World Report, September 15, 1980). Apparently, there are enough executive women and those aspiring to such positions to merit the publication of several magazines designed to appeal to their interests and needs, including help with formation of networks for mutual assistance.

Mentors for either men or women probably do not need to be attached to corporate pyramids. A look at the functions ascribed to the mentor (Levinson, 1978b) suggests that these might be undertaken with great advantage by a number of different kinds of people at different stages of life. A charismatic teacher, a remarkable grandfather, or the mother of a best friend are sometimes, for fortunate ones, present at the right time with an imperishable contribution.

One is reminded in this regard of a study by Norman Garmezy (1976) of a group of children he calls "invulnerables." These are children who have everything stacked against them: poverty, broken families, urban ghetto life, physical disabilities, unstable parents. Yet they bounce up, not only surviving, but surviving exceedingly well. They tend to be good students in school, to be well liked and admired, to have leadership qualities, and to seem to be on their way toward becoming useful, solid citizens despite the enormous odds. In the study of factors that seem to have helped these children to cope, Garmezy often found a single person, someone who had taken special interest in the child. Like the mentor of a later age, the expansive effect of having someone who really believes in you and with whom you can discuss your inner hopes and fears seems to do wonders (miracles, in these cases). Garmezy's work suggests that perhaps all of us, in addition to being parents for our own children, might assist development by mentoring some children of others.

INTIMACY

A Special Man or Woman

Erikson sets the task for this period as that of learning "intimacy." If everything has gone well, the relatively indiscriminate eroticism of adolescence has become tempered, because both the newness and the sense of personal uniqueness (as if you alone had discovered sex!) obtain some perspective as the young person passes age 18 and heads into the 20s. The adolescent's route toward this point has been somewhat perilous. Relationships with "significant others" needed to be fashioned and broken; partners and friends need to be sought and cherished without exploitation or relinquishing the self. The relationships that are close and warm must not become forced into premature commitment, an ever-beckoning temptation because of the intensity of adolescent sexual desire.

Ideally, the adolescent years are useful for exploring personal strengths and traumas in relationships. With experiences, discoveries, joys, and sorrows, there is a gradual decision-making process. The young person becomes aware of liked and disliked characteristics in others, of acceptable and unacceptable values and behaviors. Then the stage becomes set for finding the "most special" one. By this time, the adolescent is likely to be a young adult, ready for intimacy and, perhaps, for forming a marriage.

This ought not to happen too early. In any case, the marriage will have to partake of some of the left-over adolescent conflicts, including separation from parents. The earlier the marriage, the less likely will be the successful sorting out of guilts and anxieties of early sexual experiences and the less likely will the mate be seen as distinct from the childhood fantasy images of mother and father.

Levinson (1978a) points out that a man has an additional task of learning to relate to and accommodate the feminine aspects of himself, an assignment for which his childhood and adolescence are unlikely to have prepared him. It is possible to conjecture that women may have similar difficulty in accepting their own self-assertive "masculine" qualities. Women have been taught that they are chiefly responsible for the well-being of a marriage, and for many a woman this means a constant attempt to keep her husband happy, often at the expense of her own wishes and desires.

Marriage is having a rather bad press these days. One marriage in three does not last, and the ratio is rapidly approaching one in two. Even so, more than 95 per cent of the United States population marries at least once in their lifetime.

The institution of marriage in all its varying forms has long served societies as a means for rearing children, for maintaining a certain stability of sexual relationships and domicile, and for transferring property according to some socially recognized procedure. Love, as an essential ingredient, is a notion of relatively recent origin in Western culture, as is the requirement that the partners should be happy and fulfilled in the relationship. Our young people marry for psychological satisfactions; they will wish to achieve sexual

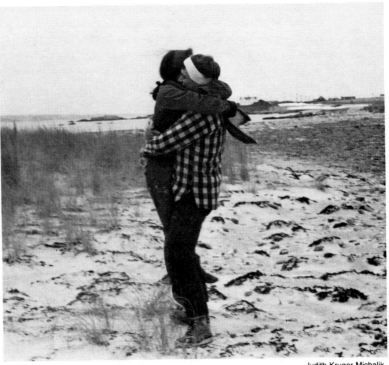

Judith Kruger Michalik

The young adult who has success-fully achieved a sense of self and identity finds the stage set for estab-lishing a relationship with a "most special" one. The young adult is ready for sharing of true intimacy.

and personal intimacy on a continuing basis. They will expect a security in commitment, sustained mutual support, and a place and a person to "come home to." The demands are high, possibly accounting in some part for the high rate of divorce as expectations go unmet. There are those who say we are making impossible demands on an institution that was not intended to serve them (Coleman, 1979).

Some young people have sought to bypass the formalized and legal bonds in favor of an informal arrangement termed "cohabitation" or, simply, "living together." This is a phenomenon of the past decade and is far different from the more casual and less respectable "shacking up" of another era. The living-together arrangements of this past decade have involved emotional commitment and tended to last from 1 to 4 years. Interestingly, cohabiting pairs express many of the problems often cited by married couples—such as jealousy, feeling cut off from friends, differing levels of sexual desire, fear of pregnancy, and disagreements about how money should be spent (Macklin, 1972).

Macklin also found that almost all (90 per cent) of the cohabiting pairs rated the experiences as successful, happy, and maturing. The practice has become fairly common. There are more than 1,500,500 such units according to United States Census estimates of 1975, with the arrangement formally identified in bureaucratic language as "persons of the opposite sex sharing living quarters." (Not all of these are young adults, it should be noted. Many elderly pairs are living together without being married so that neither loses a Social Security check.) A survey taken in 1977 (Bower and Christopherson) reported that about 25 per cent of the college students interviewed had cohabited at some point during college life. It was also found that cohabitation does not seem to dull enthusiasm for marriage. Of those who had cohabited, 96 per cent indicated their intention of being married one day (Glazer-Mabin, 1975).

In marrying, cohabiting, or participating in any of the less frequent coupling styles (such as a commune), the underlying aim is intimacy. There is a general agreement that intimacy is the most profound of relationships. For many young people, the concept has replaced the notion of "true love" because of their disaffection for the commercialization of the latter term. Ask them what intimacy means, and the answers always include such ideas as mutual honesty, sharing of innermost thoughts and feelings, erasing the facades, caring about each other's growth, understanding, and acceptance. It is possible to glimpse the terrible vulnerability that one would bring to a relationship striving for intimacy. The vital importance of having traversed the previous developmental steps successfully is pointed up. Without a solid foundation of basic trust, it would be impossible to so risk one's inner self. Without having a grasp on autonomy, initiative, and identity, there could be no independent decision to share self and life, since the capacity for decision making, and even the sense of self, would be blighted.

Delight-filled, exquisitely perceived, and especial: "Has anyone ever felt like this before?" becomes a genuine question. However, young adults need help to understand that intimate sharing cannot be sustained continuously. It is too intense. It would burn itself out. Intimacy needs ebb and flow. Individuals in an intimate relationship must have breathing room, private space. A full-time intimacy would be a crushing burden and die of its own weight.

Furthermore, true intimacy demands equality. A superior-subordinate status destroys the basic premise, which is that each chooses freely. If one partner is dependent upon the other, there is an inevitable tilt in the direction of the one-most-valued by the one who is less valued. There can be compensatory moves and trade-offs, but these are power games. A struggle for power is not compatible with intimacy.

It must be evident that an intimate relationship can never be regarded as finished or completed. It is forever changing with the transforming experiences of the participants.

Sexual Relations

Sexual union is usually thought of as the ultimate expression of intimacy. Though there is no doubt that intercourse often occurs (perhaps even most of the time) without the mutuality of emotions and sensations that we are describing, it is probably true that most partners are really searching and hoping for that ultimate fulfillment. It is also true that our generation has more actual information about sexual behavior than any other before it. This may not assist in achieving intimacy, but it assuredly can help to counter some of the old myths and tales that have colored sexuality with much unnecessary guilt and shame.

The idea that sex might be a legitimate field for scientific study was incredibly late to arrive. When Alfred Kinsey began conducting his famous surveys in the 1940s, there was almost no authentic knowledge about sexual behavior. The fact that Kinsey was inquiring into people's sexual practices was considered so shocking that the first report, *Sexual Behavior in the Human Male* (1948), almost didn't get published. Its significant and lasting contribution was that it broke the taboo and made sex a socially acceptable topic for study and discussion. The breath of fresh air was an antidote to decades of silence and unquestioned attitudes of Victorian prudishness, especially when the wide extent of many "evil habits" became known. To discover that one's own "secret vice" was not so remarkable must have offered overwhelming relief to great numbers of men and women.

Beginning in the mid-1950s, William Masters and Virginia Johnson carried the Kinsey research further. Their work consisted in actual observations of "what happens to the human male and female as they respond to effective sexual stimulation." The research was undertaken with care and sensitivity, and though there were expressions of disapproval, the general public was not as scandalized as it had been with the first Kinsey report. Their work accomplished the first systematic investigation (1966) of the physiology of sexual stimulation and orgasm and made two major contributions to understanding of sexual behavior.

The first achievement detailed the physiological reactions and progression of sexual response. More than 10,000 completed response cycles were observed, monitored, and sometimes filmed, providing the largest accumulation of empirical data up to that time.

Obviously, questions must be raised regarding the validity of the results: Do subjects who are being observed really respond in the same ways that they would if their behavior was private? However, this question of "observer effect" accompanies every investigation of behavior and should remind us that all scientific conclusions are tentative—serving until an investigator figures out a better way of observing. The Masters and Johnson work significantly advanced understanding of the nature of sexual response and was instrumental in clearing away some erroneous conclusions regarding female orgasm.

The second contribution was an outgrowth of the first. In the course of attempting to screen and select subjects capable of normal sexual activity, the researchers uncovered an enormous underground suffering because of sexual dysfunction—untreated, unacknowledged, and literally unknown before they began their investigation. They estimated (1975) that at least 50 per cent of marriages in the United States suffer from sexual inadequacy. Masters and Johnson, working together, invented a unique approach to treatment for sexual dysfunction and began to publish their findings in 1970. Since that time, they have trained many therapists for treating sexual problems. Other psychologists have elaborated and modified the Masters and Johnson procedures, and the number of "sex clinics" that have been opened attest to the fact that many people are now asking for help with their sexual lives. We will now present the Masters and Johnson findings with regard to the sexual response cycle and save the treatment of sexual dysfunction for Chapter 13.

Masters and Johnson identified four "phases" of sexual response. It must immediately be noted, however, that these are not separate and distinct. The phases are experienced as an ongoing, flowing progression. Description of the phases simply makes it easier to communicate about the process. Furthermore, the patterns of response represent a generalization of observations rather than consistent individual reactions. However, there seems to be enough predictability to warrant thinking about the response phases as "typical," providing the wide range of possible deviations is kept in mind.

Male and female sexual responses are very similar in terms of the physiological mechanisms involved, no matter what the source of arousal, whether with a partner or by means of masturbation. Two basic systemic reactions are involved—*vasocongestion* and *myotonia*. Vasocongestion is an increased flow of blood into certain tissues, engorgement of blood vessels, and a pooling or collecting of blood, particularly in the genitals. Myotonia is increased muscle tension, affecting both smooth and skeletal muscles, occurring both voluntarily and involuntarily. These two mechanisms are the source of almost all of the bodily manifestations during sexual activity. Variations in amount of blood flow, engorgement, timing, and strength of tension in the muscles account for differences in individual reactions from person to person and from occasion to occasion.

For both men and women, the phases of the sexual response cycle, beginning with "effective stimulation" and moving all the way through to climax and back to an unaroused state, seem to correspond loosely to the subjective feelings that people report of their sexual experiences. From start to finish, the four phases describe the physiological changes observed by the investigators as the sexual reactions proceed. These are as follows:

Excitement.   This phase is characterized by an increase of blood flowing into and remaining in the genitalia (vasocongestion), causing penile erection, enlarging of the testicles, swelling of the labia, and lubrication of the vagina.

Plateau Phase.   There is an increase in penile circumference, testicular enlargement, and an initial secretion from the penis (which may contain sperm). The woman shows expansion of the inner two thirds of the vagina and retraction of the clitoris under the clitoral hood (this should not be interpreted as loss of excitement). There is discoloration (frequently) of the "corona" (crown) of the penis and of the labia minora (inner lips);

flushing of the chest, breasts, and neck of the woman ("sexual flush," more common in the fair-skinned); and an increase in the respiratory and heart rates.

Orgasmic Phase. For the man, orgasm begins with contractions of accessory organs (seminal vesicles, prostate, and vas deferens), yielding the sensation that ejaculation is inevitable. Almost immediately, contractions of the muscles at the base of the penis and the penile urethra occur, at first at intervals of approximately 0.8 second, then slowing and becoming more irregular for three or four last contractions. The seminal fluid, about a teaspoonful of milky, mucoid material, is "thrown out." The subjective sensation is probably one of the most intense pleasures of life, entailing a true loss of self and time and place for the brief instant.

The physiological events during orgasm for a woman are similar. There are convulsive contractions of the congested walls of the outer third of the vagina (the *orgasmic platform*), a "tenting" of the inner two thirds of the vagina, and contractions of the uterus. The rhythm is like that of the man, about 0.8 second apart during the first intense contractions, followed by intervals more widely spaced. For the orgasmic woman, the physiological mechanisms are precisely the same, according to Masters and Johnson, no matter how the stimulation to orgasm has occurred (whether it was clitoral or vaginal). This has turned out to be a very "liberating" finding, since it dispelled the last remnants of Freud's contention that women can experience two different kinds of orgasm. One, resulting from clitoral sensitivity, was supposed to be less "mature" and to result from some kind of failure to proceed to mature sexuality. As a consequence, several generations of women were held captive by a false concept, striving for something that may not exist and feeling depressed about their defect. It means that women can now decide for themselves what constitutes "good" and "bad" for their sexual experiences without needing to live up to Freud's model.

Another myth that troubled men and women for at least a century has been the idea that women are genetically unresponsive to sexual stimuli, are aroused with difficulty, and climax rarely. The Masters and Johnson research, having selected responsive subjects, discovered fewer response failures among the women than among the men. Some of their female subjects were capable of achieving several orgasms in succession (multiorgasmic). It was thus possible to conclude that female orgasmic capacity is learned, that its repression is also learned, and that women may have a potential for "enjoying" erotic activity even more than men (Hall, 1969).

Resolution. The man shows rapid loss of pelvic vasocongestion, resulting in relaxation of the penis, scrotum, and testes. The loss seems to be less rapid for some women, which enables them to return readily to an orgasmic phase. For most men, there is a "refractory period" in which new excitement build-up is impossible. For both sexes, the return to the pre-excitement level of functioning is completed by the end of the resolution phase.

In the case of excitement sustained at the plateau level without orgasmic discharge, the resolution phase is much more gradual for both men and women. The vasocongestion dissipates slowly, giving rise to sensations of "fullness," "swelling," and "throbbing." Contrary to the widely held mythology, this is not excruciatingly painful, nor is it harmful to the individual. The engorgement can be easily and efficiently dispersed by masturbation.

Intimacy and Sex—One Last Thought

Karen Horney, the noted psychoanalyst, described the unhealthy tendency to become enslaved by mental pictures of all the things we think we ought to be doing (1950). She suggested that the anxious worrier is subject to "the tyranny of the 'should'," and she pointed out that for each of us, living up to all the "shoulds" accumulated in the course of growing up creates an intolerable burden. It robs us of spontaneity and prevents us from making decisions of our own, for ourselves. There are few areas of life in which this is more apparent than for sexual relationships.

The "sexual revolution" has brought a whole new set of "shoulds" that now trouble sexual relationships as much as the old ones. No one advocates a return to a belief that women should be passive recipients of men's uncontrollable desires. However, the current emphasis on sexual *performance* can be as dehumanizing.

The old myths about sex said that women did not have orgasms and that "good" women did not enjoy sex. Today, if you were to believe everything you read in the popular press, you would think that every woman wanted to have sex every day in every way and had multiple orgasms on each occasion. Men live with even greater oppression in regard to sexual performance. The image of the man in our society has always been one who aggressively pursues sexual adventures. In addition, today a man may fear that he has responsibility for his partner's orgasm or risks censure as unfeeling and selfish.

There is need now for another look at sexuality and a re-evaluation of these new "shoulds" and pressures. The insistence that everyone must be sexy all the time needs to change to a more relaxed acceptance of individual rhythms, inclinations, and disinclinations. "No, thank you" needs to be as legitimate a response as "yes, please." We will be closer to real sexual freedom when both men and women are free to enjoy sexual activity when and if they want to, when they don't feel pressured into any form of activity, and when they are not judged by their sexual performance.

The most important thing to remember about the sexual pressures of today is that despite the preoccupation with sex in society, having physical sex is not really the problem. Sex can be had almost anywhere. It is for sale, and impersonal sex can be had easily for free. But intimacy: that is something else again! Intimacy, as Erikson (1963) said long ago, is a relationship that is enabling, enhancing, and enriching. It is recognition of the significance of the person. It is "knowing" each other in the full Biblical sense of the term.

Erikson suggested a "shorthand" formulation of the goals for mature and growing intimacy that would include:

1. Mutuality of orgasms (note that this does *not* specify "simultaneous")
2. With a loved partner
3. Of the other sex
4. With whom one is able and willing to share a mutual trust
5. And with whom one is willing and able to regulate cycles of
   a. Work
   b. Procreation
   c. Recreation
6. So as to secure to the offspring, too, a satisfactory development.

Erikson originally wrote this definition for the 1950 White House Conference on Children and Youth. He did not then deny the possibility for emotional well-being to those who, for one reason or another, do not marry and build families. There are those today who point out that on an overpopulated planet, procreation is not the first aim of sex and therefore offspring are not necessary in order that a relationship be mature, satisfactory, and intimate. However, in 1950 and now, this formulation seems to represent a grand design, a goal for most of us, representing the innate "life force" tendencies that provide an impetus toward re-creating the families that made our own lives possible. Erikson calls this *generativity*, and it will be the main subject of the next chapter.

GLOSSARY

EXTERNALIZER One who believes that the control of one's life is largely under the direction of outside forces.

FORMAL OPERATIONS The fourth and last period, or highest order, of cognitive development, according to Piaget. It enables an objective view of the world, along with the ability to assess reality, to perform inductive and deductive reasoning, to engage in abstract thinking, to formulate and test hypotheses, to use formal logic in reasoning, and to understand higher mathematics.

GENERATIVITY Erikson's term for the seventh stage of development, the time of adulthood when intimacy deepens to the point of desire to share with the world. It is a kind of returning to the world after a period of preoccupation with the self and a beloved partner. There is the concern for establishing and guiding the next generation. Ordinarily, this is manifested in bearing and raising children, but it can also include productivity and creativity.

INTERNALIZER One who believes that the control of one's life resides in the individual.

LOCUS OF CONTROL The term used to designate an individual's perception of whether his life is at the mercy of outside forces or whether the individual, autonomously, is in control.

MYOTONIA Increased muscle tension.

ORGASMIC PLATFORM The outer third of the vagina, which narrows and tightens during the course of mounting sexual excitement.

VASOCONGESTION Increased flow of blood into certain tissues, with the engorgement of blood vessels and the collecting of blood that occur during sexual excitement.

REFERENCES

Bardwick, J.: *Psychology of Women.* New York: Harper & Row, 1971.

Bower, D. W., Christopherson, V. A.: University student cohabitation: A regional comparison of selected attitudes and behavior. *Journal of Marriage and the Family,* 39:447–452, 1977.

Carruth, J. F.: Crises: An abstract model versus individual experience. In Datan, N., Ginsberg, L. (eds.): *Life Span Developmental Psychology. Normative Life Crises.* New York: Academic Press, 1975.

Coleman, J.: *Contemporary Psychology and Effective Behavior* (4th ed.). Glenview, Ill.: Scott, Foresman, 1979.

Daniel, P., Lachman, M.: The prime of life. In Rebelsky, F. (ed.). *Life, the Continuous Process. Readings in Human Development.* New York: Alfred A. Knopf, 1975.

Dewey, J. A.: *Democracy and Education.* New York: MacMillan, 1916.

Erikson, E.: *Childhood and Society* (2nd ed.). New York: W. W. Norton & Company, 1963.

Garmezy, N., Masten, A., Nordstrom, L., Ferrarese, M.: Vulnerable and invulnerable children: Theory, research and intervention. Abstracted in the Journal Supplement Abstract Service. *Catalogue of Selected Documents in Psychology,* 6(4):96, 1976.

Glazer-Mabin, N.: *Old Families/New Families.* New York: Van Nostrand, 1975.

Hall, G. S.: *Educational Problems.* New York: Appleton, 1911.

Hall, M. H.: A conversation with Masters and Johnson. *Psychology Today,* 3(2):50–58, 1969.

Hennig, M., Jardim, A.: *The Managerial Woman.* New York: Anchor Press/Doubleday, 1977.

Horney, K.: *Neurosis and Human Growth.* New York: W. W. Norton & Company, 1950.

James, W.: *The Principles of Psychology.* New York: Holt, 1890.

Kinsey, A.: *Sexual Behavior of the Human Male.* Philadelphia: W. B. Saunders Company, 1948.

Kinsey, A.: *Sexual Behavior of the Human Female.* Philadelphia: W. B. Saunders Company, 1953.

Komarovsky, M.: *Dilemmas of Masculinity: A Study of College Youth.* New York: W. W. Norton & Company, 1976.

Krause, C. A.: *Guyana Massacre.* New York: Berkley Publishing, 1978.

Levinson, D. J.: How men grow up: The necessary search for a dream, a mentor and a special woman. *Psychology Today,* 11(8):20–31, 1978a, p. 89.

Levinson, D. J.: *The Seasons of a Man's Life.* New York: Alfred A. Knopf, 1978b.

Macklin, E.: Heterosexual cohabitation among unmarried college students. *The Family Coordinator,* 12:463–471, 1972.

Masters, W. H., Johnson, V. E.: *Human Sexual Response.* Boston: Little, Brown, 1966.

Masters, W. H., Johnson, V. E.: *Human Sexual Inadequacy.* Boston: Little, Brown, 1970.

Number of working women up in '77. Bureau of Labor Statistics. *Providence Sunday Journal,* May 14, 1978, p. B-17.

Perkins, C. S.: *Sex Discrimination and Sex Stereotyping in Vocational Education.* Washington, D.C.: Government Printing Office, 1975.

Piaget, J., Inhelder, B.: *The Child's Conception of Space.* London: Routledge & Kegan, 1958.

Piaget, J., Inhelder, B.: *Memory and Intelligence.* New York: Basic Books, 1973.

Riegel, K.: Dialectic operations, the final period of cognitive development. *Human Development,* 16:346–370, 1973.

Rotter, J.: Generalized expectancies for internal versus external control of reinforcement. *Psychological Monographs*, 80, No. 609, 1966.

Shock, N. W.: The physiology of aging. *Scientific American*, 206:100, 1962.

Suniewick, N.: Beyond the findings: Some interpretations and implications for the future. In Astin, H. S., Suniewick, N., Dweck, S. (eds.):*Women, a Bibliography on Their Education and Careers.* Washington, D. C.: Human Services Press, 1971.

Tavris, C., Staines, G., Jayarantene, T. E.: The queen bee syndrome. In Tavris, C. (ed.): *The Female Experience*. Del Mar, California: CRM Publications, 1973.

Tiger, L., Fox, R.: *The Imperial Animal*. New York: Holt, Rinehart & Winston, 1971.

Whithurst, C. A.: *Women in America: The Oppressed Minority*. Santa Monica, Cal.: Goodyear Press, 1977.

Women forge gains in banking industry. *U. S. News & World Report*, September 15, 1980, p. 81.

THE ADULT:
Generativity

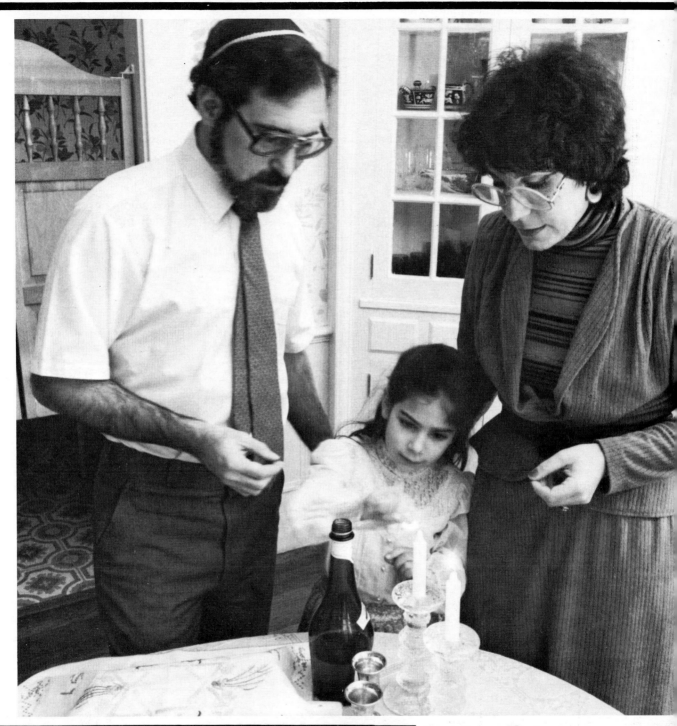

CHAPTER 13

Although young people in love usually feel that they need only each other, life's events propel them into new circumstances that require development and change. This appears to be the dialectical process, in which a comfortable state of being is upset and forces attempts to establish a new comfortable position. The dynamic was described by Klaus Riegel (1975) and discussed in Chapter 12 of this book. For the young adults, the joys of intimacy are very likely to lead to childbearing; the harmony of two turns into three, and the pattern must be reworked. The years of parenting, of responsibility, of giving, begin.

The changes in family configuration are not the whole story. There are moves to new locations with loss of old friends and gain of new ones, the striving for progress and recognition in one's chosen career, the stress of career setbacks, strains on relationships, and sometimes a severing of the bonds by divorce or death.

Adulthood is marked further by physical and social changes that attend growing older and wiser in our society. These have come to be called the "midlife crisis" by the media and dramatized (overdramatized!) as a trauma for everyone, heralded by menopause for women and anxiety about sexual dysfunction for men. However, as will become apparent, the midlife crisis turns out to be descriptive of still another set of circumstances calling for attempts to obtain a new balance and stability that can be, at best, only temporary.

In a comprehensive, long-range study that followed men from their college classes in the early 1940s through middle age, George Vaillant (1977a) discovered that for the men who were classified as "Best Outcomes" (measured on his Adult Adjustment Scale of Mental Health), this midlife period from age 35 to 55 was regarded as the happiest in their lives. Men who were classified as "Worst Outcomes," on the contrary, longed for the earlier time of young adulthood and found the later stresses both difficult and painful.

Satisfaction with life at age 55 seems to be associated with having achieved a good measure of intimacy, a gratifying and productive occupation, and a feeling of self-esteem (Vaillant, 1977a). We will use some of the findings of Vaillant's study to give form to the discussion of this period of adulthood that bridges the time from the "novice" in the early 30s to the beginning of preretirement thinking at 60.

GENERATIVITY

Vaillant (1977a) affirms Erikson's contention that this period, for which *generativity* is the key, represents the ripened, fruitful stage of human existence. Erikson (1960) coined the word "generativity," searching for a description not only of reproduction but also of the productive, creative aspects of adulthood. Its converse is "stagnation," a standing still of mentality, capability, and outlook. Examples might be the man who is still haranguing the philosophy of Franklin Delano Roosevelt and reliving the glories of his college football years, or in the woman squeezing herself into junior-miss fashions and waging frantic war on wrinkles and graying hair.

For Erikson (1963), generativity is the developmental task that follows discovery and accomplishment of intimacy in young adulthood. It involves looking up and beyond the self with desire to "rejoin the world" after the intense inward focus of early intimacy. The outward reaching can take many forms, but usually it is the birth or adoption of a child. The task of generativity, however, is much more than bringing a child into the world. Generativity also implies a warm and heartfelt welcoming of responsibilities in nurturing and caring for the young. It need not, of course, be one's own children; an adult could instruct and share with the children of someone else. The Big Brothers, the dedicated leaders of Cub Scouts and Campfire Girls, religious leaders who minister to their congregations, teachers, the medical professions, counselors . . . in every instance with the wish to assist and to help foster another's well-being, the individual is practicing generativity.

Generativity is the developmental task that often follows establishment of intimacy as a young adult. When two people become three, a fundamental change in outlook takes place; nurturing and caring for the young can bring out the best in both men and women.

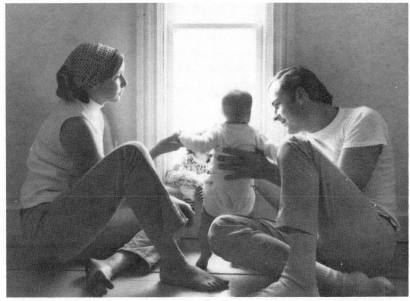

Judith Kruger Michalik

Generativity, it should be emphasized, is not likely to be a wholly conscious, deliberate activity. You are hardly likely to remind yourself, "Now I must serve the future of the race by being generative," any more than the adolescent notes, "This is the time for me to acquire identity." The "inner forces" of which Erikson speaks seem to be a combination of social influences and biological events during the life cycle. Between birth and death, an individual becomes independent, grows capable of reproduction, assumes a place in adult circles, and typically creates the socially structured family. It is usually convenient and comfortable to follow the pattern. Children of all societies are informed about what is expected of their future on every hand so that there comes a time in life when it seems expedient and "right" to step into the displayed footprints; the fact that the prospects of the race have been furthered is a happy outcome, but it has not been the primary conscious motivation. To deviate from the prescribed path, even in these days of easier acceptance of different kinds of lifestyles, probably requires more active deliberation than following the typically unexamined love-marriage-baby sequence.

Becoming a Parent

Pregnancy and childbirth immensely change the lives of those involved with the new baby. During the next several decades, parents will have intrusions and joys, worries and hopes, problems and excitements as a direct consequence of the offspring. By the time children are grown, parents are very different people than when the firstborn entered their lives.

Being a parent is a role for which there is little explicit preparation in our society. The main source of "instruction" is your own family. There is evidence that parents tend to reproduce the conditions of their own rearing quite faithfully, especially (unfortunately) in use of physical punishment and violence (Straus et al., 1980).

There has been a long-standing tendency, even in textbooks, to idealize parenthood and family life. Until very recently, children's primers depicted a family so stereotyped that few children could identify with it—a suburban home with a white picket fence, father going off to work with a briefcase in hand, mother in an apron making cookies, brother Dick climbing a tree to rescue sister Jane's kitten, sister Jane looking adoringly at the skillful rescuer. Now efforts are being made with some success to broaden the content so that there are black families, working mothers, urban housing, and heroic sisters for children to read about.

In the same vein, many of today's families are very different from those in the Norman Rockwell pictures that tend to come to mind. It is not that all families were ever alike, but, rather, there are now even greater variations. More importantly, these need to be recognized. There has been a fair amount of effort, with good results, toward accepting and, indeed, celebrating the different ethnic backgrounds and customs. It can be suggested that perhaps we need some of the same kind of positive regard for the new circumstances of child rearing. Certainly the single mother (or, increasingly, the single father), who is undertaking alone what is a difficult task for two parents, needs social support rather than disapproval and more hurdles. We should be as ready to honor the generativity of an unmarried parent, a late-in-life parent, a foster or adoptive parent, or a "house parent" for troubled children, as that of a traditional pair.

Similarly, discussions of "successful" parenting have tended to promote the notion of idealized practices and to popularize the presumption of parents-to-blame for undesirable child behaviors. There is little public acknowledgment of the fact that being a parent is enormously trying and that the best of parents become exasperated and unreasonable. The several studies of the impact of children upon parents' lives have findings that are surprisingly negative. One (Skolnick and Skolnick, 1971) suggests that marriages without any children at all seem happiest, and others (Burr, 1970; Dytrych et al., 1975) find couples reporting the most happiness before children come and after they leave home. It is becoming clear that in order to speak credibly about parents, we need to know much more about the differences in adult lives, including individual reactions to the situations in which the child is to be reared.

So it is with parenting. It is one thing if you are half of a loving couple. It is another if you are a deserted spouse. It is one thing for a first child, another for the sixth. It is one thing if you have a steady income and bright promise, another if you are unemployed and unskilled. It is one thing if you have a backlog of golden childhood memories, but another, as we mentioned, if childhood was filled with fear and pain. It is different at

Being a parent can be trying, especially if the child's push toward independence comes at the same time the parent is facing the problems of middle age.

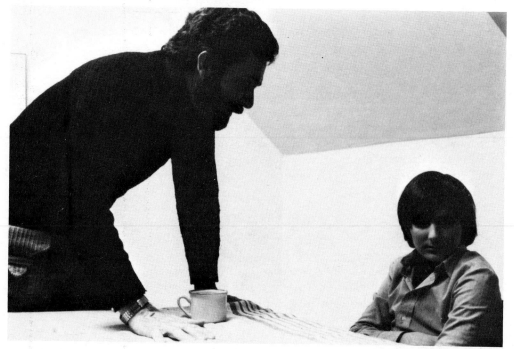

Judith Kruger Michalik

age 33 than at age 23. The criterion for successful generativity, therefore, must necessarily be a relative one. It all depends: One way or another, a new generation must be readied to carry humankind forward.

Diana Baumrind (1980), speaking of the research that attended principally to how this might best be done, suggests that the great portion of it (including her own work) may have been too narrowly conceived. Especially as studies incorporated the researchers' own "built-in" viewpoints with regard to what mothers do and what fathers do, they simply reflected existing views of men as action-oriented initiators and women as emotion-oriented placaters. The new studies, Baumrind feels, will have to take the changing social environment into account and will have to pay much more attention to changing gender roles and to the developmental stages of children.

Baumrind (1980) also argues that child-rearing practices must be evaluated in terms of some understanding of the environments in which the children will be living out their lives. In this regard, her earlier findings (1971) seem to be holding up. Children will need to learn, ideally, to become self-reliant and successful in performance, to engage with others in reciprocal relations that are moral and mature, and to gain a measure of resilience or flexibility that will accommodate change. Most important of all, she suggests, children must learn tolerance of human frailty and imperfection. This can best be taught, according to Baumrind (1980), by parents who see the child as maturing through ages and stages and who are able to transfer power and endow responsibilities appropriately, as the child's behavior warrants. Such parents further understand their own role in encouraging, instructing, and modifying the maturational process. This is a description of the *authoritative parent*, first discussed in Chapter 8. Baumrind contrasts this type of parental approach with that of the *permissive parent*, who views children as having adult rights and assigns few responsibilities (thereby failing to assist children's learning to be competent), and with the *authoritarian parent*, who views children as having responsibilities similar to adults but few rights (thereby teaching injustice and damaging the sense of reciprocity).

Implicit in these descriptions is the premise that the rational, self-confident, judicious authoritative parents must themselves have developed a solid foundation of basic trust, autonomy, initiative, industry, and intimacy in order to function effectively. The further implication—that it is possible for parents to be unerring in deciding each child issue—needs to be tempered by Baumrind's own statement (1980) that she is attempting to describe what could be, rather than what is.

In sum, generativity is seen to be the push toward the future of another person (or entity) who is propelled forward to proceed where we cannot. With whatever gifts the parents have managed to offer, the child (or creation) goes on, carrying that part of us along. By this means, to be generative is to achieve a kind of everlasting life.

Love and Work

There is a story, probably apocryphal, told of Sigmund Freud, that bears recounting. It is said that he was walking one evening with a young student who inquired earnestly, "What is required for happiness?" Freud is supposed to have answered cryptically in his native tongue, *"Lieben und arbeiten."* Happiness is to love and to work. The importance of love to human life—including the love in glowing young romance, the devotion during "sickness and health" of committed partners, the wonder of sharing with children, the warm affection between friends, the empathy for the distressed, and the good will toward humankind—has been discussed in previous sections and will be further considered ahead.

As for work: Both Vaillant (1977b) and Levinson (1978) affirm its vital place in the adult life. Both speak of the fortunate men in their samples who were able to discover their own best talents and devote these to a career that was both absorbing and challenging. That ideal is not available to everyone. Indeed, a number of the men in Levinson's study were from families and backgrounds with limited opportunities and expectations. The several case histories depict men who, with varying degrees of success, had to make some sort of peace with their work as a necessity for survival and whose satisfactions are derived from other sources. One managed to transfer his Dream (of becoming a professional athlete) into avocational coaching and following sports with something of the avid intensity that he might have brought to his life's work had he been able to merge Dream and occupation.

There is a general recognition that our work contributes to the very sense of "being," that we would "go crazy" without a job. However, Terkel (1974), who has given us a vivid picture of how workers in a wide variety of occupations feel about what they are doing, reports a disquieting sense of grievance (p. xxii): "It is a daily circumstance, an awareness of being hurt and an inordinate hunger for 'another way'." One of his interviewees, a young editor, said (p. xxiv): "I think most of us are looking for a calling, not a job. Most of us, like the assembly line worker, have jobs that are too small for our spirit. Jobs are not big enough for people." Such dissatisfaction is corroborated by a survey indicating that about half of all blue-collar workers are unhappy with what they are doing and that three quarters would attempt to choose something else if they were able to "start all over again." White-collar and professional worker responses were only slightly more favorable, with almost one half suggesting that they would wish for another line of work if they were to do it over again (*Science News*, May 8, 1976).

The loss to individuals and to society is incalculable. The generative aspect of adulthood must extend to include a sense of meaning and productivity from a job; a dead-end occupation is as suffocating as a stagnant personal relationship. The fact that much work is "too small for the spirit" has been noted by an industrial psychologist (McGregor, 1960, 1975). He proposes a "humanistic" theory of work ("Theory Y")—that when workers are clearly respected and valued, they respond with enthusiasm, take pride in their efforts, initiate ideas for improvement, show high morale, and have little job turnover and absenteeism. Upholding this view is a study of worker motivation showing that workers favored opportunity for assuming responsibility and being recognized for achievement ahead of all other possible improvements. Such job enrichment weighed more heavily than fringe benefits, shortened work periods, company-sponsored counseling, and even increased wages in terms of sustained effect (Herzberg, 1968).

Work and Stress

The importance of work in adult lives is manifested by another kind of impact during these middle-life years. The facts that stress-related circulatory disturbances begin to show up, especially for men, and that these are apparently related to inner pressures for achievement and success have been documented (Friedman and Rosenman, 1974).

"Coronary-prone" behavior, described as "Type A" by these investigators, is associated with seven times the incidence of heart disease as the behavior of "Type B" individuals. Type A people are "go-getters," highly competitive, aggressive in action and speech, energetic, and generally hostile in attitude. Their chief characteristic, however, is a sense of time pressure; inevitably they schedule more activity than the hours can contain and attempt to cram 30 hours into 24. They are always scrambling to meet deadlines, many self-imposed, and operate under a feeling of unrelenting demand.

All this sounds much like the high-powered executive with little time for family, becoming richer by the moment but only in money. It is also a behavior pattern that, at present, is more characteristic of men than women and may contribute substantially to the fact that men have a mortality rate during these midlife adult years that is 60 per cent higher than that of women (Waldron, 1976). Waldron points out that the qualities of men in our society are idealized as tough, decisive, impatient, and fearless and that Type A men seem to be running frantically in an attempt to live up to that ideal.

However, there have been highly successful efforts to retrain Type A individuals. Sometimes a heart attack that is not fatal offers a "second-chance" reassessment of lifestyle. Sometimes a dramatic family event brings about the series of self-questions. In any case, it is possible for Type A people to learn a more relaxed, less time-pressured existence (Glass, 1977).

Work—In the Lives of Women

The place of work in a man's life seems to be inextricably tied to his feelings about himself and what he thinks about his life. As we have seen, for men, "who you are" is, in large part, based on "what you do."

How is it for women? The fact is that little is known about the meaning of work to women. One can venture to guess that women's attitudes will be much more varied because large socialization changes have taken place with regard to women's roles. Today's women tend to perceive that they have choices and therefore adopt attitudes to justify the selection, whether traditional or new.

Certain generalizations can be made about the work of women, however, whether it takes place within the home as full-time mother and housekeeper, or whether it includes outside work for pay. In both instances, at least at present, the work has been undervalued not only by society but also by women themselves. "Just a housewife" is underscored by laws that have counted the full-time homemaker's contribution to the family financial position as nothing. A widow has to pay taxes on her husband's estate if she did not work outside the home, even if her thrift and sagacity made much of the accumulated savings possible. But if she dies first, her husband would pay no tax because the estate is presumed to be his to begin with. The Social Security statutes and income tax rules have regarded the full-time homemaker as dependent and noncontributory. Furthermore, women have accepted the unjust status with relative passivity, often feeling that being protected and cared for made it a fair trade.

Women's work has been similarly undervalued in the "marketplace." Whether she is working outside the home because she is achievement- and career-oriented or because she must, and though the Equal Pay Act of 1963 has been a law for 20 years, a woman earns, on the average, 57 per cent of a man's wages. The quick response that this wage gap represents women's lack of education is simply not true. Women's educational levels, in general, are as high as those of men. But women who have completed 4 years of college earn less than men who have completed only the eighth grade. Nor can this gap be attributed to women's lack of job experience. Single women who have never left the workforce and whose work profile is much like a man's still demonstrate greatly reduced earnings, spread over a lifetime of work (Sawhill, 1973). Sawhill's startling conclusion is that if all women workers were to remain on the job during their full life histories, they would still make 43 per cent less than men who were their equals in age, education, and experience.

The reason is that most women chose or find themselves only able to enter occupations that are dominated by women. Twenty-five per cent of all working women hold jobs that are almost wholly (95 per cent) female-dominated, and half of all employed women hold jobs that are at least 70 per cent female-dominated. The occupations have come to be called "female ghettos." The upshot is that "equal pay for equal work" rules are not applied, because there are too few men in the occupationally segregated areas doing comparable work. Employers pay "what the market will bear," and there has been almost no organized resistance among women to the fact that these jobs are the lowest-paying on the job ladder (Blau and Jusenius, 1976). Employers routinely channel entry-level women into dead-end positions where training and advancement are denied, using the justification that women will not remain long enough to make training and promotion "pay off" (Kahne and Kohen, 1975). The dynamics of a self-fulfilling prophecy is clear.

The psychological effect on women is a perpetuation of the traditional make-the-best-of-it outlook. Women are trained to smile and accept, to refrain from "making waves," to avoid controversy. It is taken for granted that secretaries and clerical workers, nurses, social workers, and schoolteachers are all paid "less than they are worth," but few inquire how much less. Or why. For example, a contract for registered nurses was negotiated at $7.60 per hour, a rate that is almost what local high school boys were charging for mowing the lawn (*Newsweek*, Sept. 22, 1980).

An expanded concept of "equal pay for equal work" is beginning to creep into the consciousness of those who are concerned about the well-being of women. It suggests that equal pay ought to be accorded for work of "comparable worth." This means that jobs would be evaluated in terms of education or training necessary, skills, and responsibilities entailed. Nurses, for instance, would no longer receive less money than janitors or maintenance men and many a secretary might receive equity with management personnel. A full-time homemaker would have her own Social Security and vested pension benefits; moreover, a certain proportion of the family income that her housekeeping and child care assists would be hers by law.

The "comparable worth" idea, according to Eleanor Holmes Norton in an address at a conference on equity for women (Bennetts, 1979), is ". . . a true sleeping giant . . . the issue of the 1980's." If the concept is accepted by the courts and implemented, it is estimated that it will cost employers billions of dollars. These are dollars that are being withheld from present-day women while they continue to carry workloads equal to and beyond those of many men. This is particularly true of the women who shoulder household responsibilities as well as those of an outside job.

This section began with a question about the place of work in a woman's life. It might be more sensible to inquire about what women want: What is the content of a woman's Dream? Men's Dreams consist in some kind of personal achievement that will bring honor, success, acclaim, and money. The motive to achieve has been studied extensively for men (Atkinson, 1964; McClelland, 1958) and is defined as the desire to be competent in a situation in which standards of excellence exist. Situations in which standards of excellence exist are usually categorized as intellectual, athletic, mechanical, and artistic. Studies of achievement strivings in women seem to indicate that, in contrast to men, these areas do not tend to arouse images of being successful or experiencing a great sense of accomplishment. It was this fact that made Atkinson give up on his attempts to include women in his study; they are represented by only a footnote in his book, *Motives in Fantasy, Action and Society* (1958). Later investigators, however, suggested that it is not the actual motivation that is different for men; rather, it is expressed in different areas by women. Thus, Lipinski (1966) found her women subjects stressing desire for success in achieving satisfactory relationships with family and friends, wishing for achievement of maturity and independence, and hoping for favorable outcomes for their roles in clubs and organizations. Almost 10 years later, practically identical findings were reported by Friedrich (1976), suggesting that women were most likely to express achievement motivation in areas defined traditionally as feminine, particularly social skills and interpersonal relations.

This seems to mean that, at least up until now, women have not regarded work as the most important feature of their lives. Rather, they have tended to choose the "affiliative motives" and to strive for interpersonal success with the same kind of persistence and focus that men devote to their achievement goals (Deaux, 1976).

Bardwick (1971), after surveying several studies, concludes that there may be a two-step motivational process for women: an early preoccupation with affiliative motives and then, 10 to 15 years later, a surge of achievement motivation that is vocational or career-oriented and therefore similar to that of men. Bardwick suggests two possible explanations. One possibility hypothesizes a real difference in developmental timing for women, with achievement motivation emerging later; the other suggests that women tend to defer their basic achievement motivation in favor of affiliation during a certain stage of life; when affiliation is secure, the achievement images can re-emerge.

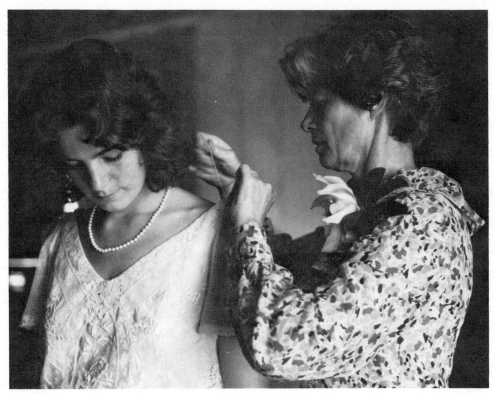

Achievement, success, and accomplishment for many women in society today are still inextricably bound up with the family.

Judith Kruger Michalik

There is also the inescapable fact that having a baby is an intensely creative process for many women, a unique and highly personal achievement. It establishes identity and status. It can be a tremendous source of self-esteem and serves as a focus for energies and commitment, in quite the same way as building that bridge or perfecting that product does for someone else. Although the new socialization practices may change some of these outlooks as parents try to rear girls and boys with equal emphasis upon potential and choices, the fact of maternity may be one reason why many women do not feel the intense pressure for "success" that characterizes most men.

However, the lessons of development teach that the assets of one period become the liabilities of the next. The identity so fiercely secured during adolescence simply will not do for age 40 and must be restructured. The achievement-motivated successes may come to seem too expensive in terms of some other values. The patience and self-sacrifice invested in children and other relationships create a vulnerability that is almost an invitation to hurt. It is the dialectical process (Riegel, 1975) by which each stable state (a "thesis") is eventually shattered by events and inherent contradictions ("antithesis"), resulting in formation of a new stability ("synthesis") that can, at best, be only temporary. The period of midlife change has been called the "midlife crisis."

THE MIDLIFE CRISIS

The idea of a crisis in people's lives when they're between 40 and 50 years old has been given delighted currency by press and popular media. The best-known version is the man who turns his responsible and conventional life topsy-turvy, suddenly taking to fast sports cars and young movie stars, leaving a wife of 25 years in shock and despair. The other half of the crisis is the menopause, typically pictured as the transformation of the normally well-functioning woman into a shrill, hysterical, emotionally volatile harridan.

As with many myths, it is the glimmer of recognition that perpetuates its existence. Marriages we all thought unusually solid break up. Men and women we thought we knew well engage in some inexplicable behavior. Aha! Midlife crisis! The midlife crisis has become a facile means of referring to the changes of middle adulthood. The objection to the term is that its implications are ominous and negative. There is a tendency to await the onset of "middle-age madness" as if it were foreordained, like puberty. However, the changes that come about at this stage of life are not necessarily larger or more drastic than those of any other life period. And we do not ordinarily dread the time of puberty or the changes promoted by entering school. To change is to grow. To fail to change is to stagnate. Levinson asserts that the men in his sample who drifted through this period, refusing to deal with its questions, became "weighted" and lost the vitality that would be needed for continuing development during the remainder of their lives (Levinson, cited in Sheehy, 1976, p. 363).

The events of this period are set off, for both men and women, by confrontation with the reality of their own mortality. The death of a parent or, more especially, of a surviving parent or of a contemporary necessitates coping with death and its meaning. It can, indeed, bring about some bizarre "denial" behavior—frantic body-building exercises, engaging in extraordinary death-defying activity, or a search for lost youth by "falling in love" with partners young enough to be one's children. Sheehy (1976, p. 443) comments, in describing men boasting about the young women they are bedding down, ". . . the female is narrowed to one dimension; she is an age."

However, Sheehy (1976), Vaillant (1977b), and Levinson (1978) all point out that this time of reassessment can be remarkably "generative," leading to a real renewal of energy and purpose. For many, there is a mid-career shift, sometimes with sacrifice of income and security, in favor of something closer to one's Dream. It may be that this desirable option will become a lively possibility for more men as women take up some of the economic support functions and enable men to feel less "trapped" by family responsibilities and therefore less required to remain in the "rat race."

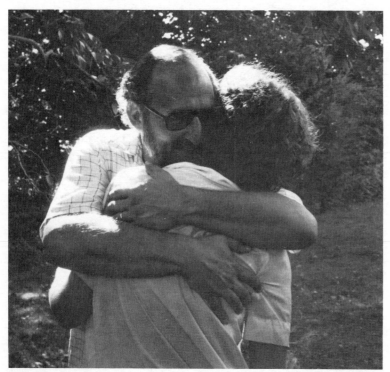

Each adult deals differently with the physical changes that are seen so clearly in the face and hairline. Some try to deny, others to delay, changes with makeup or surgery. Some are so busy with life they don't even notice the evidence of time passing.

Judith Kruger Michalik

Vaillant's study, focused on adaptation to life's crises, especially suggests that the mechanisms of adjustment and defense might be likened to the means by which an oyster, irritated by a grain of sand, protects itself by constructing a pearl. From the turmoil and mental anguish, creative solutions can emerge that permit a better survival and future resilience. As Vaillant proposed (1977a, p. 110), ". . . the human ego grows in adversity as well as prosperity."

Sex and Pleasure Over Time

Changes in Sexual Responsiveness

Impotence! A terrible word, calculated to strike at the heart of every living man. It is derived from the Latin, meaning "without power" or "to be rendered helpless." For almost every man, this is the clear definition of erectile difficulties. Men who are anxious about their ability to become erect feel that nothing less than their identity, their total manhood, is at stake.

The fact is, however, that it would be difficult to find a man who has not experienced failures to respond sexually (Kaplan, 1974). If the event can be accepted as a happenstance of little consequence, it becomes exactly that, without importance. On the other hand, especially for one who has concerns about aging, the failure is seen as the dread signal . . . the beginning of the end.

Often the scenario is one that is played out after a heavy dinner and several drinks. There is a gradual dawning of the horrible certainty that the penis is just going to remain flaccid. The partner offers some half-hearted reassurance, but she has raised worried questions in her own mind. Is she no longer desirable? So the next session will find the pair, literally, with both sets of eyes focused on the offending part, a situation that could not be better contrived to guarantee failure.

The basic ingredients of this "crisis" are several. One is the fact that the mental picture of masculine sexuality is that of the young adolescent, at his peak of sexual capability, stamina, strength, and arousal (Zilbergeld, 1978). As a standard of comparison, this ideal is impossible to measure up to after a man is past the mid-20s. Midlife men who are self-aware will know that their erections have not been as firm for well over a decade, but this is usually easier to ignore than to accept.

The second ingredient is that adults in general do not understand processes of changing sexual responsiveness with age. Sexual activity has been widely regarded as an all-or-nothing reaction. The possibility of obtaining authoritative information is, as we have seen, a comparatively recent outcome of the Masters and Johnson (1966) research and studies that have followed.

The really good news first: Adult human beings are capable of sexual desire and sexual pleasure for as long as they live. As was true of their early sex lives, older adults will differ greatly, one from another, with regard to how the desire is expressed and the sexual behavior for expression.

Both sexes will find that the responsiveness slows with age; it takes longer for women to lubricate and for men to become erect. If both can accept this "fact-of-life" in order to engage in erotic, sensitively prolonged lovemaking, sexual pleasure can be better than ever. Both sexes will tend to have full resolution after climax, with a refractory period that inhibits subsequent response to stimulation for a longer period than when younger. It can be a warm, sensuously relaxed time, if partners permit—as rewarding as a second climax if messages of intimacy, caring, and delight are reciprocated.

The "midlife crisis" precipitated by sexual fears and anxiety does not need to happen. Persistent sexual difficulties should be regarded as a symptom of serious communication problems between partners and therefore as a signal that something is indeed wrong. But the better part of wisdom in any instance when relationships seem to have hit a snag and ordinary remedies do not serve is to seek professional help.

Help for Sexual Problems

Fortunately, the new openness with regard to sexuality has helped people to begin to look at their sexual relations more honestly in spite of backgrounds that tended to make sex a shameful or guilt-ridden aspect of life. Fortunately, also, Masters and Johnson were pioneers in offering a new approach to therapy for sexual dysfunctions (1970). They provided training for a large number of therapists so that sex clinics offering specific treatments are now widespread.

Sex therapy has become so commonplace, however, that some caution must be advised. Potential clients ought to investigate the qualifications of those who conduct the therapy in a sex clinic. If the therapists are qualified, there will be no difficulty in learning about the educational background and training. If questions are greeted with hostility or if the professional societies cannot supply the information, it would be best to look for another resource.

The key to the Masters and Johnson therapy for sexual dysfunction (1970) is their proposition that behavior causing trouble can be replaced by behavior leading to the greatest of all reinforcements—sexual pleasure—through a series of straightforward learning exercises. Contary to seeing sexual problems as having deep roots in psychosexual fixation needing years of intensive work, Masters and Johnson suggest that expectations and beliefs, nurtured in an unwholesome climate of taboos, produce behavior that confirms the beliefs, therefore perpetuating them.

For example, a widespread presumption is that after several years of marriage sex becomes, at best, a pleasant but boring routine. Add this to another pervasive belief—that women are not as interested in sex as men—and the decline of excitement and joyful sexual experience after marriage is assured. The assumptions can be undone quickly and effectively *if* (a big "if!") the partners are truly committed to each other and wish to grow in their relationship. Says Virginia Johnson (1976, p. 114), "Nothing good is going to happen in bed between husband and wife unless good things are happening between them before they got into bed."

The therapy invented by Masters and Johnson differs from traditional therapy in several important aspects. First of all, a sexual problem is regarded as "belonging" to both partners—a kind of "no fault" approach. Second, therapists work as a team, male and female, so that each partner has a "friend in court." The aim is to prevent any possiblity of assigning or accepting blame for problems that have mutual origin. Third, the therapy is short and intensive. Clients are typically instructed to set aside 2 weeks of uninterrupted time that can be devoted to the new learning. Lately, the original prescription of 2 solid weeks has been modified considerably by many practitioners, but the focus is still concentrated and the number of therapy sessions is limited (Sarrel and Sarrel, 1979). Contrasted with this are the many months, perhaps years, of therapy required by the conventional psychiatric treatment. Last, although a sexual history provides information with regard to how the client grew up sexually, the emphasis is firmly on the present. New learning is to take place in the here-and-now, and what has happened before is important only for a modest perspective (and research purposes).

An early focus of the new learning turns on "pleasuring"—the experience and realization that being together can yield many different kinds of sensual pleasure that are not necessarily genital. Masters and Johnson (1976) suggest that the sense of touch is a vastly underrated and underutilized source of sensation in spite of the fact that it is probably the first and most fundamental of the sensations. Watch the mother animal caressing her newborn with her tongue: The bonding that is created by touch is clear.

Clients are instructed in how to give each other nongenital pleasure—stroking, patting, and gently massaging and caressing each other's body surfaces. One gives and the other receives, taking turns. The only obligation is to inform the other if a certain activity is not acceptable. Such information is especially important, since most of the couples are not accustomed to talking freely about sexual feelings and desires and feel especially reticent about saying a particular practice hurts or could be improved. The Masters and Johnson therapeutic instructions for pleasuring anticipated one of the messages of the Hite Report (Hite, 1976), which clearly depicted the importance to the female respondents of noncoital touching and caressing.

A second objective of the therapy is to abolish the sense of "performance." The very idea of "successful sex" carries an achievement orientation that can turn the participant into a spectator who worries about "How am I doing?" As another team of sex therapists, the Sarrels (1979), point out, sex is not like other kinds of endeavor: Trying harder does not help but, rather, will actually hinder full response. The new learning involves enjoyment of all sensual pleasures and permitting the natural sexual energy to emerge. With some basic instruction in male and female anatomy and physiology, the partners can help each other learn how to best please and to become joyfully involved in whatever happens.

A third emphasis is as important for successful relating in any phase of life and with anyone, as it is for good sex. It teaches partners to stop attempting to read each other's minds and to stop assuming that the other is a mind reader. In other words, each must become responsible for communicating feelings to the other and for owning the feelings. "I feel . . ." is the format for this. It is an entirely different message from the one that begins, "You always make me feel . . .," placing the recipient immediately on the defensive. A corollary of the stress upon effective communication of feelings is that these messages must be received without criticism or judgment. None of us can tell others how they ought to feel. A feeling exists and therefore may be pleasant or unpleasant to its owner and of concern to an involved other person. But the *existence* of the feelings is not legitimately open to discussion. "Feelings are facts," is the way Masters and Johnson (1976) phrase it. You cannot quarrel with facts, though you may decide to attempt to deal with them.

Earlier in this section, we mentioned the decline of delight in sex after some years of marriage. Is it inevitable? The Masters and Johnson answer to that question would clearly be, "No way!" Listen to their description of one of the couples who came for therapy (1976, pp. 283–284):

Although almost thirty years had gone by during which intercourse had taken place infrequently and generally unsatisfactorily, the husband and wife had remained affectionate and close. Their faith in each other apparently sustained them in a way that permitted them both to be more sad than angry over their sexual frustration. Most important, the wife never mocked or attacked her husband for his inadequacy in bed—she said that she always knew that he felt miserable enough about it without her saying a word.

In coming for help, this couple, with their high degree of mutual caring, exemplified the meaning of commitment. Thirty years of deprivation had not embittered them, nor had it extinguished for either partner a genuine desire to find sexual happiness together. Their decision to try therapy was a way of telling each other, without saying a word, 'Sex matters to me and you matter to me—and I want everything to be as good for both of us as it can possibly be.'

In treatment they followed their therapists' directions and almost immediately discovered the pleasure derived from the opportunity to touch each other in ways they had never before permitted themselves. The husband was one of a myriad of men who have grown up believing that there must be something wrong with them if they need 'help' from a woman in order to become physically aroused. Once released from the bondage of ignorance, he reacted to his wife's hands on his body much as an adolescent might have—and both he and his wife eagerly took turns pleasuring each other.

And finally, in sum (p. 285):

This does not mean that every sexual embrace is a transcendent experience. On the contrary, precisely because both partners are under no pressure to perform or pretend, any sexual embrace can be as casual as a good-night kiss, if that is what both partners want or if that is what one of them needs and the other is pleased and privileged to provide. Moreover, in such a relaxed atmosphere, each has earned emotional credit in the other's bank. If, as it occasionally must, sex proves unsatisfactory or disappointing or even frustrating to either husband or wife, their security as a committed couple lies in knowing that there is always tomorrow.

Menopause and Depression

The myths that shroud menopause create the same psychological climate for women as the ideas about impotence do for men. Few women escape the tales of unbearable hot flashes, painful sexual activity, and the "dowager's hump" of osteoporosis. Hardly anyone has heard menopause described as a marvelous time of blooming, when vibrant energy and a sense of freedom characterize functioning, when one is ready and willing to take some risks and try a little adventuring, when the burden of caring what other people think lifts, or when it is possible to have an uninterrupted conversation with a partner or plan a spur-of-the-moment trip without rounding up babysitters and making endless preparations to be absent from the family.

Well, which picture is the most accurate? Weideger (1977) points out that it is virtually impossible to separate the actual experience of menopause from the social evaluation that has been placed upon it. In our society today, like in ancient days when the "horror" of menstruation meant that women were isolated as "unclean," menopause is linked to many of the old superstitions. Menstruation had been regarded as getting rid of "poisons"; therefore, the menopausal woman was believed to be retaining those poisons and thus became even more dangerous. A "crone" is an older woman, past menopause; the "witches" who were hung, burned, drowned, and racked were almost all older women.

However, it is not really necessary to call upon the persistence of ancestral fears to account for the negative imagery surrounding menopause. Our society is notorious for its double standard of aging (Sontag, 1979). Just as the adolescent young man serves as the standard for male sexuality, the adolescent young woman represents the standard of beauty for women. However, women are progressively devalued in terms of their age far more rapidly and obviously than are men. Women are regularly congratulated upon "not looking" their age. To ask a woman her age is often considered insulting. The French say discreetly, ". . . of a certain age." Sontag writes (p. 474): "Aging in women is a process of becoming obscene sexually, for the flabby bosom, wrinkled neck, spotted hands, thinning hair, waistless torsos and veined legs of an old woman are felt to be obscene. . . . There is no equivalent nightmare for men." The undeniable signal of menopause is that of bodily aging, and unless the woman has made her peace with the inexorable cycles of life, it will be viewed with dread and alarm.

The physiological changes do not explain menopausal symptoms very well. It is true that estrogen production drops off. However, there seems to be considerable redundancy in the human system, according to Dr. Estelle Ramey of Georgetown University (1980), so that a back-up system (the adrenals) begins to produce hormones very much like estrogen as the regular estrogen level decreases. The level seems to vary from woman to woman, though, and the need for good research regarding estrogen replacement therapy (ERT) is critical. The various replacement therapies have been implicated in increased breast and endometrial cancer (Weideger, 1977), but there are numerous flaws in the research. There are also studies suggesting that replacing estrogen will delay osteoporosis and will provide relief from hot flashes and emotional whiplash. Ramey insists that use of ERT is an unsolved problem of "great magnitude" and that a major project for the immediate future should be finding out how to use it and how to protect women from unfavorable effects.

In addition to ushering in a new chapter for her physical self, menopause is also coincidental with a number of other changes in a woman's life. Her responses to these will inevitably be entangled with her attitudes toward menopause. One problematic event occurs when children move up and out of the household and "Supermoms" are suddenly unemployed. Pauline Bart (1972) found that women who were heavily involved in the lives of their children suffered more depression than those who did not put their children ahead of all other life activities. Suggesting that the depression is associated with loss of primary role, Bart points out that the symptoms seemingly characteristic of menopause are missing in societies where the climacteric brings increased status rather than decline.

For every man diagnosed as suffering from depression, there are two to six times as many women (*Newsweek*, September 8, 1980). Furthermore, a study of four groups of men and women undergoing major life changes (adolescence, newlywed, middle-age "empty nest," and preretirement) found that middle-aged women were the most distressed group (Lowenthal, et al., 1975). They were the lowest in life satisfaction, the most pessimistic, the highest in existential despair, and the most negative toward their spouses. They were depressed. Perhaps there are other sources of psychological pain in the lives of women in mid-adulthood that can help to account for such startling statistics.

Martin Seligman (1975) believes that depression develops in women at this age because they have become very dependent upon the approval, regard, and support of others for all of their feelings about themselves. The depression sets in when the dependency is threatened or when the support is lost. A paralysis of will that Seligman calls "learned helplessness" is the chief characteristic, resembling the inability of laboratory animals to take "obvious" means to protect themselves from electric shock if they have been prevented from previous practice in coping. Such animals refuse to step over a barrier to a safe zone even after being led through the procedure. Seligman suggests that women who have spent much of a lifetime "protected" from the outside world become passive and timid, exhibiting a kind of hopelessness about their capabilities and future. When, as a therapist, he points out routes to independence, such women erect all kinds of mental barriers to effectively prevent any such possibility.

Barnett and Baruch (1979) suggest further that "locus of control" theory (see Chapter 12) can be added to the idea of learned helplessness, with depression and lack of self-esteem stemming from a sense of not being able to control the events in life. Maggie Scarf (1980), also looking at the lopsided statistics, suggests that women are biologically more responsive to emotional bonding and therefore more devastated when bonds are fractured.

But it does not seem necessary to invoke a genetic bonding mechanism. Seligman (1975) offers an optimistic note that every small success in managing and coping that can be introduced into the "helpless" woman's life has the effect of an energizing, revitalizing injection. In locus of control terms, when a woman can be assisted in some way to take charge of a portion of her own life, she gains a new stature in her own eyes. She becomes a problem solver. She learns something about her potential.

The reality of women's lives needs to be based on the fact that most will spend a significant portion of time without someone upon whom to depend because of divorce, widowhood, or single status. That time will be less destructive as women come to look upon themselves in terms of an inner worth that is not derived from someone else, and as they begin to consider themselves competent defenders and problem solvers. When menopause no longer signifies "uselessness," it is likely to have far fewer repercussions, either psychological or physiological. It will be another milestone that each of us must pass. All of us can assist ourselves and each other by valuing every age period. This will help to ensure that a new view of menopause, with its sense of renewed zest and liberation, becomes the most typical experience for women at midlife.

GLOSSARY

GENERATIVITY Erikson's term for the seventh stage of development, the time of adulthood when intimacy deepens to the point of desire to share with the world. It is a kind of returning to the world after a period of preoccupation with the self or a beloved partner. There is the concern for establishing and guiding the next generation. Ordinarily, this is manifested in bearing and raising children, but it can also include productivity and creativity.

TYPE A   A type of individual who is highly competitive, who tends to be hostile to a world that doesn't move fast enough to suit, and who feels under constant "time pressure" with not enough hours in the day to accomplish everything that has been scheduled. This type is considered to be coronary-prone.

TYPE B   A type of individual who, in contrast to type A, is easygoing, patient, and relaxed. Tomorrow, in their view, is always available to accomplish what doesn't get done today. This kind of individual has been found to have only half the rate of heart attacks as Type A individuals (Rosenman, 1975).

REFERENCES

An acute shortage of nurses. *Newsweek Magazine*, September 22, 1980, pp. 93–95.

Atkinson, J. W.: *Motives in Fantasy, Action and Society*. Princeton, N.J.: Van Nostrand, 1958.

Atkinson, J. W.: *An Introduction to Motivation*. Princeton, N.J.: Van Nostrand, 1964.

Bardwick, J.: *Psychology of Women*. New York: Harper & Row, 1971.

Barnett, R., Baruch, G.: Women in middle years: Conceptions and misconceptions. In Williams, J. (ed.): *Psychology of Women: Selected Readings*. New York: W. W. Norton & Company 1979.

Bart, P.: Depression in middle-aged women. In Bardwick, J. (ed.): *Readings on the Psychology of Women*. New York: Harper & Row, 1972.

Baumrind, D.: Current patterns of parental authority. *Developmental Psychology Monographs* (Monograph I), No. 4, pp. 1–103, 1971.

Baumrind, D.: New directions in socialization research. *American Psychologist*, 35:639–652, 1980.

Bennetts, L.: Male-female wage gap is as wide as ever. *Providence Sunday Journal*, Nov. 4, 1979, p. E-15.

Blau, F. D., Jusenius, C. L.: Economists' approaches to sex segregation in the labor market: An appraisal. *Signs*, 1(3, pt. 2):181–199, 1976.

Burr, W. R.: Satisfaction of various aspects of marriage over the life cycle: A random class sample. *Journal of Marriage and the Family*, 32:229–237, 1970.

Campbell, A.: The American way of mating: Marriage, si; children only maybe. *Psychology Today*, 8(12):37–43, 1975.

Deaux, K.: *The Behavior of Men and Women*. Monterey, Cal.: Brooks/Cole, 1976.

Dytrych, Z., Matejcek, Z., Schuller, V., David, H. P., Friedman, H. L.: Children born to women denied abortion. *Family Planning Perspectives*, 7(4):165–171, 1975.

Erikson, E.: *Childhood and Society*. New York: W. W. Norton & Company, 1950, rev. 1963.

Erikson, E.: Youth and the life cycle. *Children*, 7 (March–April):43–49, 1960.

Erikson, E.: Youth, fidelity and diversity. In Erikson, E. (ed.): *Youth, Change and Challenge*. New York: Basic Books, 1963.

Friedman, M., Rosenman, R. H.: *Type A Behavior and Your Heart*. New York: Alfred A. Knopf, 1974.

Friedrich, L. K.: Achievement motivation in college women revisited: Implications for women, men and the gathering of coconuts. *Sex Roles: A Journal of Research*, 2:47–62, 1976.

Giele, J. Z.: *Women and the Future*. New York: Free Press, 1978.

Ginsberg, G., Frosch, W., Shapiro, T.: The new

impotence. *Archives of General Psychiatry*, 26:218–220, 1972.

Glass, D. C.: *Behavior Patterns, Stress and Coronary Disease*. Hillsdale, N.J.: L. Erlbaum Associates, 1977.

Herzberg, F.: One more time: How do you motivate employees? *Harvard Business Review*, January–February 1968.

Hite, S.: *The Hite Report*. New York: Macmillan, 1976.

Institute for Social Research. Education and job satisfaction. *Science News*, May 8, 1976, p. 297.

Kahne, H., Kohen, A.: Economic perspectives on the role of women in the American economy. *Journal of Economic Literature*, 13:1249–1292, 1975.

Kaplan, H. S.: *The New Sex Therapy: Active Treatment of Sexual Dysfunctions*. New York: Brunner/Mazel, 1974.

Levinson, D. J.: *The Seasons of a Man's Life*. New York: Alfred A. Knopf, 1978.

Lipinski, B.: Sex role, conflict and achievement motivation in college women. In Bardwick, J.: *Psychology of Women*. New York: Harper & Row, 1971, p. 171.

Lowenthal, M. F., Thurnher, M., Chiriboga, D.: *Four Stages of Life*. San Francisco: Jossey-Bass, 1975.

Masters, W. H., Johnson, V. E.: *Human Sexual Response*. Boston: Little, Brown, 1966.

Masters, W. H., Johnson, V. E.: *Human Sexual Inadequacy*. Boston: Little, Brown, 1970.

Masters, W. H., Johnson, V. E.: *The Pleasure Bond*. New York: Bantam, 1976.

McClelland, D. C.: The importance of early learning in the formation of motives. In Atkinson, J. W. (ed.): *Motives in Fantasy, Action and Society*. Princeton, N.J.: Van Nostrand, 1958.

McGregor, D.: *The Human Side of Enterprise.*, New York: McGraw-Hill, 1960.

McGregor, D.: Theory Y. The integration of individual and organizational goals. In U.S. Military Academy (ed.) *A study of Organizational Leadership*. Washington, D.C.: Office of Military Leadership. 1975.

Pearlin, L. E.: Sex roles and depression. In Datan, N,, Ginsberg, L. H. (eds.): *Life-Span Development: Normative Life Crisis*. New York: Academic Press, 1977.

Ramey, E. Personal communication. October 23, 1980.

Riegel, K. F.: Adult life crisis: A dialectic interpretation of development. In Datan, N., Ginsberg, L. H. (eds.): *Life-Span Developmental Psychology*. New York: Academic Press, 1975.

Rosenman, R. H.: Coronary heart disease in the Western collaborative study: A final follow-up experience of 8½ years. *Journal of the American Medical Association,* 233:872–877, 1975.

Sarrel, L. J., Sarrell, P. M.: *Sexual Unfolding: Sexual Development and Sex Therapies in Late Adolescence.* Boston: Little, Brown, 1979.

Sawhill, I. V.: The economics of discrimination against women. *The Journal of Human Resources,* 8 (Summer):383–395, 1973.

Scarf, M.: *Pressure Points in the Lives of Women: Unfinished Business.* New York: Doubleday, 1980.

Seligman, M. E.: *Helplessness:* On Depression, Development, and Death. San Francisco: W. H. Freeman Company, 1975.

Sheehy, G.: *Passages.* New York: Bantam Books/EP Dutton, 1976.

Skolnick, A., Skolnick, J. (eds.): *Family in Transition.* Boston: Little Brown, 1971.

Sontag, S.: *No Longer Young: Occasional Paper in Gerontology.* No. 11, Wayne State University, 1975.

Sontag, S.: The double standard of aging. In Williams, J. H. (ed.): *Psychology of Women: Selected Readings.* New York: W. W. Norton & Company, 1979.

Straus, M., Gelles, R. J., Steinmetz, S. K.: *Behind Closed Doors.* New York: Anchor/Doubleday, 1980.

Terkel, S.: *Working.* New York: Random House, 1974.

Vaillant, G. E.: The climb to maturity: How the best and brightest came of age. *Psychology Today,* 11(40):34–41; 107–110, 1977a.

Vaillant, G. E.: *Adaptation to Life.* Boston: Little, Brown, 1977b.

Waldron, I.: Why do women live longer than men? *Journal of Human Stress,* March 1976, pp. 2–13.

Weideger, P.: *Menstruation and Menopause.* New York: Dell, 1977.

Why women are depressed. *Newsweek,* September 8, 1980, p. 81.

Zilbergeld, B.: *Male Sexuality.* Boston: Little, Brown, 1978.

HEALTH CONCERNS IN THE ADULT

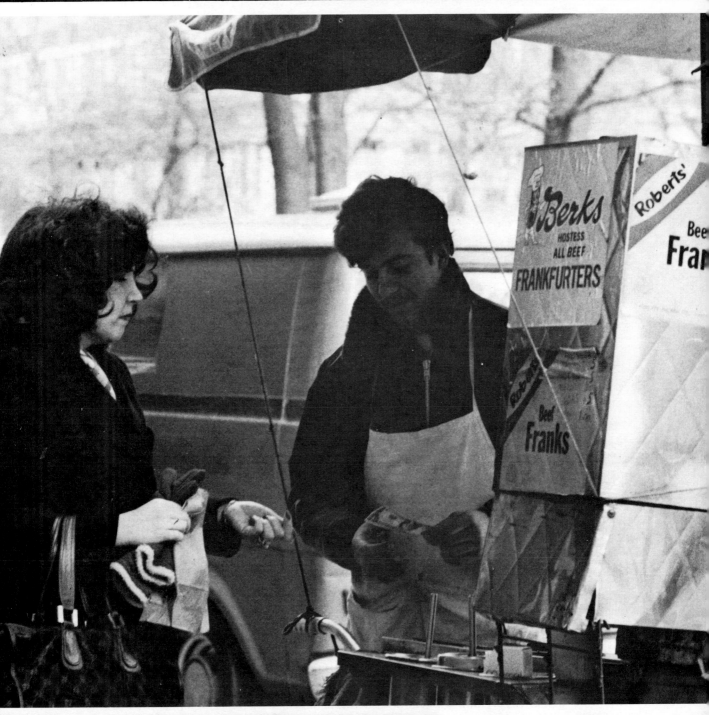

CHAPTER 14

Childhood and adolescence are times of discovery, of attaining social skills, of growing up. Adulthood—young adulthood and middle age—is a time of settling in and of assuming responsibility for independent living, consistent work habits, steady, satisfying relationships, marriage, and childbearing, *i.e.*, stability.

All these tasks must be managed during a time in our society in which the threat of nuclear disaster, economic crises, overpopulation, pollution, and shrinking natural resources make the prospect of a successful, fulfilling existence more problematic than at any time in recent history. The transition from dependency to emancipation may take longer than anticipated as many young adults, anxious to strike out on their own, find jobs scarce and financial security tenuous. At a time when their own parents are anxious to have fewer parenting responsibilities, they may find themselves having to ask for more assistance, thus delaying their independence and often causing stress within the family. If the transition to a self-sustained existence has been successful, the middle-adult years—from 40 to 65—should then be a time of solidification of values, self-enrichment, and relationships that are constant and enduring.

The health issues facing adults are generally those associated with lifestyle choices and changes, the emergence of what may become chronic conditions, and the diseases that are most prevalent in the population over 45 years of age. To provide a way of understanding the aging process, we have divided this chapter into two main sections: Young adulthood (20 to 40 years of age), and middle age (from 40 to 65). In each section, the content will emphasize:

1. Physiological changes.
2. Health maintenance and prevention of disease.
3. Lifestyle decisions that have an impact on health.

YOUNG ADULTS

Like healthy adolescents, young adults generally do not have a well-established relationship with the medical establishment and tend to seek assistance only when confronted with an illness. The inclusion of health insurance in a work-benefit package does enable many young adults (some for the first time) to have access to medical facilities and professional health care. The rise in prepaid health maintenance organizations (HMOs) has further provided many thousands of people the benefits of comprehensive, on-site medical, surgical, laboratory, pharmacological, and psychological assistance. In effect, HMOs are one-stop medical settings with good quality control of services and expenses and with follow-up procedures to ensure that recommendations will be implemented. These organizations also tend to employ the services of a growing group of professionals—physicians' assistants, nurse practitioners, and surgical technicians. These professionals, working closely with specific physicians, have the opportunity to develop long-lasting relationships with their patients and thus the potential of making a greater impact on the patient's life.

Often, these professionals may be working with and advising people close to their own age who are likely to be experiencing similar stresses, lifestyle issues, and health concerns. Health workers benefit the patient not by imposing opinions, but by offering options and alternatives. It is appropriate and ethical for health professionals to refer patients to other personnel for assistance if situations arise in which individual moral judgments could interfere with objective helping of the patient in the decision-making process.

Physiological Changes

Physical maturity occurs early in young adulthood. Growth rates for both young men and young women either cease or slow down to the point of very small changes. Muscle tone and coordination are at their peak. Menstruation should be well established in women. The respiratory and circulatory systems should be working at optimal levels, with cell replacement and tissue repair at peak efficiency. Muscle mass has stabilized, and physical strength and endurance are optimal. Few of the degenerative changes that may become evident in middle age are apparent in early adulthood, but the aging process has already begun. This process will be more fully explored in the section on middle age.

Relevant Health Issues

The health issues confronting young adults tend to revolve around modern living habits, health maintenance, and disease prevention. Decisions made during this time of life have long-range and, frequently, adverse effects on the rest of life.

Smoking

In 1880, the patent on a cigarette-rolling machine was awarded James A. Bonsack from Virginia. Although he has not been remembered as a major American inventor, the effects of his invention have reverberated through the years.

In 1979, 704 billion cigarettes were smoked in the United States by some 54 million adults and 5 million adolescents. Smoking is today the largest preventable cause of death in the United States. Smoking has been implicated as a major cause of coronary heart disease, cancer, ulcers, and, as previously mentioned in an earlier chapter, perinatal problems in the newborn. Bennett (1980) states: "As a rule of thumb, each cigarette smoked knocks about 5 minutes off the smoker's life. For an average habit, that adds up to 6 or 7 years."

The effects of smoking are generally related to the amount of the tar and nicotine inhaled. Nicotine is addictive. As the nicotine-loaded blood is carried to the heart, the heart pumps about 15 per cent of the inhaled dose within 7 seconds to the brain, where it produces a generally pleasurable sensation. Once addicted, a smoker finds it increasingly difficult to cease because the effects of withdrawal are very unpleasant. However, since 1973, there has been an annual decrease in per capita consumption of cigarettes. Warner (1981) believes that this decrease may be due, in part, to the increase in antismoking activity by nonsmokers. His research indicates that without this activity, consumption would have exceeded the 1978 level by more than one third.

Smoking and Cancer. The relationship between smoking and cancer has long been a focus of medical attention. In 1974, warnings were required to appear on cigarette packages to alert smokers to the potential for harm. This warning was based largely on statistics showing that a large proportion of people who died of lung cancer were smokers. Hammond and Seidman (1980) report:

> Based on mortality studies of over one million Americans who have been followed in an epidemiologic study since 1959, it is estimated that from 25 per cent to 35 per cent of cancer mortality in the United States male population and from 5 to 10 per cent in the female population are mainly due to smoking of tobacco products and cigarettes.

Smoking and Cardiovascular Problems. There is also convincing evidence of a link between smoking and cardiovascular disease. Friedman (1980) reports on a study in which 4,004 middle-aged smokers, nonsmokers, and ex-smokers were followed with periodic health assessments over an 11-year span. Forty-eight variables were considered, including marital state, age, sex, race, serious disease, exposure to harmful chemicals, medicinal drugs, and questionnaire items. It was found that the death toll from heart disease for smokers was 2.1 times higher than that for nonsmokers. He suggested that the only true way of establishing direct correlation between smoking and coronary disease is to follow a large number of young smokers throughout their lives.

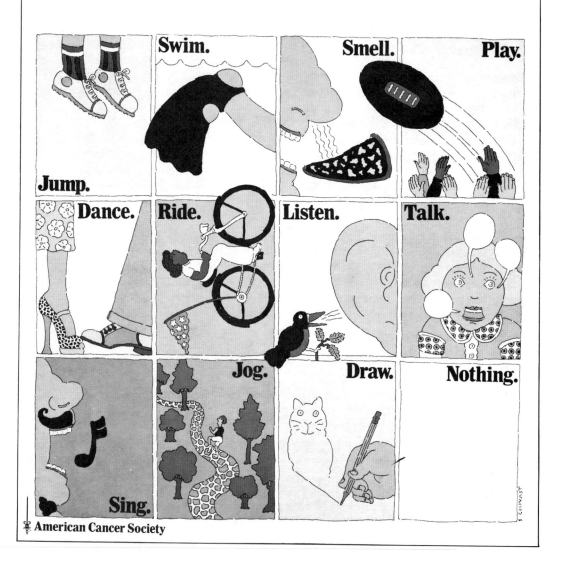

12 THINGS TO DO INSTEAD OF SMOKING CIGARETTES.

Swim. Smell. Play. Jump. Dance. Ride. Listen. Talk. Sing. Jog. Draw. Nothing.

⚕ **American Cancer Society**

Nutrition

The food fads that are evident in adolescence tend to become more patterned in young adults. Away from parental pressure and influence, many young people try a variety of eating patterns and dietary regimens; some become "natural food" experts, and develop an interest in cooking as well as eating foods perceived as beneficial to overall health. Many also wish to learn about the correlation between food and coronary heart disease.

According to Stamler (1978), there are several risk factors associated with coronary heart disease, not the least of which is diet. He sees a "rich" diet, one that is heavy in saturated fats, as a primary, essential, necessary cause of premature degenerative diseases of the blood vessels. He further implicates high intakes of salt and alcohol and a low intake of complex carbohydrates, particularly pectin, which is found in fruit. Add to these risk factors an imbalance between caloric intake and energy output—the result being obesity—and the risks rapidly escalate for young and middle-aged people.

In an effort to determine the correlation between obesity and mortality from cardiovascular disease, Noppa (1980) reviewed findings of several extensive studies done in the United States as well as other countries. He concludes, in part, that population studies indicate an excess overall mortality from all kinds of cardiovascular diseases that appears to be connected with extreme obesity and extreme thinness. According to his findings, there is a further connection between some kinds of heart disease and other risk factors, including smoking. Weight reduction seems to be beneficial in reducing most risk factors. However, long-term preventive studies would be important in order to establish the specific connection between reduced obesity and the reduction in morbidity and mortality from cardiovascular diseases.

Thus, prevention of obesity is a primary goal for health maintenance. Nutritional counseling can help the obese person, with emphasis placed on menu planning, caloric intake, and, especially, motivational aspects of overeating. Young adults who are cooking for themselves for the first time are frequently interested in recipes, menus, and cooking hints. This offers an ideal situation for enlisting their attention to principles of sound nutrition, which could provide life-long benefits.

Alcohol

Alcohol consumption tends to peak among young adults. According to Hagen (1977), the total number of drinkers in the United States has increased dramatically: "Now figured at 96 million," he states, "more drinkers are consistently found among young adults." According to the Commission on Marijuana and Drug Abuse, 10 per cent of the 96 million drinkers in the United States are compulsive drinkers, with serious consequences in terms of social functioning, job stability, and accident rates. As noted in a previous chapter, alcohol is a factor in 50 per cent of all highway deaths, and 50 per cent of all homicides (Smith, 1978).

Alcohol has a cumulative effect on body organs, the most dramatic of which impact on the central nervous system, as evidenced particularly in behavior changes. Though low blood alcohol levels may produce a sense of relaxation, higher levels appear to produce reactions of aggressiveness and suspension of ordinary judgmental processes and may progress to stupor, disorientation, uncoordination, and confusion. These symptoms are caused by the depression of brain centers that inhibit such behavior.

In addition to these effects, there are other medical consequences. Liver damage is the foremost cause of alcohol-related incapacitating illness and death. When liver cells die, scarring occurs. These fibrous scars distort and constrict the liver tissue, causing obstruction of blood flow in the liver and eventually death. Hagen (1977) also observed that, in large urban areas, liver damage (also called *cirrhosis* of the liver) is the fourth most common cause of deaths from alcohol.

Cancer and Alcohol.   During the past few years, research has been undertaken into the incidence of cancer and alcohol abuse. Several areas have been studied, including the irritating effect of alcohol on mucosal cells, malnutrition associated with alcoholism, the effects of smoking and drinking (which combine two toxins acting together and are thought to increase the incidence of cancer), and the process of regeneration of liver cells (Hagen, 1977). Some of this research is also attempting to examine the correlation between drinking, smoking, and cancer of the mouth, pharynx, larynx, and esophagus.

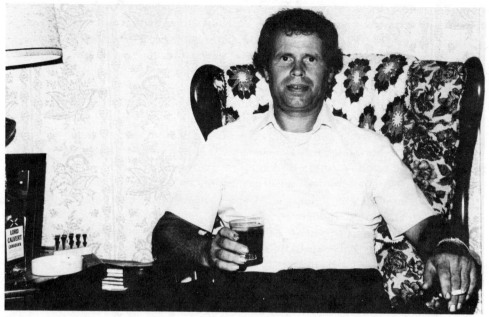

Alcohol and tobacco can be part of an adult's world, but they cause many health problems. Smoking is the primary cause of preventable death, according to the Surgeon General of the United States

Rothman (1980) speculates that approximately 3 per cent of all cancer deaths in the United States can be attributed to alcohol. The figures for cancers of the mouth and pharynx jump spectacularly when the patient is both a heavy smoker and a drinker. Rothman states that the proportion of cancers of the mouth and pharynx attributable to alcohol and tobacco together has been estimated to be about 75 per cent in American men; those attributable to alcohol alone, approximately 50 per cent. He further indicates that antismoking campaigns are probably more effective than antidrinking campaigns because of the relationship of tobacco and alcohol.

As long as young people associate independence, success, and acceptability with alcohol consumption, the toll in sickness will be heavy. It might be helpful for people to understand their drinking habits and to be aware of the stages of alcoholism, which follow:

1. *Early stage.* Heavy drinking, "blackouts," loss of control, some attempts at abstinence.

2. *Crucial stage (middle).* Excuses for drinking, drinking alone, antisocial behavior, acute hangovers, morning drinking, health symptoms, job problems.

3. *Late or chronic stage.* "Benders," deficiency diseases, loss of tolerance for alcohol, delirium tremens, or withdrawal symptoms.

Referrals are needed for any patient whose drinking patterns fit any of these categories. Self-help groups, clinics designed specifically for alcohol-related problems, and individual psychological counseling all play a role in helping the drinker resolve the problem.

Physical Activity and Coronary Health

Americans are exercising more frequently and more vigorously, and in a greater variety of modes. Centers abound that specialize in aerobic dancing, racketball, handball, fencing and martial arts, weight lifting, swimming, and general physical fitness. The controversy over whether exercise can prevent coronary disease has continued on many fronts. Froelicher (1980) reviewed studies dealing with the more recent investigations of the health benefits of regular *aerobic* exercise. Aerobic exercises are those that raise the pulse rate significantly for a specific period, usually 20 minutes, and then progress to a gradually lower rate while exercising continues. On the basis of surveying studies involving 14,000 patients, Froelicher concluded:

1. There is no evidence linking inactivity to the development of atherosclerosis (hardening of the arteries).

2. Physical activity may offer protection from the manifestations of coronary artery disease and from its complications.

3. Individuals with increased physical activity have lower mortality from coronary disease.

4. Exercise training may play an important role in the primary prevention of coronary disease and may improve the outcome for patients with the manifestations of this disease.

Froelicher believes that it is prudent for all people to engage in regular physical activity. Such activity probably helps reduce the risks of coronary disease. He suggests that more work will have to be done to determine the specific effectiveness of exercise in relation to the prevention of primary and secondary coronary disease. Young adults should be encouraged to set aside some regular time for exercise that is pleasurable. The regularity appears to be the important factor. Any activity that offers a change of pace, some physical exertion, and recreation brings physiological and psychological benefits.

Sexuality

Chapter 11 presented the various methods of birth control and common gynecological problems. For the young adult, establishing a sexual identity that is comfortable and satisfying is important. Many individuals now engage in a variety of sexual practices that until very recently were considered perversions, or at least abnormal. In the last few years, for instance, there has been a remarkable shift in attitude toward people whose sexual practices depart from what has been considered "normal." Although the majority of people identify themselves as being exclusively heterosexual, there are other who consider themselves homosexual or bisexual. Just as heterosexuals differ in their sexual styles, so do homosexuals and bisexuals. A health professional can be of value by remaining open and nonjudgmental. All people, whatever their sexual orientation, will have questions and need medical attention from time to time. Health workers, by knowing about human sexual response, can dispel the myths that still accompany all sexual activity, and can make appropriate referrals if the need arises.

Murray and Zentner (1979) list some of the basic facts concerning human sexuality:

1. In men, sperm are produced in optimal numbers when ejaculation occurs two or three times weekly.

2. In women, spontaneous ovulation may occur during intercourse at any time in the cycle, probably as a result of extreme excitement or a high emotional state.

3. Premenstrual tension is a group of symptoms associated with the retention of fluids prior to menstruation.

4. Most women need some clitoral stimulation in order to achieve orgasm (Masters and Johnson, 1966).

Human Sexual Response

Chapter 13 discussed the importance of the Masters and Johnson (1966) findings on physiological changes accompanying sexual activity. These findings revolutionized our understanding of human sexuality and, in the process, enabled both lay and professional people to dispel anxieties concerning their sexual functioning. Table 14–1 charts the sexual response cycles for both men and women.

Dysmenorrhea

Dysmenorrhea has long been thought to be a psychological problem manifested by physical symptoms. Recently, research studies have been conducted to determine why as many as 30 to 50 per cent of American women suffer from symptoms ranging from

TABLE 14–1 HUMAN SEXUAL RESPONSE CYCLES

Women	Men
Phase 1. Excitement	
Vaginal lubrication	Blood pressure and pulse rise
Vulva becomes reddened	Respirations increase in quantity
Labia begins to swell	Penis becomes erect
Clitoris becomes erect	Scrotal sac elevates
Nipples become erect	
Breasts become larger	
Blood pressure and pulse rise	
Respirations increase	
Phase 2. Plateau	
Vulval tissues become more engorged	Penis increases in circumference
Inner labia become two or three times thicker	Cowper's glands produce droplets of fluid, which might contain some spermatozoa
Clitoris retracts under the clitoral hood	Testicles increase in size by 50%
Uterus moves up in the abdomen and increases in size	Skin flush on face and extremities may occur
Upper two thirds of vagina balloons out ("tenting")	Increased sensation of inevitability of ejaculation occurs
Lower third of vagina swells	
Skin flush may occur on face and extremities	
Phase 3. Orgasmic	
Lower third of vagina contracts	Ejaculation occurs through contraction of penile muscles
Uterus contracts	
Phase 4. Resolution	
Return to pre-excitement phase with potential for subsequent orgasms	Penis loses erection
	Testicles drop down and become smaller
Phase 5. Refractory	
—	Evident in men. During this time, erection and orgasm are not possible

cramps to nausea, vomiting, headaches, and excessive fatigue. Research now indicates that dysmenorrhea does have a physiological basis—the overproduction of prostaglandins by the uterus (Marx, 1979). Prostaglandins cause the smooth muscles of the uterus to contract. In those women who suffer from these symptoms, relief is available in the form of drugs that inhibit excessive production of prostaglandins.

Contraception

During adolescence, the need for consistent birth control may be sporadic. As young adults become more sexually active, the need for safe, reliable birth control becomes more urgent. In Chapter 11, we outlined the risks associated with many of the most common forms of birth control, urging teen-agers to use nonsystemic methods. Although more and more adults are using these methods, there are still millions of women who employ birth control pills as the method of choice. For this reason, it is important to review the hazards associated with the use of pills, particularly for women who are 35 years of age and older. Blood clotting disorders are significantly more common in women over 35 who take high-estrogen pills, who smoke, and who use the pill for more than 5 years. Stewart (1979) observed that the risk of death from a circulatory disease for women in the 30- to 39-year-old age group using the pill is 1 in 50,000. If the woman smokes, the risk rises to 1 in 10,000. For women under 35, the risks associated with childbirth are generally considered greater than the risks associated with the use of oral contraceptives. After 35, however, the risks reverse, with the use of the pill becoming more of a hazard. Health professionals should be able to discuss the options available to women in this age group, including sterilization, which will be covered in a subsequent section.

Infertility

According to Mazor (1979) "infertility is generally defined as the failure to achieve a successful pregnancy (*i.e.*, leading to a live birth) following a year of regular relations without contraception." In about 70 per cent of all couples who have been investigated for infertility, an organic problem can be found. In 50 per cent of these couples, the problem resides with the woman; in 30 per cent, with the man; and in 20 per cent, with both.

Problems in Women.   Infertility problems in the woman can be grouped under the following categories:

Mechanical Barriers.   Infection of the pelvic organs causes scarring of the fallopian tubes, ovaries, or uterus. Common sources of infection are venereal disease, septic abortions in which all the products of conception are not removed, and a ruptured appendix, which causes a leakage of fecal material from the digestive tract.

In endometriosis, tissue that is normally found only in the lining of the uterus starts to grow in the abdominal cavity or in the fallopian tubes and around the ovaries and uterus. This tissue bleeds at each menstruation, causing inflammation and eventual scarring. Endometriosis is most common in women over 30 who have never had children.

Last, there may be a situation in which sperm either are prohibited from moving freely into the uterus or are destroyed before they can reach the uterus because of some abnormalities in the mucus of the cervix.

Endocrine Disorders.   Dysfunction of the pituitary, thyroid, or adrenal glands may cause a variety of symptoms, many of which are related to problems in ovulation, implantation of a fertilized ovum, or maintenance of the egg after it has been implanted in the uterus.

Structural Disorders.   These disorders may include abnormalities or malformation of the uterus, fibroid tumors of the uterus, or a cervix that cannot stay closed for the duration of the pregnancy, leading to spontaneous abortion (Mazor, 1979).

Problems in Men.   There are several factors associated with infertility in men.

Sperm Production.   Sperm may not be produced in adequate numbers as a result of infection associated with high fever, mumps (which can permanently damage the testicles), exposure to radiation, certain drugs, industrial chemicals, excessive smoking and alcohol consumption, and undescended testicles that have not been corrected.

Sperm Motility.   Sperm motility, the rate at which sperm move through the cervix, into the uterus, and out into the fallopian tubes, can be affected by disease, hormonal problems, prostate disorders, or, in rare cases, antibodies produced by the man that attack his own sperm.

Sperm Transport.   The conduction of sperm can be hindered by scarring from venereal disease, accidental injury to the *vas deferens* (the tubes that carry the sperm), or vasectomy.

Support for Couples.   Infertile couples are faced with a barrage of feelings, medical examinations, physicians who pry into their sexual lives, directions on how and when to have sexual relations, and health personnel who may appear to be insensitive to the anguish produced by the process and the condition. Health professionals can benefit couples who are seeking help by being extra supportive and available, offering explanations for procedures and helping the couple to become active participants in their own care and treatment. Often, it is appropriate for couples concerned with fertility to seek help from specialists in the area. The specific research, specialized tests, and sensitive procedures are perhaps best carried out by someone whose entire practice and orientation are focused on dealing with this problem.

MIDDLE-AGED ADULTS

Middle age is not a static period of time, but one in which productivity is high, family and social life tend to be stable and satisfying, and adaptation to change is still relatively easy. In this section, we will discuss the physiology of aging, the physical changes associated with the aging process, and the health and medical issues confronting those who continue through this phase of the life span.

The Aging Process

Aging is a complex series of events still not yet wholly explained by the several theories invoked to account for the process. These include the theory that aging is the disorderly accumulation of random errors and damage secondary to living, and another theory that aging is an orderly, genetically programmed developmental event, essential for the preservation of the species (Calkins, 1981).

There is agreement, according to Calkins, that the process of aging is under genetic control with a correlation between life span of parents and offspring; the aging process is also recognized as part of developmental progression. Some scientists have theorized that the harmful effects of aging occur in cells that stop dividing and reproducing. Cells in the central nervous system and in major blood vessels do not have the capacity to regenerate. If, for example, brain cells did constantly divide and regenerate, the functions of memory and imprinting from early childhood would be lost. Furthermore, there appears to be a limit to the ability of any population of cells to double, even under prime laboratory conditions. In addition to this doubling limitation, there is some indication of degenerative change in the basic cell structure of some of the building blocks of tissues.

All theories agree that there seems to be a maximal normal life span for all species, including humans (Calkins, 1981). This aging process affects all body systems to some degree and begins shortly after sexual maturity is reached. Of particular interest is the way in which the aging occurs. Calkins cites research that carefully noted the exact number of cells in a very small section of skin. Over the years, the numbers of cells were recounted, with a regular decrease in the numbers being shown as each year went by. Other cells from other parts of the body have been studied with similar results.

Bone density, an indication of the numbers of cells in a particular segment of bone, can be measured and bone age determined. Bone minerals start to decline, cell wear decreases, and cell solids diminish with age.

Although many of these changes are not apparent, there are physiological changes that do occur during the middle years that are more evident. Because of the decrease in bone density, a gradual compression of vertebrae occurs, and people begin to "shrink." Since many tissues do not regenerate, the wear and tear on the surviving tissue cause the aches and pains of age, with the complaints of "arthritis." As people get older, they expend less energy and therefore need fewer calories. Most people, however, do not limit their caloric intake and "middle-age spread" becomes apparent. Coupled with a decrease in the capacity for strenuous exercise, this has a bearing on lung capacity, which also declines.

Health Issues and Health Maintenance

Many of the concerns of young adulthood, such as alcohol, smoking, exercise, and nutrition are also the concerns of middle-aged people. In addition, there is the factor of the increase in cancer in this age group. Cancer accounts for almost 25 per cent of all deaths during the decades of the 40s and 50s. There are particular neoplasms that are more common in women, namely cancer of the breast and uterus, whereas some are more common in men, particularly cancer of the colon and lung. According to Smith and colleagues, (1978), the prevalence of a variety of disorders in essentially healthy people who participated in a screening examination study, ranged from obesity in 16.3 per cent of all people examined, to osteoarthritis in 4.4 per cent, and anemia in 3.1 per cent; diabetes, deafness, and eye problems were also present. Instruction, information, support, and understanding from health workers can assist patients through the transition of the life span and help to maintain their self-esteem and to promote their sense of fulfillment. In the next section, we will discuss those health issues that have a direct impact on the ability to manage these transitions.

Sexuality

Sexual activity during middle age is often considered the most satisfying of all. If the people involved have established a sense of what constitutes good sexual experiences for themselves, are able to express their needs, are responsive, and have no underlying physical or emotional disorders that prevent sexual activity, these may be the years of the freest expression. There are hormonal changes that occur in both men and women, but, contrary to age-old myths and legends, these do not necessarily deter and may even enhance enjoyment.

Contraception

Contraception for middle-aged women presents different problems than for those who are younger. As women get older, final decisions about childbearing have to be made. If the decision is to have no more children, anxiety over birth control could have an adverse effect on sexual activity and responsiveness. Finding the safest and most reliable method of birth control becomes imperative. As stated earlier, the continued use of birth control pills after the age of 35 is considered risky. Other methods, though physiologically safer, do not offer the same margin of protection. For these reasons, more and more women are choosing sterilization as a permanent method of birth control.

Sterilization

Sterilization is considered an irreversible form of birth control. It is legal in all states (Boston Women's Health Book Collective, 1979) but there may be restrictions as to age, numbers of existing children, and marriage state.

Tubal Ligation. This procedure, the most common method of sterilization for women, can be done under local or general anesthesia on an outpatient basis. Called a "mini-laparoscopy," the procedure entails making a small incision under the umbilicus. A small tube is then inserted through which carbon dioxide gas is pumped. The gas pushes the intestines into the upper abdomen so that the uterus and fallopian tubes can be seen. Another tiny incision is made, and a narrow instrument containing lights, mirrors, and cautery is inserted. The physician locates, cuts, and removes a small section of each fallopian tube and cauterizes (burns) the ends. The operation effectively prevents the sperm and egg from meeting in the fallopian tube.

Another more experimental technique calls for bands or rings to be placed around the fallopian tubes and tightened. Eventually, the tight bands cause scarring of the fallopian tubes, which closes them.

Still another technique involves putting a small amount of silicone with a string attached in each fallopian tube. The silicone, which does not react with body tissues, can remain in place until a time when the woman wishes to conceive. The physician can then pull the strings and the plugs will come out (Brozan, 1982).

All these techniques have been made possible because of new instrumentation employing fiberoptics, which allows the physician to perform exacting procedures with excellent visibility, using small, precise tools. Sterilization does not alter a woman's ovaries, uterus, vagina, or hormones. Some women may experience a brief period of discomfort in the shoulder area after a tubal ligation, from the carbon dioxide gas, which rises.

Women requesting a tubal ligation need an opportunity to discuss their feelings about not having any more children and the permanence of the operation. Medical personnel can be helpful in providing descriptions of the procedure by using pictures, as well as by showing the instruments that will be used. If the procedure is to be done in a hospital setting, health workers can play a supportive role if they avoid referring to the patient as a number or a procedure. In a rushed atmosphere, there is always the risk of impersonal attention. For a woman who is making an irrevocable decision, a few moments of quiet consideration and kindness can do a great deal to make the procedure easier and less traumatic.

Vasectomy. In this sterilization procedure for men, the testicular ducts (vas deferens) are cut and tied or cauterized. These ducts are tubes that carry sperm from the testicles, where they are produced and mature, to the prostate, where they mix with seminal fluid before ejaculation.

Vasectomy does not alter sexuality, hormone production, or ability to achieve orgasm. In a society that equates masculinity and success with sexual performance, some men may harbor unexpressed fears that a vasectomy will somehow prevent them from being fully "masculine." In a study done at Saint Paul–Ramsey Medical Center (Cass, 1979), attention was focused on the kind of preoperative counseling offered to men about to undergo vasectomy. Men who returned with problems after the surgery were found to be suffering from a variety of psychosexual complaints, including loss of erection, loss of libido, guilt feelings on the part of religious wives, and guilt because of their own religious beliefs. As a result of the study, more intensive preoperative counseling was instituted to allay fears about sexual performance and to address issues that could have an impact on the men's lives after the surgery. In many clinics, men are instructed to have at least one and possibly two counseling sessions, and they may be asked to have their wives participate.

As with female sterilization, techniques are being tried that will eventually make the procedure reversible. Work has begun with gold valves, placed in the vas deferens, that can be turned on and off; the use of silicone plugs; and an operation that reattaches the ends of the tubes, even after the initial surgery.

Because the prostate gland can store live sperm for several weeks, vasectomized men need to have sperm counts done on a regular basis, usually monthly, until the sperm count is zero. This may take as long as 3 months, depending on the frequency of orgasm. During this time, they and their partner should be advised to use some form of birth control. A careful explanation of the procedure, diagrams, and a matter-of-fact attitude on the part of health workers are helpful for both partners.

Menopause

Perhaps the most profound change that occurs during middle age is menopause. Men as well as women experience hormonal changes as they get older. Because the changes are more abrupt and occur over a shorter period of time, women tend to report more specific symptoms. Menopause has been shrouded in misconceptions, the subject of anxiety-producing myths, and can generally become the focus for a number of psychosocial symptoms.

Menopause can be defined as a period of time during which menstruation ceases. In effect, menopause is assumed to have occurred only after one full year has elapsed without menses. The process may take several years. Although the average age of menopause in the United States is 49 years, many women continue to menstruate well into their 50s.

Menopause occurs in three stages. The *premenopause* is the period of time in which the woman begins to notice a change in her menstrual cycle; it is sometimes late, sometimes early; and sometimes the flow itself is scanty, sometimes prolonged and excessive. For this reason, every woman having a checkup should be asked questions about her periods and perhaps be given a menstrual cycle chart to keep a more precise record.

Menopause, referring to the complete cessation of menses, can be pinpointed only after it occurs. *Perimenopause* is a period of time, generally 2 years, occurring after menstruation stops. Contrary to popular assumptions, there is no correlation between age of menopause and age of the beginning of menstruation, age of last pregnancy, or numbers of pregnancies (Kemmann and Jones, 1979).

Endocrine Changes.   During menopause, estrogen levels in the blood decrease and the levels of *gonadotropins* (follicle-stimulating hormone [FSH] and luteinizing hormone [LH]) rise. These two releasing hormones are secreted in response to the levels of estrogen. As estrogen levels go down, these hormones are secreted in greater quantity in an effort to make the estrogen level rise. There has been speculation that this imbalance in hormones may be the reason for the "hot flashes" experienced by many women, but research to date has not been able to pinpoint the cause.

Approximately 70 per cent of all women experience some physical symptoms during the menopausal period, although only 25 to 30 per cent are so adversely affected that they require medical intervention. Following are some of the more common symptoms.

Vasomotor Instability ("Hot Flashes").   According to Perlmutter (1979), this is the most common sign of approaching menopause. It has been described as the sudden onset of a feeling of warmth that starts on the chest and progresses to the face, where the skin becomes reddened and flushed. The flush may be accompanied by profuse perspiration. Some women complain of awakening at night, drenched with sweat, making it impossible to sleep and necessitating a change of night clothes and bed linens. The flashes may occur at any time and may fluctuate in intensity, ranging from a few seconds to more than 30 minutes. These flashes may begin some time before actual menopause takes place, increase in intensity during menopausal changes, and usually wane the following year. It is possible for women to have symptoms for as long as 5 years.

Atrophic Changes.   Several changes occur in the skin and underlying tissues as people age. All people begin to notice that their skin no longer is as firm as when they were younger, but seems to sag a bit. With the hormonal changes that occur during menopause there is also a loss of natural moisture in certain tissues that hastens the aging apperance of some women. Skin may begin to appear more wrinkled and dry. For women with naturally dry skin, these changes may cause itching and burning. Women should use a good moisturizing cream regularly.

Cervix and Uterus.   The uterus shrinks in size, and the cervix will cease to produce mucus. For women who have fibroid tumors of the uterus, menopause may mean that they may not have to undergo surgical removal of the tumors, which are benign and which shrink as the uterus diminishes in size.

Vagina.   The vagina is generally a moist, flexible organ. During menopause, the mucous lining may become thinner, drier, and less flexible, causing painful intercourse. Because the vagina does not lubricate as readily during sexual arousal as before menopause, a longer period of foreplay is required to prevent discomfort. It is interesting to note that the studies done by Masters and Johnson (1966) point out that women who remain sexually active, having intercourse once or twice a week, suffer less from reduced lubrication and elasticity than those whose sexual activity has decreased a great deal. As the hormonal balance changes, so does the pH balance, and the vagina then becomes the site of "senile vaginitis." This infection is caused by organisms that normally do not grow in a youthful vagina but gain a foothold in older women. If the infections persist, hormonal therapy may be indicated.

Other Body Changes. In addition to the more obvious changes during menopause, other parts of the body show signs of aging, particularly the external labia and internal pelvic organs, which may start to relax owing to a lessening of internal muscle tone. This relaxation may cause a prolapse (the structures fall forward, protruding into the vagina). When this happens, women complain that they lose urine when they exercise, sneeze, jump, or laugh. Women can deal with this embarrassing problem quite easily by learning some specific exercises designed to strengthen the muscles surrounding the urinary opening.

Estrogen Replacement Therapy. This approach is aimed at alleviating menopausal symptoms associated with hormonal loss. Since only 30 per cent of women suffer severe symptoms, the use of estrogens should be considered only in the most difficult cases. Some women should not take estrogens at all, particularly during menopause. These include women who have a history of cancer, any circulatory problems, liver or kidney disease, or any diagnosis of fibroid tumors or endometriosis. For these women, other medication will have to be used to help relieve symptoms.

Perhaps the best treatment of menopause is a supportive, understanding family. Menopause comes at a time in a woman's life when many things are changing. Children are leaving home, roles are being questioned, physical energy may be decreasing, and their own parents are becoming old. For women who have never worked, the issues of what to do once the "nest" is empty reflect real problems. In an environment that stresses youth, good looks, and sexual allure, women need added support. Health workers may lend strength if they help to redefine "femininity" in the context of aging when counseling women.

Notman (1979) summarizes several studies that discuss symptoms reported by a variety of women. In many of these studies, it is suggested that middle-class women who perceive that they have options and opportunities beyond mothering and homemaking suffer less from depression than women whose lives have been completely child oriented. In another study, Maoz and associates (1978) interviewed 1,148 Jewish women in the Middle East who came from a wide variety of ethnic and socioeconomic backgrounds. They found that European Jewish women who had worked before the onset of menopause suffered the fewest symptoms before and after the onset of the menopausal period, but Persian Jewish women who had never worked had no symptoms. The investigators concluded that the suggestion to all women that they "go to work" and find something to do might not necessarily be the most therapeutic advice.

The Male Climacteric

Just as a woman goes through a change in hormonal levels and influences, so do men, although to a lesser degree. Men experience a gradual decline in the effective levels of circulating testosterone and an increase in pituitary gonadotropins. This decrease in testosterone that results from aging is caused by two factors: One, the testicles produce less testosterone, and two, the amount of hormones available to tissues also decreases (Witters/Jones, 1980). This change in hormonal influence is generally not enough to cause any sexual dysfunction. Men have the same life issues to contend with as women and suffer the same fears of aging and loss of physical agility.

Prostate Problems.　There is one very common problem associated with aging in men, gradual enlargement of the prostate gland. Ten per cent of all men have evidence of enlargement by age 40 and 50 per cent by age 80.

The prostate gland, situated in the pelvis and surrounding the urethra, provides seminal fluid to carry sperm. As the gland enlarges, it can compress the urethra, causing difficulty in urination. The prostate has two lobes; the anterior lobe is the one most often associated with benign or nonmalignant enlargement, and the posterior lobe is the one most often the site of cancer of the prostate, the second most common form of cancer in men. When the prostate gland enlarges so much that urination becomes a real problem, a partial removal of the anterior portion becomes a necessity.

Some men may equate a prostatectomy with inability to remain sexually active, but the operation itself has little effect on potency. What men experience, even without prostatic enlargement, is an increase in the time to achieve and maintain an erection, some slowing of libidinal drive, and a somewhat extended period of time before ejaculation. In the latter case, this may bring added pleasure for the sexual partner who enjoys the longer period of foreplay.

Summary

It appears that for both men and women, continued sexual activity on a regular basis is the best way to forestall many of the problems linked to middle age. For health personnel, an understanding of the transitions in the lives of their clients, knowledge about the aging process, and a matter-of-fact approach to sexual issues will encourage openness and communication. Middle age can be a liberating, satisfying period, with both partners realizing individual and collective goals, together with optimism about the future. It is imperative that attention be focused on this process as the age shift in the American population becomes evident.

REFERENCES

Bennett, W.: The cigarette century. *Science 80,* 1(6):36–43, 1980.

Boston Women's Health Book Collective: *Our Bodies, Ourselves,* rev. ed. New York: Simon and Schuster, 1979.

Brozan, N.: Sterilization without surgery has promise. *New York Times,* Sept. 6, 1982.

Calkins, E.: Aging of cells and people. *Clinical Obstetrics and Gynecology,* 24(1)165–179, 1981.

Cass, A.: Unsatisfactory psychosocial results of vasectomy resulting in modification of pre-operative counseling. *Urology,* 14(6):588–590, 1979.

Friedman, G.: Cigarette smoking and coronary heart disease. *American Heart Journal,* 99(3):398–399, 1980.

Froelicher, V., Battler, A., McKirnan, M.: Physical activity and coronary heart disease. *Cardiology* 65:153–190, 1980.

Hagen, B.: *Alcohol, the Crutch That Cripples.* St. Paul, Minn., West Publishing Company, 1977.

Hammond, E., Seidman, H.: Smoking and cancer in the United States. *Preventive Medicine,* 9:169–173, 1980.

Kemmann, E., Jones, R.: The female climacteric. *Archives of Family Practice,* 20(5):140–151, 1979.

Maoz, B., et al.: The effect of outside work on the menopausal woman. *Maturitas,* 1:43–53, 1978.

Marx, J.: Dysmenorrhea: Basic research leads to a rational therapy. *Science,* 205:175–176, 1979.

Masters, W., Johnson, V.: *Human Sexual Response.* Boston: Little, Brown & Company, 1966.

Mazor, M.: The problem of infertility. In Notman,

M., Nadelson, C. (eds.): *The Woman Patient.* New York: Plenum Press, 1979.

Murray, R., Zentner, J.: Nursing assessment and health promotion for the young adult. In *Nursing Assessment through the Life Span.* Englewood Cliffs, N.J.: Prentice-Hall, 1979.

Noppa, H., et al.: Obesity in relation to morbidity and mortality from cardiovascular disease. *American Journal of Epidemiology,* 111(6):682–690, 1980.

Notman, M.: Midlife concerns of women: Implications of the menopause. *American Journal of Psychiatry,* 136(10):1270–1274, 1979.

Perlmutter, J.: A gynecological approach to menopause. In Notman M., Nadelson, C. (eds.): *The Woman Patient.* New York: Plenum Press, 1979.

Rothman, K.: The proportion of cancer attributable to alcohol consumption. *Preventive Medicine,* (9):174–179, 1980.

Smith, D., Bierman, E., Robinson, N. (eds.): *The Biologic Ages of Man.* Philadelphia: W. B. Saunders Company, 1978.

Stamler, J.: Lifestyles, major risk factors, proof and public policy. *Circulation,* 58(1):36–43, 1978.

Stewart, F.: *My Body, My Health: The Concerned Woman's Guide to Gynecology.* New York: John Wiley & Sons, 1979.

Warner, K.: Cigarette consumption. *Science,* 211(4483):729–731, 1981.

Witters/Jones, P., Witters, W.: *Human Sexuality: A Biological Perspective.* New York: Van Nostrand, 1980.

THE OLDER ADULT:
Integrity

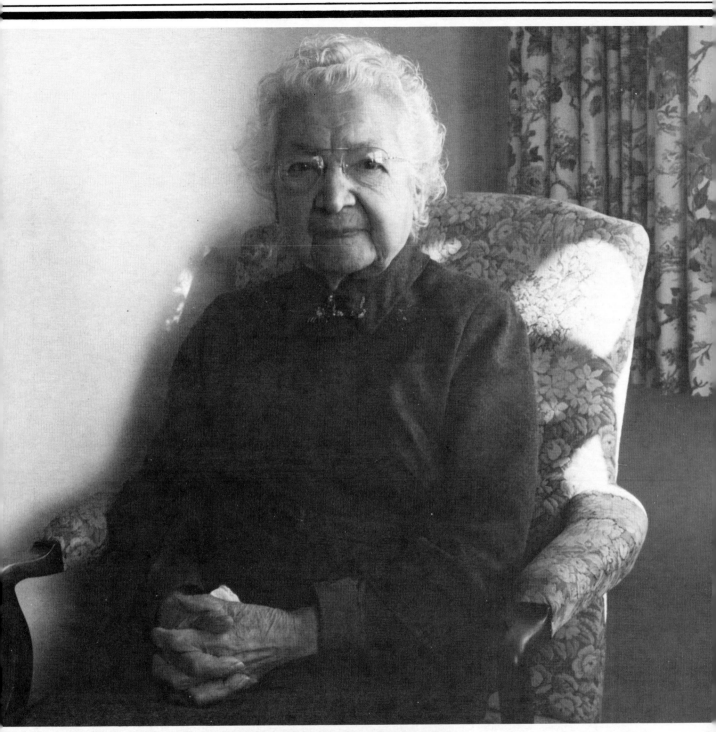

CHAPTER 15

"Grow old along with me . . ., The best is yet to be."

The poet expresses a hope that (examine your true reaction!) most of us don't really believe. Yet, with the life expectancy in the United States hovering around an average of 72 years (approximately 69 for men and a little over 76 for women), the majority of individuals reading this sentence will be likely to reach the time of life that is considered "old."

There is little doubt that regard of the elderly in our midst is, on the whole, negative (Nardi, 1973). Part of the disaffection can be attributed to the heavy emphasis in our society upon independence and productivity. The old are typically seen as dependent and nonproductive. Furthermore, their "uselessness" is more apparent in a society that is changing so rapidly that the store of information and knowledge held by the elderly is considered out of date. Additionally, the mobility of the nuclear family often removes its members from close contact with family elders. This means that many of us do not have fond memories of grandparents to carry forward into thinking about old age.

Still another significant factor is the general lack of definitive information about aging. Though research findings have begun to be substantial, these have not been widely disseminated. Media attention has usually focused on the "horror stories"—the poor conditions in nursing homes, criminal attacks on elderly women, or elderly people freezing to death because of lack of money for heat.

An added circumstance is the fact that, until relatively recently, there have not been many aged people visible in our society. At the beginning of the 20th century, life expectancy had not reached 50 years, and there were only 3 million Americans over age 65. Today some 10 per cent of the population is past 65 years of age. By the year 2030, it is estimated that more than a quarter of the population (28 per cent) will be 55 and older, with 17 per cent past age 65 (*Facts about Older Americans*, 1976a).

In effect, the elderly have been increasing rapidly in number during the time when publicized theories and studies were concentrating on younger age groups. We tend to know quite a good deal more about the first 18 years of life than we do about the next 50.

So, stereotyped thinking abounds. "Old" is associated with watery eyes, a quavering voice, a faltering step, sagging jowels, irascibility, failing memory, poor judgment and thinking processes, senility, dependence, and death. With such a catalogue, it is no wonder that most of us are reluctant to look seriously at age and aging. Like Scarlett O'Hara, we are more comfortable in deciding to "think about that tomorrow." Moreover, most of us have someone in mind to fit the stereotype: An impoverished widow living only in her memories, or an old man who no longer recognizes members of the family and cannot control his bodily functions. Although it is also possible to point to vigorous and articulate elderly citizens who are active in community and social circles, they are often considered to be rare exceptions.

The facts, however, contradict the outmoded images and point to changes in society that are now being only dimly perceived. An ever-increasing proportion of the elderly indicates that the "youth culture," which has been characteristic of the past, is bound to give way to a more "adult-oriented" point of view. This change is just beginning to be manifested—in products designed to appeal to older people; in movies and television shows with elders playing leading roles (for instance, George Burns, Henry Fonda, and Katherine Hepburn); in new ideas in housing, such as the condominium; in streams of "how-to-do-it" books and magazines directed toward this population; and in an increase in the number of agencies and political organizations designed to serve this group. Perhaps growing old is not so bad after all! Let's take a look, attempting to sort out what is known, from what are persistent, but essentially false, notions.

WHO IS OLD?

The question of who is old does not lend itself to neat and tidy answers. At almost any senior citizens center, it would be possible to see two people separated in age by 20 years, the younger with deteriorating body functions and fading responsiveness and the older still lively and robust. It is clear that age alone does not provide a key. As a matter of fact, individual differences among same-age elders are likely to be greater than at any time earlier in life. This should be easy to understand.

The experiences of younger age groups are much more similar, one to another. Schoolchildren and adolescents share their common school environment; young adults become involved in jobs, marriage, and family; adults in midlife share questions about direction for themselves and about guidance for older children. However, it is difficult to make generalizations about late adulthood. By age 65, the accumulated variations in life experiences tend to create enormous differences in coping and problem solving, personality, outlook, attitudes, interests, and intellect. Life circumstances and social relations of elders are also very diverse. Widowed and living alone or widowed and remarried, maintaining close contact with adult children or being isolated, good health or poor health, optimistic or dour, poor or financially comfortable, interested or apathetic . . . in no instance is it possible to predict one's state of being from age alone.

The variations that are present across same-age groups of late adulthood make the usual form of cross-sectional research suspect. The process of obtaining an average from a group of same-age individuals, then another average from an older same-age group, and still another average from a still older group has the effect of making a difference in the averages appear to come about because of age. Moreover, if the average increases (or decreases) with the successive groups, these differences can easily be interpreted as inevitable. For example an investigation attempting to determine the numbers of denture wearers would likely find the incidence of dentures to be higher and higher for each age cohort studied. This does not mean that one is certainly going to be wearing dentures in the same way that the average number of infants walking at successive ages predicts that an infant will certainly walk during a certain age range unless something is dreadfully wrong.

Physical status undoubtedly plays a part in determining the answer to the question of who is old. But whether one looks in the mirror, inspecting the strands of gray and mourns, "I am old," or assents cheerfully, "I am getting older," is indicative of the major source of the aging experience. It is "in the head," placed there in large part by the circumstances of one's life. Even socioeconomic status exerts an influence on "the picture in the head" of what it is to be growing old. Neugarten (1968) found that upper-middle-class people generally agreed that middle age begins around 50, and old age, at about 75; lower socioeconomic classes felt that middle age starts at age 40 and old age, correspondingly earlier.

Neugarten and Datan (1973) underscore the importance of the socialization process in designating who is old. They describe three dimensions of time that need to be considered with regard to any portion of the life cycle, including that of aging.

1. *Life time*, or biological time, is most predictive early in life and least predictive in later years.

2. *Social time* refers to the manner in which each society defines and regulates the various ages (and which we consider far more significant in dictating the shape of the experiences of a particular age than chronological age).

3. *Historical time* is specific to a given society and interacts with social time to give an individual consciousness of his or her generation. For example, those who experienced the Depression, World War II, or Vietnam share much more than a biological age; rather, the particular age group is distinguished by the historical events experienced during a particular period in their lives.

This is not a wholly new concept, of course. The times in which one lives and the social specifications for various roles have always been reckoned in our accounting for personality development. What is new is that the expectations of social time for the elderly have not yet caught up with reality and are no longer valid. For example, there are entire new family-cycle rhythms under way—such as the trend for grown, sometimes divorced, children to move back in with parents (*Time*, October 13, 1980, p. 118)— for which there is no role preparation or practice. Elders must find their own way, and the rocking chair does not seem to be a viable option.

Historical time for the elderly, too, is changing before our eyes as older people become, by sheer weight of numbers, more visible and important. With the slogan "Senior power!", organizations of elders are amassing for political action and aggressive lobbying. The Gray Panthers have had as their leader a dynamo in her seventies named Margaret Kuhn. The National Council of Senior Citizens has nearly 4 million members. These are unprecedented developments, certain to change ideas about what it is to be old.

Changing social definitions will buttress changing psychological definitions of who is old. Although self-appraisal will continue to be affected by circumstances such as illness or death of the life partner, it begins to look as though there may be pretty good times ahead for those growing older.

INTEGRITY

It would be difficult to imagine a more ideal psychological definition of late age than *integrity*, Erikson's (1950) eighth task for the "last of life." Integrity has the notion of "wholeness" about it; it signifies an inner assurance of order and meaning in the total scheme of things. It not only looks back without regrets but, more importantly, looks forward with optimism and enthusiasm. No matter what one's political outlook is, it would be hard to deny that Ronald Reagan's election to the Presidency and his remarkable recovery after a gunshot wound served as a tremendous example of enthusiastic old age.

Integrity also brings perspective and therefore and a special kind of wisdom. There is some interesting evidence that much of the reminiscing of the elderly is useful to obtain this sense of relationship to and proportion for the past. It serves the purpose of getting a lifetime in order, placing life events along a "time line," weaving together the old strands, tying up loose ends, and making peace with bygone sorrow and disappointments. Kastenbaum (1979) terms this the *general life review* and suggests, in addition, four types of reminiscing that he calls *retrospective modalities*.

Retrospective Modalities

Validation

Kastenbaum (1979) suggests that the recollections of the elderly are not aimless and meandering, but, rather, are likely to have pattern and purpose. Sometimes the older person is seen to be searching the past for courage to face the present. Many older people can sustain themselves with a self-reminder of previous competence. "I did it before and I can do it again!"

Boundary Setting

Psychological boundaries are the "don't cross over" markers that we carry around in our heads. For the elderly, the markers are likely to be erected thick and fast, many imposed from the outside. Some of the reminiscing seems to be the effort to adjust to new boundaries, a kind of "working up to it," as it were. One older man would describe his beloved summer home in Vermont, often and in detail, obviously relishing every word. He always added that the home had been sold because he was no longer able to travel and there were no heirs to take over. It seems clear that the recital was more for himself than for his listeners—it was a way of saying good-bye to the cherished place in Vermont and he was managing gallantly. As Kastenbaum notes (p. 616), one is forced to look at the older person with a new appreciation when the tremendous demands of boundary setting are recognized and understood.

Perpetuation of the Past

Sometimes, the older person literally carries the past into the present (Kastenbaum, 1979). Often such a person is very isolated, with little happening in any day to persuade in favor of present reality. It is important to be reminded here that the dynamic at work is quite the same as that in our own occasional perpetuation of the past. If you have ever wept a few tears over a baby shoe (its owner now stands 6 feet tall), kept a summer camper's room exactly as she left it for several days, or talked to a photograph, then you can feel for those who are keeping their past alive because it was the best part of their lives.

Replaying

The tendency of the elderly to retell the same anecdotes over and over again is probably one of their best-known characteristics, often tolerated with little grace by the captive audiences. Regularities can be observed in this phenomenon, just as in other types of recollecting (Kastenbaum, 1979). One of the distinctive features of "replaying" is that the experience is one with a strong emotional attachment. It has a great deal of meaning for the recounter. Kastenbaum likens it to pulling a favorite record out of the collection and experiencing it again and again. Replaying, like the other retrospective modalities, is not uniquely the province of the old. Each of us has favorite stories that are told to any available listener; however, most of us remain relatively aware of those who have already heard the account. Furthermore, with the presence of a full and active life, we probably manage to replenish our stock of tales quite regularly. As the events of one's life become more restricted, adding new effective experiences is more difficult. Parenthetically, in this regard, one of the important contributions of a readily accessible senior citizens center is that of bringing increased variety in the lives of the participants. It would be worthwhile to investigate whether the amount of "replaying" decreases as the life of the older person becomes richer and more interesting.

It took a dramatic and moving television series, "Roots," to make us think about our own "roots," and to acknowledge the great store of family history that exists only in the memories of family elders. Some families have set about preserving the heritage with benefit to the storyteller (there is absolutely nothing more stimulating than an interested listener) and, equally, to the listener who is sharing in another time in a way that, for the family, will season and enhance all time to come.

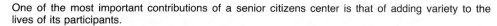

One of the most important contributions of a senior citizens center is that of adding variety to the lives of its participants.

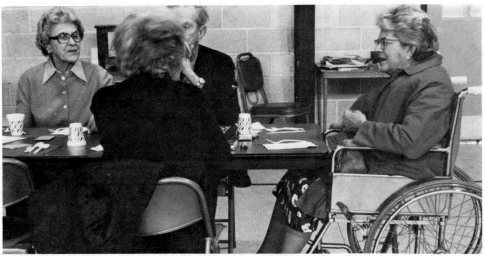

Judith Kruger Michalik

Although the retrospective modalities can be thought of as assisting the older person in a number of adaptive ways, such a happy outcome is not evitable. Often, to be sure, a memory is bittersweet. But memories can also stir anger, shame, or regret. None of us escapes segments of life during which we behaved less than admirably, in which we wronged others, made ridiculous decisions, should have known better, looked downright foolish. If the individual is not able to accommodate human frailty and mistakes in the life review, the result is not integrity, but its counterpart, *despair*. The usual components include a feeling that life has been and is futile and that the time is now too short to take any other paths; there is also considerable anger directed vaguely at "ingratitude" or "the unfairness of it all."

Despair

Erikson's description of despair tends to attribute it to a failing of the inner resources that should have been built up and strengthened during each of the developmental tasks. As with every stage of life, the lessons of the preceding periods play an important part. Early vulnerabilities affect later relationships, which, in turn, determine something of the quality of later years. A preoccupation of youth may be carried forward as a strength (a satisfying occasional pastime then, a deeply engaging focus of interest now) or become a debilitating rigidity (a mild prejudice once, fierce hostility and suspicion now). Attitudes toward love, work, and the self have origins in the past. Problem solving and coping need to have been practiced in other days. It is evident that much of the pattern for later years is woven in earlier ones and that impoverishment of spirit while young leads toward a drab and bleak old age.

However, lest an "only himself to blame" attitude be adopted toward a despairing elder, it is necessary to understand that not all of the determinants of late-life satisfaction or unhappiness are under individual control. Palmore (1968) and Schonfield (1973) both found that activity level, in terms of sustained and future commitments, correlated significantly with expressed satisfaction and successful aging. However, Schonfield discovered another variable linked to the activity index—that is, the ease of transportation—pointing up the fact that mobility is an additional critical factor in whether or not the older person can maintain social contacts and interests.

Other studies (Cutler, 1973; Edwards and Klemmack, 1973) find that socioeconomic status (especially family income) and physical health are significantly associated with life satisfaction. Availability of transportation, economic aspects of late adulthood, and the status of one's physical being are not wholly self-determined, and despair in the face of isolation, poverty, and poor health is no stranger to the aged. Suicide rates peak for white men after the age of 75, becoming four times the national average (Resnick and Cantor, 1970). Rates are higher for those living alone and for those who are seriously ill, these authors report. Another finding from the same study is more helpful—that the suicide rates have declined about 25 per cent for both men and women over age 65 in the United States with a similar decrease noted in England, Norway, and Denmark. The authors attribute the drop to lessened economic distress because of more adequate Social Security coverage.

Despair versus integrity. Integrity versus despair. The developmental task for late life points up, once again, the complex relationship between internal and external, between the shaping processes of the past and how we have reacted to them, between what we bring to the situation and the situation itself. Although it is necessary to insist that society make an honored and useful place for its elderly citizens, it is up to each of us to strive to truly have something to contribute when our time comes. People should be helped to take early steps toward providing themselves with income and interests for later years; at the same time, an array of support services could offer help and authoritative information.

Integrity, the quality of vision that recognizes and accepts the continuity of the life

The task of coming to terms with life, in dignity and with self-respect, is a challenge to test the mettle, courage, and humor of the best of us.

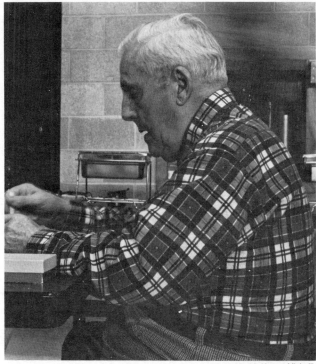

Judith Kruger Michalik

tapestry, does not seem to be a characteristic that one could develop by one's self, alone. Indeed, the concept of the outstretched hand, thankfully accepted and warmly offered, should come to be appreciated by elders as never before. The task of coming to terms with life, in dignity and with self-respect, is a challenge to test the mettle, courage, and humor of the best of us.

We all need to be grateful to present-day elders who are tackling the route, showing us how to do it!

PHYSICAL STATUS

The state of physical functioning for the aged is important, not only in terms of life satisfaction (Edwards and Klemmack, 1973), but also for longevity predictions (Palmore, 1969). However, the general good health at the initial interview of the longitudinal studies to be described was the most important factor in predictions.

The interesting fact about the physical changes that are associated with aging is that we are not wholly clear about the "cause." The quick and pat response that age in all organisms brings progressive deterioration and, finally, death is not adequate. Such a theory does not account for the tremendous variations between individuals of the same age or even differences with regard to decline of organ structures for the same person. Popular thinking about age, however, continues to make comparisons of mental ability between 20-year-old college students and the individuals seen on the porches of homes for the aged, thereupon pointing to the "ravages of age." The performance careers of Martha Graham and Margot Fonteyn are dismissed as miraculous and of no significance for the ordinary individual.

Actually, it is only a little more than 20 years since the beginning of the first systematic gathering of information about aging. It was not until the data began to come in from the Gerontology Research Center (Shock, 1968), from the National Institutes of Health (Birren, 1964, 1974), and from the Duke University Center for the Study of Aging (Palmore, 1970, 1974)—all longitudinal studies—that a clearer picture of the functioning during late adulthood began to take shape

The problem that investigators have been trying to track down by means of the longitudinal studies is what portion of physiological change can be linked to other life events such as disease or malnutrition and what portion seems to be "programmed" (built into the biology of the cells). The answers are not yet clear, but at least we now understand enough so that *age per se* is not seen as the unrelenting crippler and destroyer of function. These first answers also begin to explain the great observable difference between individuals of the same age.

Stress

One of the key concepts emerging from the research is the suggestion that aging brings about an increased vulnerability, including diminished capacity to "snap back" in the face of stress (Shock, 1974). Hans Selye (1956, 1973), who has spent more than 40 years studying the psychobiological effects of stress, suggests that a long lifetime of repeated arousal to deal with demands will eventually result in a lowered level of resistance and, sometimes, what he terms the "adaptation diseases"—high blood pressure, arthritis, and cardiovascular changes (1970).

Selye views stress as the nonspecific response of the body to any demand made upon it (1973). The demands can be pleasant or unpleasant, great or small. Each and every demand calls forth a degree of biological response. Selye describes a three-stage reaction, the *general adaptation syndrome*, which mobilizes the body's resources to meet an injurious agent or set of circumstances. The *stressor* (potential injury) could be physical (excessive fatigue, drugs, burns, malnutrition) or psychological (death of a loved one, losing a job, being criticized, being frightened).

The first stage, the *alarm reaction*, calls up the body defenses through activity of the sympathetic nervous system and hormones from the adrenal glands. The second stage, *resistance*, is called into operation if the threat continues; the body must both repair and maintain its first-line defenses. Increased levels of hormones from the anterior pituitary (ACTH) and the adrenal cortex (cortin) enable the individual to continue the aroused reaction and often to seem to resume normal functioning. However, if the emergency continues for too long, all of the reserves available may be used up and an overwhelming counterreaction may occur. This is termed the *stage of exhaustion*. The hormonal level drops, the body is no longer able to adapt, body functions are slowed dramatically, and death may ensue.

The increased vulnerability can be manifested in several ways. One is the presence of some sort of chronic illness. About 85 per cent of the individuals over age 65 report at least one persisting ailment, and about half of these individuals indicate that their activities are somewhat curtailed because of the chronic disorder (Hendricks and Hendricks, 1977). The most common conditions are arthritis and rheumatism, high blood pressure, obesity, abdominal cavity hernia, cataracts, hemorrhoids, prostate disorders, and orthopedic impairments (U.S. DHEW Publication, 1976b). Approximately 25 per cent of the elders over age 65 are likely to be hospitalized for a period of time during any given year (compared with the rate of about 15 per cent of the age 45- to 64-year-olds). When acute illness occurs, it tends to require more time for recovery for the older person.

There is, too, the fact that the heart rate and blood pressure may be comparable with that of a younger person, but only at rest (Weg, 1975). Responses to demands are not as extensive or intense as those that were possible when younger. Increased time is needed to return to the prestress level. This adjustive capacity decline also shows up in the fact that homeostatic regulation of the body to environmental temperature change is less efficient. The elderly "feel the cold" more quickly and become chilled more readily. Shawls, sweaters, head coverings, and foot warmers are welcomed in weather that younger folk find only a little cool. Similarly, the body's cooling system does not operate as well for older people, and a prolonged summer heat wave poses a definite danger, especially for the poor without fans or air conditioning.

The increased vulnerability and lessened adaptation to stress are accompanied by another tendency that needs to be recognized and accommodated. It is the general slowing of the psychomotor skills. This becomes especially noticeable to an observer if some degree of speed is required for a reaction. The time pressure is likely to undermine the quality of the response as well as point up its lagging execution. The slowing down varies from task to task and, according to Hicks and Birren (1970), ranges from a decrement of about 20 per cent to a decline of more than 100 per cent of the speed of a younger person. However, as you can probably guess by this stage of your study, the onset of appreciable slowing, the reactions affected, and the implications for the life of the older person are all highly individualized matters (Bromley, 1974). A constant barrage of admonitions to "take it easy," "don't try to do too much," or, worse, "let me do that for you" is practically guaranteed to slow the elder even more. In many instances, the slowdown can be offset by increased ability to concentrate, so that a worker can give better attention to accuracy or quality. For example, a 92-year-old woman regularly wins a Scrabble game over her daughter (author Dennis) because she studies the board very intently, never failing to pounce on the most obscure possibilities for combinations.

Even though the increased vulnerability, lessened capacity to respond to stressful demands, and slowing down of psychomotor skills seem to be rather securely established "facts" of aging (Weg, 1975), still at issue are which portions of the changes are inevitable (if any) and which portions represent the end result of lifelong habits known to be "hazardous to one's health." As a matter of fact, smoking supplies a ready example. Almost any listing of biological and physiological changes occurring in later life will include decreased lung capacity, lessened elasticity of the bronchioles, and functional shortness of breath. Each of these conditions is typically noticed in a smoker of a much younger age; but if the smoker has survived, the coughing, wheezing, and painful breathing of emphysema are almost sure to be present in the elderly person. The symptoms are not as predictable for a nonsmoker (Rockstein, 1975). Are the symptoms attributable to age? Or smoking?

Obesity is another carryover from a more youthful time. Its association with diabetes, high blood pressure and other cardiovascular problems, varicose veins, and kidney and gallbladder disorders is well known. If a major portion of lifetime nutrition has been invested in too much of the wrong kinds of food, the consequences are likely to become observable eventually, but the age of the individual seems to be apart from but still attached to the process.

Mention might be made of the various industrial and environmental hazards that could well catch up and overtake an individual as long periods of time pass. Asbestos is known to have a lengthy "inactive" period before its effects are manifested. Miners can work for a number of years before being felled by "black lung." It is possible that some of the often-cited respiratory problems of the aged might be caused by the pollutants in the air, including the smoke of other people's cigarettes.

Any diminished physiological functioning is likely to have a deleterious effect on activity. There is a tendency to reduce motor action to a minimum in the face of pain or difficulty. The lowered activity level leads to rapid loss of muscle strength and further decreases in use. Add to this the fact that even many midlife individuals are less active than is desirable, that most of us ride when we should be walking, that we use elevators too readily and engage in too many sedentary pursuits in any case, and the unsteady gait, stiffened movements, and quickened fatigue of the aged can thus be explained without the invocation of age.

Exercise

The importance of exercise for the elderly is emphasized in studies by DeVries (1975). He demonstrated that an exercise regimen lasting to 8 weeks for men, age 50 to 87, provided significant improvement in oxygen transport and vital capacity, reduction in

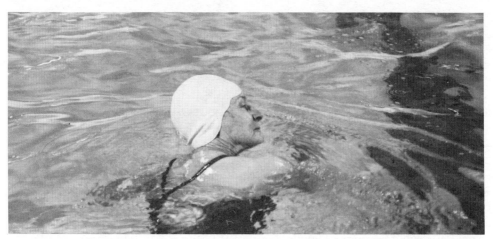

The importance of exercise for the elderly has been pointed out by numerous studies. It not only affects physical condition but can improve a person's psychological outlook profoundly.

Judith Kruger Michalik

percentage of body fat, increase in physical work capacity, and more favorable systolic and diastolic blood pressures. Another group of men, who had been placed on a modified exercise program because of existing cardiovascular problems (they walked instead of jogging), showed a pattern of improvement remarkably similar to the harder-exercising normal subjects. DeVries concludes that older individuals can be benefited even if they are not in "good condition" and that the amount of improvement is entirely comparable to that of the young. He suggests that vigorous physical conditioning of healthy older subjects can bring about marked improvement in the cardiovascular and respiratory systems musculature and in body composition, resulting in a more vigorous individual who is able to relax more efficiently.

Environment and Nutrition

In light of the DeVries studies and others, Weg (1975) feels that even present knowledge would permit encouraging of a more optimal physiological aging. She points to the many environmental factors that are known to have an association, if not a causal relationship, with a number of the physiological dysfunctions of the elderly that might be modified if we cared enough. Intervention with proper nutrition is an obvious possibility that might combat not only obesity but a host of allied disorders including the periodontal diseases that have seemed inevitable for those who are growing older. Denny (1975) points to studies that suggest a dietary component in the formation of "age pigment" deposits in aging cells. Lutwak (1969) suggests that proper intake of dietary calcium may be effective in preventing loss of bone tissue in osteoporosis.

Health Awareness

An immense public health mission, waiting to be undertaken, seems to be that of educating Americans about the steps that are within the reach of most people but are not recognized clearly as vital to one's own positive elderhood. For example, although the number of joggers and bicyclers on any road attests to an increased consciousness regarding the need for exercise, the awareness needs to be extended to even greater numbers. Exercise periods built into agency, factory, business, and corporation workdays is not too far-fetched an idea. Present-day young people need to become convinced that they must carry their exercise programs into old age, and present-day elders should be encouraged to engage in systematic vigorous activity.

The possibility of living out one's life in relative good health may be more than an empty promise. It is given substantiation from what is known about the groups of long-lived individuals who exist in small groups over the world. Even with some skepticism about how records are kept, the people of the Abkhasia of the Georgian Soviet Republic are noted for their vigorous long life (Leaf, 1973). Each individual is expected to contribute to the life of the community with work that characteristically demands a high level of physical activity. Their diet is low in calories, sugar, and saturated animal fat, and high in fruits and vegatables. Obesity is unknown. Homemade wine and a little vodka are used in moderation, and there is very little smoking.

The professions concerned with human development and with promoting optimal human development logically should be the banner carriers of the message that successful aging is under our own control to a great extent. There are measures that can be put into operation now for ourselves and our loved ones with regard to diet, exercise, smoking, and ecology to contribute to an energetic and sturdy old age. Of the responsibilities for health education that fall to those associated with the health services, this must be a major one.

REMEMBERING AND FORGETTING

"Grandma! Your eyeglasses are up on your forehead!"

The children are always delighted when Grandma forgets where she has placed something even though she knew where it was but a moment before. The functioning of memory is often a frustration to all of us (wishing to remember a name that escapes at an embarrassing moment, for example). Such episodes seem to occur with more frequency as we grow older. D. O. Hebb, the former president of McGill University and a noted psychologist, in a poignant essay about growing older (1978), recounts the "instant" that he was forced to acknowledge his own aging. He was reading a professional journal, becoming more and more excited about an especially fresh and intriguing article. Suddenly, to his horror, he encountered some penciled notes in the margin—his own writing, though he had absolutely no recollection of having read the article before.

The Memory Process

Research on memory indicates that remembering is not a single process, but a complex system of processes. There seem to be three stages to the ultimate storage of material in long-term memory.

Sensory Memory

This process is used for an initial screening of incoming information. It registers with extreme rapidity, preserving perception of the stimulus just long enough to be judged by the brain as possibly useful, to be passed on for longer processing, or to be judged unimportant, to be discarded. The sensory memory seems to have tremendous capacity, but the registering persists for only 0.25 to 2 seconds (Craig, 1977; Murdock, 1967).

Short-Term Memory

If the information is deemed valuable, the individual attends to it and thereby transfers it to this second memory system. At this stage, the information undergoes further processing. It is inspected, sorted out, classified, and acted upon, if necessary, and another judgment is made with regard to whether it needs to be retained longer. All of this takes place in a matter of seconds. Furthermore, processing of a number of items may be taking place simultaneously. You have just looked up a telephone number and are in the process of dialing it when a television commercial within your range of vision and hearing reports a sale of winter coats that you decide to attend, and simultaneously the sound of the children outside reminds you to speak to your neighbor about a PTA committee. By this time, the number has been dialed and your phone call proceeds.

It is this system with which older people seem to have the greatest amount of difficulty. It looks as though they are vulnerable to distraction between perception and recall (Craig, 1977). However, there is some research suggesting that it is the perception (or registration) process itself that determines whether the short-term memory is activated and that it, in turn, depends upon how important or relevant the information appears to the individual (Botwinick and Storant, 1974). Some diminished perception could be due to failing hearing or eyesight. Some might be due to a kind of "disengagement" or withdrawal so that fewer experiences seem needful of attention. However, there is evidence that, for some of the elderly, significant short-term memory loss occurs much later, if at all, than has been considered typical (Horn, 1970).

Long-Term Memory

At the third stage of memory processing, material for long-term storage is transferred from short-term memory by means of techniques that have served, more or less efficiently, in the past. This form of memory seems to hold up well for many older individuals, provided the general physiological functioning of the nervous system is in good order. There is some indication that elders can be assisted in memory if cues are provided; in other words, it is a more successful process if recognition is required rather than straight recall (Schonfield and Robertson, 1966). This tends to be true of younger subjects as well; however, an older person can be greatly benefited by learning to write notes of reminder about the things that must be remembered.

Memory and Learning

Many of the tasks set to test memory are learning tasks, and it is impossible to speak of one without involving the other. Clearly, one must learn in order to remember, and memory is called upon to demonstrate the learning. Some of the problems that older people perceive with their memories seem to come from inefficient learning strategies. Hulicka and Grossman (1967) point out that present-day older subjects tend to have had less formal education and therefore less opportunity to "learn how to learn" and that this is reflected in their recall ability.

The psychomotor slowing, as we mentioned earlier, could account for some of the difficulties. Hulicka and Weiss (1965) found that older subjects were not able to remember as well as younger subjects when both were given equal time for learning. However, when the older subjects were permitted to learn at their own speed, they recalled as much as the younger. It would probably be well for all of us to see which time pressures might be lightened, but especially for the elders, environments need to be designed to be more in harmony with their own rhythms.

Help for Memory Problems

There have been some studies directed at helping older people to overcome or prevent memory problems. One of the most interesting, with controversial results, is the use of oxygen twice a day for 15 days (90 minutes each session for a total of 3 hours per day) for elderly patients who were exhibiting memory deficits. In contrast to a control group who received no oxygen, all of the subjects in the experimental group demonstrated large improvements on the Wechsler Memory Scale and other test scores. When the control group was later given the oxygen treatment, they too showed the same significant improvement (Jacobs et al., 1969). The results did not receive support, however, in a replication of the procedure several years later (Goldfarb et al., 1972). Not only did the latter investigation fail to verify the previous results; it was reported that the patients themselves expressed great dislike for the treatment, with six of them terminating before the procedure was complete. The striking discrepancy between the two studies calls for further investigation.

Kastenbaum (1979) suggests that the elderly might be instructed in how to talk to themselves. Though this kind of behavior has been regarded as evidence of mental peculiarity, he points out that to repeat the information to one's self involves an active rehearsal—the best technique for keeping information firmly anchored and ready for retrieval.

Age As a Factor in Memory

A summary statement regarding declining memory function for elders is similar to the other assumptions for aging. It does not appear that age is as important as what has gone on before (including the individual's previous capabilities for learning and memory, previous level of education, physiological status, and motivation); pace of the learning task; and even the distractions in the individual's life and environment. These variables are also significant in the memory function of younger individuals, but in such instances we tend to study individual differences in memory prowess, rather than age-17 abilities versus age-25 abilities.

This is not an attempt to propose that all elderly persons operate as effectively as when they were younger; rather, we suggest that many of the "of courses" apply only to certain older people (and might apply equally to some individuals who are quite young!). It is, in effect, a plea for a much more individualized approach to elders that will assist their own regard of themselves as individuals and lessen the tendency for resignation and passive acceptance of ageism (negative stereotypes) when it is not necessary.

Instructive in this regard is the study of centenarians, people age 100 and older (Beard, 1968). The group, all at least 100 years old, was compared with a group age 95 to 99. Among the interesting findings, individuals age 103 and beyond remembered recent events better than those who were "only" age 100. Furthermore, all of the centenarians recalled more events of national importance than the younger subjects in their 90s. Level of education had a significant effect on the test results, and people who performed well on one memory test tended to perform well on others. The investigator also found a remarkable number of the sample playing chess, bridge, and checkers, keeping their own financial records, doing their own shopping, and engaging in dressmaking and carpentry!

LATE-AGE INTELLIGENCE

Is it really impossible to teach an old dog new tricks? Do human mental powers decline with age? There was a time when the answers to those questions were considered settled. You did not attempt to teach an old dog anything new, and human intelligence presumably reached its peak at age 16, thereupon declining gradually and deteriorating rapidly in late years. Documentation for the latter assertion was easy to obtain. Administer intelligence tests to successive age groups, and observe the fact that the average score will be lower for each cohort as age increases. However, the cross-sectional method, as we have seen, becomes less and less valid for assessing age differences as the gap between the various ages grows larger. It is one thing to look at children of the same generation (age 1 versus age 3). It is quite another to look at age 20 versus age 70, when all of the changes experienced by different generations need to be taken into account (Schaie, 1975).

Another problem with cross-sectional testing is that older subjects may obtain averages that are spuriously low because of a phenomenon that has come to be known as *terminal drop*. Testing and retesting a large number of subjects, Riegel and Riegel (1972) (the former is the same Klaus Riegel who proposed the idea of dialectical processes in development) discerned a sudden drop in intellectual performance shortly before death. They suggested that the decline in test scores of older samples of cross-sectional studies may be reflecting this terminal drop.

In addition, there are some problems with the test situation itself that may also contribute to the lower scores observed by the early investigators. Some factors have been demonstrated to influence performance on the tests that have nothing to do with intelligence. For example Birkhill and Schaie (1975) show that the cautiousness with which elderly persons approach test items and their reluctance to "take a chance" on an uncertain answer may significantly lower test scores. Some of this hesitancy could be due to lack of appropriate skills. We have already noted that the present group of Americans beyond age 65 were much less schooled than subsequent generations, less than half having completed high school (U.S. Bureau of the Census, 1972).

Lack of school-related skills and general unfamiliarity with test situations can result in inhibiting motivational barriers. Neugarten (1977) has pointed to the unconscionable amount of ageism in our society, the term referring to negative stereotypes that are applied to the elderly and that they come to believe about themselves. If elderly subjects are quite aware that an investigator "knows" they will do poorly on a task, the performance is prejudiced from the beginning. A "cautious" approach to test items is likely to be even more evident if decades have passed without exposure to similar material.

Is it true, then, that there are no appreciable intellectual changes that come about because of age? When the question is phrased that way, the answer is almost an unequivocal "yes." As a matter of fact, several longitudinal studies (Bayley, 1968; Owens, 1966) suggest the possibility of an *increase* in scores on tests taken as college freshman and again at age 61, and for midlife adults over their scores as adolescents. Schaie (1975), reviewing his own years of investigating adult intelligence, believes that there is very little age-related decrement in intelligence in functions that do not require speed of response.

The present thinking, articulated by the American Psychological Association Task Force on Aging (Baltes and Labouvie, 1973), is that any observed decline in intellectual functioning among the aged is attributable to poor health, reduced environmental opportunity, social isolation, economic privation, limited education, lowered motivation, and other variables not intrinsically related to aging.

The issue of what it is that intelligence tests are measuring was raised in Chapter 6 and should remind us that whatever the score, test scores represent only a small portion of the individual's competence. In this regard, a recital of some notable accomplishments by elderly people could be enough to make the ordinary youthful mortal feel very raw and inept:

Pablo Picasso	Continued to paint and design pottery until his death at age 91
Sigmund Freud	Wrote his last book at age 83
Artur Rubenstein	Performed in a remarkable concert at Carnegie Hall at age 89
Jean Piaget	Active, lecturing, and writing until his death at age 84
Grandma Moses	Was still painting at age 100
Benjamin Franklin	Served as a member of the Constitutional Congress at age 81
Frank Lloyd Wright	Completed the Guggenheim Museum at age 91
Arthur Fiedler	Led the Boston Pops in a triumphant Fourth of July concert at age 83
Margaret Mead	Lecturing and writing until death at 77

Goethe	Completed *Faust* while in his 80s
Thomas Jefferson	Writing and inventing until his death at 83
Eubie Blake	Charming audiences in a play about his life and music while in his 90s
Winston Churchill	Wrote the four-volume set, *A History of the English Speaking People*, at age 82
Golda Meir	A leader in the Israeli government until her death at 80

WIDOW AND WIDOWER: DEATH AND GRIEF

A surviving spouse experiences one of life's greatest emotional and social losses. Even a long-lasting marriage with some sense of good fortune for many years does not offer protection from the shattering emotional experience. There does not seem to be any practice for being grief-stricken.

The anguish is undoubtedly increased by a general taboo against discussion of death. Partly because of greatly reduced mortality rates at all younger ages, many of us are left protected from a personal encounter with death until late in life. The fact of dying is cloaked with euphemisms—"passed away," "the departed," "gone to the great beyond," "the big sleep." Only toilet functions and sexual matters in our society are similarly surrounded by anxious whispers, the exclusion of children from straightforward explanations, and a steadfast refusal to admit the topic into everyday life, as if not looking might make it go away.

To our great advantage, Kubler-Ross (1969, 1974, 1975) has accomplished for death and dying some of the legitimizing for study and discussion that Kinsey (1948) did for sex. Kubler-Ross's psychiatric work with the dying and their families led her to suggest a pattern of reactions both for those confronting their own death and for those coping with the death of a loved one. The cycle of "stages" is necessary and seems to be predictable, dealing with a series of themes that Kubler-Ross would have us regard as a developmental *life-process*. As a matter of fact, the title of one of her books is *Death: The Final Stage of Growth* (1975). Ideally, each phase of coping with grief ought to be completed, but can easily become short circuited, leaving the "grief work" unfinished.

The Process of Dying

Shock and Denial

The first reaction may consist of a refusal to admit that one is dying, or, for the widowed, there are some disturbing episodes of "hearing" or "seeing" the lost partner. Both patient and widowed partner need the steady support of other people during this period. A patient should be reassured that everything possible is being done, that hope is never surrendered, and that he or she will not be left to suffer alone, ever. A widowed partner in the initial shock of experiencing the loss of a loved one needs the physical presence of others.

Anger

Following the shock and denial, there is typically a stage of anger. "Why me?" is the unanswerable question of both the dying and the survivor. "Why do I have to die?" or "Why did I have to be left alone?" It is often a troubling source of guilt as intense anger of a dying person is directed at loved ones for being alive and healthy, or by a grieving spouse, toward the one who "went off and left me with all these problems." Anger spills over onto the medical staff for fancied neglect, onto the caring friends for not being able to "know how it is," onto the whole world for going about its business as if nothing had happened. A devastating sense of unfairness and injustice predominates. For those who are attempting to offer support, the essential knowledge is that this stage must be expressed and worked through. There are no answers to the questions raised; each of us must find answers for the self, but a hand to hold and an ear to listen can help.

Bargaining

This stage is likely to follow, a poignant time of "if only." The patient begins to come to grips with the reality and wishes for a little more time—to see a son graduate, to share a holiday. For the bereaved, this is a stage of inexpressible longing and regret. "If only I had tried harder to make him happy." "If only she could return for just a little while."

Depression

This stage represents the grief and sorrow about the loss. For the patient, there is need to mourn, which is no less keen than that of a survivor. The sense of hopeless despair is likely to come in great waves (Schneidman, 1971); there is the feeling that one will never be happy again. It is a difficult period to attempt to assist. All of us become anxious about our inability to set things right in the face of death and its heavy emotion. This makes it hard for dying patients or for surviving partners to obtain the quiet empathy and companionship that are so desperately needed. Grief is too often a lonely road because those who could help do not realize that they don't have to do anything except *be* there. One of Kubler-Ross's good contributions has been to teach the importance of "living through" the various stages so that others become more knowledgeable and can better sustain those who are grief-stricken.

Acceptance

Finally, after the emotional storms (provided these have been expressed and experienced fully), there will come a reintegration, an acceptance. The patient often enters a quiet tranquility, reaffirming life as good, with a good end. For widows or widowers, there will be a glimmer of the fact that one has survived and life is still waiting to be lived. It will not be the same, of course; it is unlikely that mourning the death of someone you love ever ceases entirely. But the process of experiencing loss and facing your own mortality is a basic aspect of life itself—a necessary reminder of our relatedness and need for each other as humans, embarked on the same journey, each toward the same destination.

Because of the disparity in mortality rates, most surviving spouses are women. A study of 300 widows living in the Middle West, all past age 50 (Lopata, 1973) revealed an almost universal sense of loneliness among them. They described the loss of social role and disruption of social relationships, feeling like a "fifth wheel" among coupled friends. The possibility of eventually "re-engaging" the social world seems to depend primarily on both personal and circumstantial factors. Some were able to build a new lifestyle with considerable support from family and friends. These women tended to be the best educated of the sample. Some accepted a "widow status," usually in the group of married couples, whereas some retreated into a more constricted existence. For the most part, the "reduced-life" individuals were the least educated and lowest on the socioeconomic scale.

Lopata (1973) suggests that those who wish to help a new widow need to be able to listen to her grief, attempt to include her in activities, and act as a sounding board for decisions that must be made. These ought to be "walked through" verbally many times before any major change is put into effect. Lopata believes that at least a full year should pass before actual implementation of such a change as a new location. By that time, a widow's outlook and status will have stabilized and become more comfortable, enabling her decisions to be better considered.

The loss of a spouse is sometimes thought to be more traumatic for men than it is for women. Men see fewer of their friends losing wives to death and are therefore even less prepared for the occurrence than women. An older man is unlikely to have acquired homemaking skills, and even the task of making breakfast may seem wholly impossible. Widowed men do not tend to stay widowed for long, however. They remarry at six times the rate for widowed women (Treas, 1976). Some of this difference is due to the fact that there are nine times as many women as men who have lost their mates (Duvall, 1971). Another factor is the tendency for the men to select younger brides: 20 per cent of the remarrying men over the age of 65 selected women who had not yet reached their mid-40s (Treas, 1976).

Remarriage

Remarriages contracted late in life tend to be very successful, despite the fact that society is not wholly approving. McKain (1969) located 100 Connecticut remarriages in which the wives were at least 60 years old and the husbands at least 65 at the time the marriage was formalized. The marriages were followed for 6 years with regularly scheduled interviews. The variable that was shown to be most significantly related to the success of the marriage was the approval of children and friends. Other variables that figured significantly were the partners' having known each other for some length of time ("the longer the better"), having sufficient income, and possessing two personality structures that complemented each other in terms of reactions to aging and to their life together.

HOW FARE THE ELDERS OF OUR LAND?

Better, it appears, than some of the ageism-provoked expectations, but still with too many areas of concern and worry. Of all older Americans, 14 per cent are living below the poverty level: This is somewhat better than the 20 per cent who fell below the official low-income mark in 1971, but still an unfortunate statistic when we consider that many of these people retired thinking they would be financially comfortable, only to see their income eroded by inflation (*U.S News & World Report*, September 1, 1980). The majority of the elderly poor are women living alone. Current estimates count about 5 million women past the age of 65 with yearly incomes below $3000 (Porter, 1980a). For these women and the 6 per cent of elderly men who live alone, isolation is a major problem. Another concern is the constant fear of becoming a victim of crime (Cutler and Harootyan, 1977).

A happier set of statistics suggests the fact that the elders as a group are healthier and more active than ever before. Since 1950, life expectancy for an individual who had become 50 years old has increased by more than 3 years. The death rate for those age 85 and older has declined even faster, falling 26.3 per cent between the years 1966 and 1977, a drop that is steeper than the 6.5 per cent mortality rate decline during the same period for persons aged 25 to 34 (*Providence Journal*, October 9, 1980).

Only a small number of the elderly are institutionalized, and even that proportion has decreased. In 1971 about 7.6 per cent of the older men and women were living in homes for the aged today only some 5 per cent of the aging population live in institutions. These elders typically have no family whatsoever; almost 80 per cent of the home health care given to noninstitutionalized elderly people is provided by their own families (Porter, 1980c).

Another factor leaning toward positive outlook is the fact that the elders are achieving some political power in the same way that other groups have had to bid for a voice in decisions that affect them—by banding together and making certain that elected officials know their potential impact at the polls. In state after state, legislation with regard to help with utility bills, reduced property taxes, transportation to shopping, senior citizens centers, and medical clinics has been enacted with the help of "gray power." On the national level, the new law that forbids forced retirement at 65 because of age came about in response to extensive lobbying by seniors. They have also successfully headed off proposals to cut into the size of Social Security benefit increases that are tied to the rate of inflation.

REQUIREMENTS FOR SUCCESSFUL AGING

A study of aging at Duke University (Palomar, 1974) found four important predictors for satisfactory last years:
1. Maintaining a role in society.
2. Holding a positive view of life and positive self-image.
3. Maintaining moderately good physical health.
4. Being a nonsmoker.

The last three requisites seem to be primarily personal and individual matters. The first, however, implies a certain amount of societal "permission." A ban on mandatory retirement at age 65 is certainly a great step in the direction of ensuring a continuing posture of productivity and worth for those who choose to continue to work. (The congressman who was instrumental in obtaining this important piece of legislation, Rep. Claude Pepper of Florida, was himself 78 when the bill was passed.)

There are those who look forward to early retirement, according to some surveys taken in the early 1970s. However, they seem to be, for the most part, individuals in dead-end jobs that they dislike (Kreps, 1971; Pyron and Manion, 1970). Other studies have found that the "work ethic" is still important. Wertheimer (1973) found that 90 per cent of the men and 82 per cent of the women interviewed (ages ranging from 46 to 71) indicated that they would continue working if permitted even if financial circumstances allowed retirement. Another study of leisure-time activities (Pfeiffer and Davis, 1974)

Maintaining a useful role in society and being permitted to work are central to an older person's ability to remain healthy and happy.

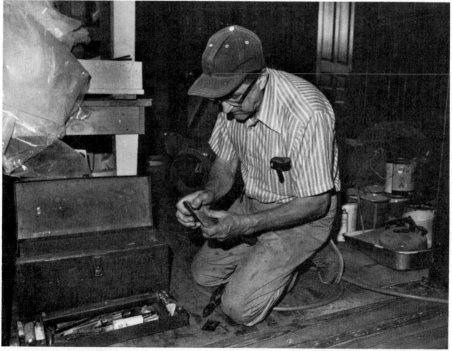

J. V. Barry

concluded that the subjects, aging and in good health, reported deriving more satisfaction from their work than from any of their leisure activities and expressed wishes to continue working as long as they possibly could.

With this kind of emphasis upon work and its place in one's life, it seems clear that it will take more than the usual "getting ready for retirement" seminars to prepare elders for relinquishing their jobs. Perhaps the preparation ought to be directed toward ways of obtaining new kinds of jobs rather than leisure-time occupations. Some communities are already engaging the talents of retired people in a variety of social service efforts ranging from day-care centers to hospitals. Individualized contacts with other seniors who need a helping hand would be another creative outlet. If such efforts can lead to full-fledged part-time jobs for pay, so much the better. Sylvia Porter (1980b), the financial columnist, insists that part-time employment is one solution to the inflationary drag on incomes of the elderly. Of equal importance, perhaps, would be the possibility of fulfilling a meaningful role in the community and providing necessary services. Especially as seniors are incorporated into care-giving for others who are less able, it would become possible for larger numbers of elderly to remain in their homes.

Another major contribution to the seniors' role in society and their positive views of life and self could come from educational institutions. This is not a new idea, of course. Large numbers of older students are being welcomed to colleges and universities these days. To share notes with someone old enough to be your grandparent is becoming fairly commonplace for many college students. However, there is need for a much broader effort in this regard. The elders now in college are those for whom money and transportation do not raise problems. Institutions could reach many more by sending teachers out to senior centers, retirement villages, and neighborhoods. Colleges and universities might begin to use television as the educational medium it once promised to be for senior instruction and might also explore the possibility of promoting senior housing and retirement centers on campus, especially as the numbers of younger students dwindle.

Our society has always counted on education to bridge other developmental hurdles. So it might look to education to assist with a number of the problems of elders, from economic to psychological. As funds have been solicited for the education of younger, they could also be solicited for the education of older students. The coming "lean years" for higher education would seem to be an ideal time for fostering a new mix of students, the younger and their elders. The two age groups could have much to teach and learn from each other!

GLOSSARY

ALARM REACTION   The first stage of the general adaptation syndrome, during which the body defenses are activated by the energy of the sympathetic nervous system and hormones of the adrenal glands.

BOUNDARY SETTING   A retrospective modality (a form of reminiscing) by which an elderly person seems to be attempting to adjust to new limits and psychological boundaries.

EXHAUSTION   The third stage of the general adaptation syndrome. If an emergency continues long enough, all available resources are depleted and an overwhelming counter-reaction may occur, leading to general collapse and even death.

GENERAL ADAPTATION SYNDROME   The term used by Hans Selye to describe a three-stage reaction that mobilizes the body's resources to meet an injurious agent or set of circumstances.

GENERAL LIFE REVIEW   Kastenbaum's term for the function of reminiscing by elders, suggesting that it serves the purpose of getting a lifetime in order.

HISTORICAL TIME The events that occur during a particular lifetime in a society. In part, these events give an individual consciousness of his or her generation.

INTEGRITY Erikson's description of the "ripening of the fruit of the seven (previous) stages." It is the acceptance of one's one and only life cycle and is characterized by emotional integration and dignity, without fear of death.

LIFETIME The biological dimension of the life cycle.

PERPETUATION OF THE PAST A retrospective modality (a form of reminiscing) that enables the elder to relive selected events of the past, usually those with an emotional content.

REPLAYING Kastenbaum's term for the tendency of an elder to tell a favorite anecedote over and over again, enjoying it each time.

RESISTANCE The second stage of the general adaptation syndrome. It is characterized by continued arousal, during which body repairs are effected and defenses are maintained.

RETROSPECTIVE MODALITIES Forms of reminiscing that seem to serve a purpose in the lives of elders.

SOCIAL TIME The way in which societies define and regulate the various ages of the life cycle.

VALIDATION A form of reminiscing (a retrospective modality) by which the elder seems to search the past for courage to face the present, looking for instances in which one was successful before.

REFERENCES

Bayley, N.: Cognition and aging. In Schaie, K. W. (ed.): *Theory and Methods of Research on Aging.* Morgantown, W. Va.: West Virginia University, 1968.

Baltes, P. B., Labouvie, G. J.: Adult development of intellectual performance: Description, explanation and modification. In Eisdorfer, C., Lawton, M. P. (eds.): *The Psychology of Adult Development and Aging.* Washington, D.C.: The American Psychological Association, 1973.

Beard, V. B.: Some characteristics of recent memory of centenarians. *Journal of Gerontology,* 23:23–30, 1968.

Birkhill, W. R., Schaie, K. W.: The effect of differential reinforcement of cautiousness in intellectual performance among the elderly. *Journal of Gerontology,* 30:578–585, 1975.

Birren, J. E.: *The Psychology of Aging.* Englewood Cliffs, N.J.: Prentice-Hall, 1964.

Birren, J. E.: Translations in gerontology—from lab to life: Psychophysiology and speed of response. *American Psychologist,* 29:808–815, 1974.

Botwinick, J., Storant, M.: *Memory, Related Functions and Age.* Springfield, Ill.: Charles C Thomas, 1974.

Bromley, D. B.: *The psychology of human aging.* (2nd ed.). Middlesex, England: Penguin, 1974.

Craig, F. I. M.: Age differences in human memory. In Birren, J. E., Schaie, K. W. (eds.): *Handbook of the Psychology of Aging.* New York: Van Nostrand Reinhold, 1977.

Cutler, N. E., Harootyan, R. A.: Demography of the aging. In Hulicka, I. M. (ed.): *Psychology and Sociology of Aging.* New York: Cromwell, 1977.

Cutler, S. J.: Voluntary association participation and life satisfaction: A cautionary research note. *Journal of Gerontology,* 28:96–100, 1973.

Denny, P.: Cellular biology of aging. In Woodruff, D. S. Birren, J. E. (eds.): *Aging: Scientific Perspectives and Social Issues.* New York: Van Nostrand, 1975.

DeVries, H. A.: Physiology of exercise and aging. In Woodruff, D. S., Birren, J. E. (eds.): *Aging: Scientific Perspectives and Social Issues.* New York: Van Nostrand, 1975.

Duvall, E. M.: *Family Development* (4th ed.). Philadelphia: J. B. Lippincott, 1971.

Edwards, J. N., Klemmack, D. L.: Correlates of life and satisfaction: A re-examination. *Journal of Gerontology,* 28:497–502, 1973.

Erikson, E.: *Childhood and Society.* New York: W. W. Norton Company, 1950.

Goldfarb, A. I., Hochstadt, H. J., Jacobson, H. H., Weinstein, E. A.: Hyperbaric oxygen treatment of organic mental symptoms in aged persons. *Journal of Gerontology,* 27:212–217, 1972.

Hicks, L. H., Birren, J. E: Aging, brain damage and psychomotor slowing. *Psychological Bulletin,* 74:377–396, 1970.

Hebb, D. O.: Watching myself get old. *Psychology Today,* 12(6):15–23, 1978.

Hendricks, J., Hendricks, C. D.: *Aging in a Mass Society.* Cambridge, Mass.: Winthrop, 1977.

Horn, J. L.: Organization of data on life-span development of human abilities. In Goulet, L. R., Baltes, P. B. (eds.): *Life Span Developmental Psychology: Research and Theory.* New York: Academic Press, 1970.

Hulicka, I. M., Grossman, J. L.: Age-group comparisons for the use of mediators in impaired-associate learning. *Journal of Gerontology*, 22:46–51, 1967.

Hulicka, I. M., Weiss, R. L.: Age differences in retention as a function of learning. *Journal of Consulting Psychology*, 29:125–129, 1965.

Jacobs, E. A., Winter, P. M., Alvis, H. J., Small, S. M.: Hyper-oxygenation effect on cognitive functioning of the aged. *New England Journal of Medicine*, 281:753–757, 1969.

Kastenbaum, R.: *Humans Developing: A Life-Span Perspective.* Boston: Allyn & Bacon, 1979.

Kinsey, A.: *Sexual Behavior in the Human Male.* Philadelphia: W. B. Saunders Company, 1948.

Kreps, J.: *Lifetime Allocation of Work and Income. Essays in the Economics of Aging.* Durham, N.C.: Duke University Press, 1971.

Kubler-Ross, E.: *On Death and Dying.* New York: Macmillan, 1969.

Kubler-Ross, E.: *Questions and Answers on Death and Dying.* New York: Macmillan, 1974.

Kubler-Ross, E.: *Death: The Final Stage of Growth.* Englewood Cliffs, N.J.: Prentice-Hall, 1975.

Leaf, A.: Growing old. *Scientific American*, 299(3):44–53, 1973.

Life begins at fifty five. *U.S. News & World Report*, September 1, 1980, p. 50–61.

Lopata, H.: Living through widowhood. *Psychology Today*, 7(2):87–98, 1973.

Lutwak, L.: Nutritional aspects of osteoporosis. *Journal of the American Geriatric Society*, 17:115, 1969.

McKain, W. C.: *Retirement Marriages.* Storrs, Conn: Storrs Agricultural Experimental Station. University of Connecticut, 1969.

Murdock, B. B.: Recent developments in short-term memory. *British Journal of Psychology*, 58:421–433, 1967.

Nardi, A. H.: Person-perception research and the perception of life-span development. In Baltes, P. B., Schaie, K. W. (eds.): *Life-Span Developmental Psychology: Personality and Socialization*, New York: Academic Press, 1973.

Neugarten, B. L.: Adult personality; Toward a psychology of the life cycle. In Neugarten, B. L. (ed.): *Middle Age and Aging: A Reader in Social Psychology.* Chicago: University of Chicago Press, 1968.

Neugarten, B. L.: Personality and aging. In Birren, J. E., Schaie, K. W. (eds.): *Handbook of the Psychology of Aging.* New York: Van Nostrand Reinhold, 1977.

Neugarten, B., Datan, N.: Sociological perspectives of the life cycle. In Baltes, P. B., Schaie, K. W. (eds.): *Life-Span Developmental Psychology: Personality and Socialization.* New York: Academic Press, 1973.

Owens, W. A.: Age and mental abilities: A second adult follow-up. *Journal of Educational Psychology*, 57(6):311–325, 1966.

Palmore, E.: The effects of aging on activities and attitudes. *Gerontologist*, 8:259–263, 1968.

Palmore, E.: Physical, mental and social factors in predicting longevity. *The Geronologist*, 9:103–108, 1969.

Palmore, E.: Predicting longevity: A new method. In Palmore, E. (ed.): *Normal Aging, II.* Durham, N.C.: Duke University Press, 1974.

Palmore, E. *Normal Aging.* Durham, N.C.: Duke University Press, 1970.

Pfeiffer, E., Davis, G. C.: The use of leisure time in middle life. In Palmore, E. (ed): *Normal aging.* II. Durham, N.C.: Duke University Press, 1974.

Porter, S.: Number of seniors to grow in future. *Providence Journal*, July 28, 1980a, pp. A–12.

Porter, S.: Elderly may find that only solution to inflation is to go back to work. *Providence Journal*, July 29, 1980b, p. A–13.

Porter, S.: For most elderly, quality of home care is the key. *Providence Journal*, July 30, 1980c, pp. A–12.

Pyron, H. C., Manion, U. V.: The company, the individual and the decision to retire. *Industrial Gerontology*, No. 7, 43–44, 1970.

Resnick, H. L. P., Cantor, J. M.: Suicide and aging. *Journal of the American Geriatrics Society*, 18:152–158, 1970.

Riegel, K. F., Riegel, R. M.: Development, drop and death. *Developmental Psychology*, 6:306–319, 1972.

Rockstein, M.: The biology of aging in humans: An overview. In Rockstein, M. (ed.): *The Physiology and Pathology of Human Aging.* New York: Academic Press, 1975.

Schaie, K. W.: Age changes in adult intelligence. In Woodruff, D. S., Birren, J. E. (eds.): *Aging: Scientific Perspectives and Social Issues.* New York: Academic Press, 1975.

Schneidman, E. S.: You and death. *Psychology Today*, 5(6):43–45, 1971.

Schonfield, D.: Future commitments and successful aging. *Journal of Gerontology*, 28:189–196, 1973.

Schonfield, D., Robertson, B. A.: Memory storage and aging. *Canadian Journal of Psychology*, 20:228–236, 1966.

Selye, H.: *The Stress of Life.* New York: McGraw-Hill, 1956.

Selye, H.: Stress and Aging. *Journal of American Geriatrics Society*, 25(3):262–264, 1970.

Seyle, H.: The evolution of the stress concept. *American Scientist*, 61:692–699, 1973.

Shock, N. W.: Age with a future. *The Gerontologist*, 8:147–152, 1968.

Shock, N. W.: Physiological theories of aging. In Rockstein, E. A. (ed.): *Theoretical Aspects of Aging.* New York: Academic Press, 1974.

The return of the prodigals. *Time*, October 13, 1980, p. 118.

The very old living longer. *Providence Journal*, October 9, 1980, p. A–6.

Treas, J., VanHilst, A.: Marriage and remarriage among older Americans. *The Gerontologist*, 16:132–136, 1976.

United States Bureau of the Census. *Educational Attainment:* March 1972. Washington, D.C., 1972.

United States Department of Health, Education and Welfare. National Clearing House on Aging. *Facts About Older Americans*, 1976. DHEW Publications, No. (OHD), 77–20006, Washington, D.C., 1976a.

United States Department of Health, Education and Welfare. *Health, United States*, 1975. DHEW Publications, No. (HRA), 76–1232. Rockville, Md.: National Center for Health Statistics, 1976b.

Weg, R. B.: Changing physiology of aging: Normal and pathological. In Woodruff, D. S., Birren, J. E. (eds.): *Aging: Scientific Perspectives and Social Issues.* New York: Van Nostrand, 1975.

Wertheimer, B.: A pilot center for workers at mid-career. *Industrial Gerontology*, No. 17, 67–71, 1973.

HEALTH CONCERNS IN THE OLDER ADULT

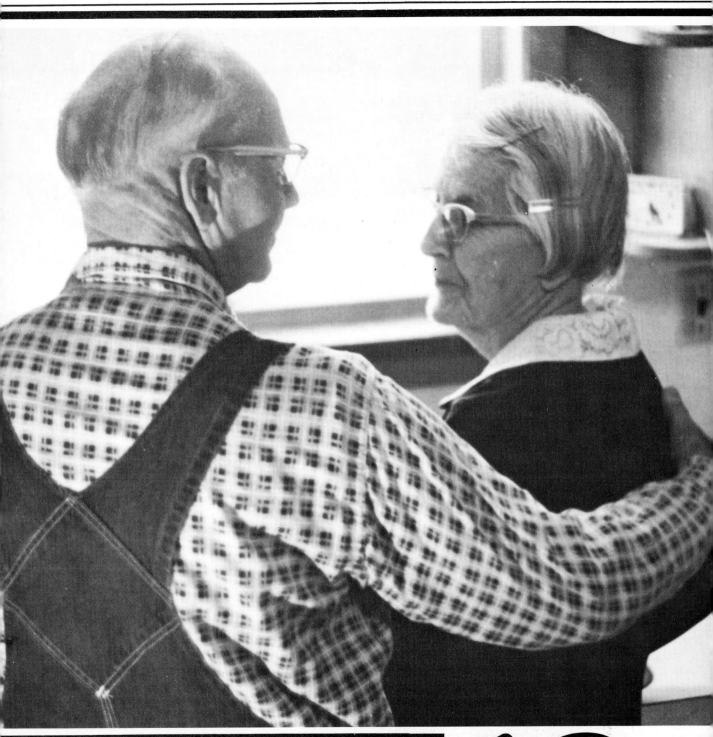

CHAPTER 16

Older people are our ties with the past, our continuity as humans, and our windows into history. When you think of old age, what enters your mind? Once you are old, are you "down the drain" or "over the hill?" Do you envision older people as frail, incompetent inhabitants of nursing homes? Does "old" necessarily mean illness, decreased functioning, and senility?

Old age is neither inherently unpleasant nor inherently trouble free. It is another stage of life, with problems, joys, and satisfactions. The way in which old age is experienced has a great deal to do with an individual's personality, expectations, physical health, financial security, earlier life experiences, medical care, support networks, and ability to accept the realities of aging and eventual death. This reality may also mean isolation, poor nutrition, instant poverty if major illness strikes, personal and physical losses, despair, and depression in a society that tends to extol its young and sometimes to ignore its elderly.

The extremes can be disconcerting. Imagine a 91-year-old woman, keen of memory and long on tales of her childhood on a large Michigan farm. Pacemaker ticking, she lives alone, with support and monitoring from family and friends. She is lucky. Picture also the "bag" people of major metropolitan areas. Frequently de-institutionalized in an effort by officials to empty mental hospitals and return their inhabitants to the "community," these people literally live on the steps of the postoffice, under the overhang of the bus terminal, or in the subways when the weather gets cold.

Relatively comfortable or destitute, active or infirm, sunny or cantankerous, together with all the variations between these extremes, the elderly are very much with us, representing a veritable population explosion in our society. Butler (1975) states that in 1975, 10 per cent of the population in the United States was over 65 years of age. When you add the 20 per cent in the 45- to 65-year age range, you can see the rationale for estimates that 15 per cent of the total population will be over 65 years of age in the year 2000.

Our concept of older people may be to see them as infirm and physically needy. On the contrary, 81 per cent of those over 65 are fully ambulatory, living independently on their own (Butler, 1975). Ninety-five per cent live in the community and, at any time, only 5 per cent are in nursing homes, chronic disease hospitals, and other institutions. For those able to remain in the community, the problems of adequate nutrition, medical care, safety, and isolation may be the stumbling blocks in the way of aging in a dignified, relatively healthy fashion.

In this chapter, we will be emphasizing the following matters:
1. Needed services.
2. Physical and physiological changes.
3. Medical issues.
4. The role of medical professionals in the care of older people.

PROVIDING SERVICES

The care and nurturing of older people can be time consuming, frustrating, and repetitive. In a medical setting, such as an outpatient clinic that is frequently rushed and impersonal, the older person may wait for what seems like an eternity for essential care, to see the doctor, to get medication, or even to talk to someone.

Older people need the same basic services needed by all of us. They must eat and must have good transportation, recreation, safety, and, in particular, readily accessible, good medical care. As Butler (1975) states: "We know what services the elderly need. The financing and logistical problems are not insoluble. When they are solved, society will save money by preventing unnecessary institutionalization."

Some of the services most essential to the elderly are described in the next section.

Referral Services

A referral service would provide the elderly and their families access to a variety of helping agencies along with information on how much they cost, their locations, and eligibility requirements. Such a referral network could be part of each Social Security or local welfare office.

Home Health Agency

A major method of maintaining independent living for older people is to help them remain at home. They may need regular medical visits, meals, homemaking help, and social contacts to fill the void left by the loss of family and friends. Homemaker and home health aides provide a variety of services, including nursing duties, cooking, laundry, and other housekeeping functions. These aides are supervised by nurses and other agency personnel. In 1971, less than 1 per cent of all medical expenditures went for home health care. Sometimes participation has been made more difficult by the reluctance of governmental funding agencies to authorize payments for these services.

Home Visits

By Physicians.   In 1972, fewer than half the physicians in the United States made house calls, and most of those who did lived in rural areas (Butler, 1975). Many physicians believe that they can provide better care in their office or in a clinic. Many elderly people, however, are too ill, too confused, or too frightened to go either to the office or to the hospital. In instances when fee-for-service house call agencies have been set up, the price per call has been prohibitively expensive for most older people.

As governmental support for medical education decreases and medical school costs continue to rise, physicians will find themselves in the position of having to work in lucrative suburban practices to pay off the staggering educational loans accumulated during their training. Under such constraints, there are likely to be fewer and fewer physicians who will be available to attend to the plight of poor elderly city dwellers or isolated rural people who have no transportation to get to medical centers. When economics do not favor sustaining human resources, it is often the least powerful in the society who suffer the most.

By Nurses.   Nurses have traditionally been the backbone of home health care. Public health nurses funded by municipal governments and the Visiting Nurse Association, a private organization, provide much of the medical support of the elderly in their homes. The pay does not keep pace with that offered by hospitals, and funding can be problematical. However, these services are essential and economically cost-efficient when compared with the cost of institutionalization. What cannot be measured in dollars is the sense of self-esteem that is fostered in people who are enabled to manage on their own when adequate support service is available.

Nutritional Services

The nutritional needs of the healthy elderly are similar to those much younger. Difficulty in maintaining nutritional standards arises when people are too ill, too frightened to go out, or too poor to afford even a minimal diet.

Meals-on-wheels and community feeding programs not only provide low-cost, nutritional meals, but also nourish with human contact. In one neighborhood of New York City, there are 37,000 elderly people. Of 2,000 eligible homebound, only 215 receive one meal brought daily to them. The average age of the recipient is 83, and 15 are over 90. All want to stay in their own homes as long as possible. Many venture out only to see a physician and make occasional visits to family members when they are able (*New York Times*, 1981).

Who will advocate for the hungry poor in our society? By becoming sensitive to those who are in need and by insisting, through political channels, that people in our affluent society should not starve, the medical worker can have an effect on the well-being and the lives of many.

PHYSICAL CHANGES

Attitudes Toward Aging

Physiological aging in the elderly is not orderly and does not affect all systems equally, either in terms of severity or sequence. Some changes are the consequence of simply growing older; others are manifestations of new diseases or the continuation and increasingly disabling effects of chronic diseases with symptoms that were present during middle age, but did not then impinge on function or *homeostasis* (physiological equilibrium). In addition, there are certain older people who perceive themselves as healthy when, in fact, they may have some biological disturbances.

Stenbach and co-workers (1978) report on a study involving 102 subjects, 31 men and 71 women, in Helsinki, Finland. All were in their 70s. They were interviewed to determine how they felt about their physical condition. Thirty-one subjects reported no chronic illness; the remaining 71 subjects suffered from 133 chronic diseases and 48 functional disturbances as diagnosed by a physician. When interviewed, all subjects were asked to identify themselves as either "well" or "sick." Wellness was defined as being well enough to do what he or she wanted to do even though ill health might be present. Of the 71 who had some chronic diseases, 40 identified themselves as "well." Six people who actually appeared sickly denied any illness. All of these people were actively engaged in social activities, were working or were otherwise very involved in the process of living. Many of the subjects considered themselves "middle aged." Almost all who identified themselves as "old" belonged to the "sickly" group. These researchers concluded that "to a considerable degree, this elderly population feels healthy and behaves that way."

This study provides an insight in assessing the health status of the elderly, for it helps put into perspective our own expectations of what "old age" is, how older people respond, how we respond to them, and how important it is for health professionals to check out their assumptions with elderly clients before labeling them as "healthy" or "ill."

Nervous System

Most neurological changes affect the central nervous system. Changes may affect balance and loss of memory for recent events and may cause some sensory deprivation, particularly in terms of sensitivity to heat and cold. Cognitive functioning, however, does not necessarily diminish as rapidly as previously thought. Ford and Roth (1977) found that the best way of assessing cognitive functioning is by longitudinal studies in which the same subjects are followed for many years. From their studies, it appears congitive functioning persists to a great extent. Also, elderly people may have increased difficulty learning new material, but they are able to retain what they learn. Older people also tend to remember events that occurred long ago better than more recent events. However, in many cases, memory defects are small in physically healthy and active elderly people. It is therefore important not to view a decline in mental ability as an inevitable consequence of aging, but to recognize that there might be some physiological reason for the decline.

Respiratory System

Changes in respiratory function that can be attributed to aging must be differentiated from those that occur in a disease process. The aging lung has reduced efficiency in expelling air (Lynne-Davis, 1977). This decrease in efficiency results in a less than complete emptying of the lungs and in reduced *vital capacity* (the maximum amount of air that can be inhaled and expelled). There is also a decrease in the ability of the lungs to exchange the gases that accumulate in them. This is probably due to a decrease in the flexibility of the chest wall, with progressive stiffening.

Cardiovascular System

The heart atrophies (gets smaller) relatively little during the aging process. Age pigments (called *lipofuscins*) that appear on the surface of the heart apparently have little effect on heart functioning. (Nejat and Grief, 1976). What seems to occur most frequently is a narrowing of the coronary blood vessels owing to fatty deposits, with subsequent reduced blood flow to and from the heart, a poorly nourished heart muscle, and an increased susceptibility to *myocardial infarction* (a loss of blood to the muscle with subsequent damage to that muscle).

Gastrointestinal System

Gastrointestinal changes in the elderly are most often manifested in a slowing of peristalsis, of elimination, of absorption of nutrients, and of enzyme action on food.

Genitourinary System

Fifty per cent of all elderly men have some *hypertrophy* (enlargement) of the prostate. This condition, in turn, may produce problems in urinating, in the retention of urine in the bladder, and in recurrent prostatic infections. In addition, there is a 50 per cent decrease in the amount of blood flowing through the kidneys as well as a decrease in the number of functioning nephrons (Boland et al., 1979).

For women, the major genitourinary problem may be a prolapse of the bladder, which is caused by pressure from the uterus with slackening uterine muscles. This prolapse may cause leakage of urine when exercising, sneezing, stumbling, and so on. Many women can help themselves to better sphincter control by consciously stopping their flow of urine for a count of 10 before permitting resumption of the flow. This exercise has brought marked relief for many cases of *stress incontinence*. Health care professionals can provide appropriate instruction if the situation warrants. In extreme cases, the bladder may actually protrude into the vagina. Corrective surgery may be required to remedy this condition.

Skeletal System

As people age, they seem to shrink. This shrinkage is due to a thinning of the discs that lie between the vertebrae of the spine. Joints may swell and become tender and painful from *osteoarthritis*. As the neck vertebrae wear and the discs thin, older people may complain of difficulty in turning their heads or of numbness in their arms when cervical nerves are pinched or become inflamed.

Skin

Some of the most obvious signs of aging occur in the skin. The skin tends to lose its elasticity and subcutaneous fatty tissue, becoming wrinkled and lined. Brown spots, larger than freckles, appear on the hands and face. Some of these brownish spots are also caused by the body's reduced ability to replace sun-damaged cells in the skin with new cells. This damage may lead to precancerous lesions, and if severe, to actual skin cancer, one of the most common forms of cancer (Tokuda and Smith, 1976).

Eyes

Eyes age internally as well as externally. Lids become baggy and lose their elasticity. Tear glands may atrophy, causing the eyes to become dry and painful. Although good vision can persist well into old age, *cataracts* are a common occurrence for many. Cataracts are thickened tissue that develops on the lens and causes visual loss.

The retina also suffers from the aging process. The most common problem is a degeneration of that portion of the retina called the *macula*. This degeneration affects 30 per cent of all people over the age of 65. In its severest form, it causes disabling blindness, with vision of 20/200 or less (Wuest et al., 1976).

Glaucoma, another condition affecting the aging eye, occurs in 13 per cent of those over 74 years of age. It is a result of thickening of the meshwork in the eye causing an increased resistance to the outflow of the ocular fluid.

Ears

Advancing age is the most common cause of hearing loss. Approximately 23 per cent of men and women between 65 and 74 and 40 per cent of those over 75 years of age report some hearing impairment (Powers and Powers, 1978). Even with some deterioration in hearing, the majority of the subjects interviewed in the Powers' study maintained an active life.

MEDICAL ISSUES

Periodic Physical Examinations

As the proportion of elderly people in the United States continues to rise, some decisions will have to be made concerning the usefulness of periodic physical examinations. Ryan (1978) concludes that people over 70 should have an annual examination with the following stipulations:

1. Cost-benefits should be considered.
2. Psychosocial assessments are as important as physical assessments.

3. Physicians should be cautious about overzealous treatment of the elderly.

4. No health examination should be time consuming, expensive, or uncomfortable for the patient.

For many older people, the discovery of yet another physical problem is not as important as whether or not they have adequate food, clothing, and security. Because so many older people have multiple medical problems, many physicians find it difficult to allow adequate time to manage each individual problem. In addition, many old people simply do not go to the physician, thus remaining at risk and perhaps eventually requiring more extensive intervention.

Home Assessments

In some countries, nurses have taken over the role of screening, evaluating, and following geriatric patients in their homes. Williams (1977) describes several such programs that utilize specially trained geriatric nurse practitioners or visiting nurses.

Using a questionnaire designed to find out information about medical and psycho-social problems, nurses involved in such a program in Iowa also have done routine urinalysis, red blood cell counts, and simple vision and hearing tests, as well as recording temperature, blood pressure, and other vital statistics. This information is discussed with the physician in charge of the program, and a nursing-care plan is drawn up. When medical problems are discovered, the patient is examined in the clinic by the physician. Community resources are mobilized according to need, and monthly checkups are initiated by the nurse.

These home visits provide much needed attention and medical supervision while focusing on specific problems in a setting that is comfortable and secure for the patient. Patients have also reported that it was easier and less intimidating for them to communicate with a nurse rather than a physician. They were pleased not to have to make an appointment or travel to a clinic except on rare occasions and to be able to ask questions and understand answers and directions.

Sensory Loss

As mentioned, many people suffer from a variety of sensory losses as they age. Memory loss may be attributed to a decrease in electrical activity within the brain. When working with people who have diminished acuity in seeing and hearing as well as a diminished sensation of pain, medical personnel should be particularly careful when giving directions for medication or for any medical procedure. Instructions should be given in short sentences, as simply as possible, and patients should be asked to repeat them. Orders should be written in large letters and brief sentences, and, if possible, should include pictures of what is intended to be done. A good example would be the directions needed to help diabetic patients administer their own insulin. Setp-by-step pictures with large, clear statements under each one can be helpful. It is essential for such patients to practice using a syringe during the office visit.

For people who have to take medication at a particular time, a small box, divided into time partitions with the specific medication in each time slot, along with clearly printed captions, can be helpful for those with a vision loss. Telephones with amplification and large numbers are available for those with seeing and hearing difficulties.

Elderly people also run the risk of burning themselves because of the loss of pain sensation. Because they frequently feel cold, many old people use heating pads and other devices that carry a risk of serious injury. Taping all but the safe setting on a heating pad might prevent such difficulty. In each case, health care workers must be innovative and sensitive to the special requirements for their patients' safety.

Nutritional Issues

Because digestive problems are common among the elderly, attention should be given to the kinds of foods that are appealing, how easy they are to prepare, whether stores are accessible, and how skillful the patient is in managing meal preparation.

Elderly persons may need to be referred to nutritionists for assistance and monitoring. Many times, complaints of tiredness, irritability, headaches, and depression can be directly traced to poor nutrition. According to Grills (1977), environmental factors such as isolation, loss of family, poor dentition, and food preferences have a great deal to do with the especially poor nutrition of many elderly women.

Calcium Deficiency

Degenerative diseases are also affected by diet. *Osteoporosis*, a disease characterized by fragile, porous, easily broken bones, is particularly common among elderly women. Low dietary intake of calcium is one of the risk factors associated with the disease. Other causes of primary osteoporosis are:

1. High phosphorus intake.
2. Vitamin D deficiency (from not enough skin exposure to sunshine).
3. Postmenopausal hormone deficiency.
4. Inactivity and bed rest.
5. Gastrectomy (removal of most of the stomach) (Jowsey, 1977).

Grill also suggests, based on studies done by several researchers, that the human body cannot adapt to less than optimal levels of calcium without risk of disabling fractures. Table 16–1 lists the foods with relatively high calcium content.

Heart Disease

Whereas men are vulnerable to coronary heart disease throughout middle age and beyond, women become more vulnerable after menopause and into old age. High intake of "empty" calories such as sugar, cookies, and pastry, as well as foods high in fat content, accompanied by diminished activity, all play a role in the rise in incidence of heart disease.

TABLE 16–1 CALCIUM SOURCES

Food	Serving Size	Calcium (mg per Serving)	RDA per Serving* (%)
Cheddar cheese	2 oz.	450	56
Yogurt	1 cup	300	38
Milk (either whole, buttermilk, or 2% skim)	1 cup	290	36
Salmon, canned with bone	3 oz.	220	28
Custard	½ cup	145	18
Pudding made with milk	½ cup	145	18
Greens, cooked	½ cup	125	16
Ice cream	½ cup	100	13
Nuts, chopped	½ cup	60	8
Cottage cheese	¼ cup	50	6
Egg, whole	1	30	4
Peanut butter	2 tbsp.	20	4

*RDA = Recommended daily allowance.

Anemia

Elderly people also tend to eat less meat; this lowers the iron content in the diet, resulting in a common form of anemia. Another cause of anemia is the overuse of aspirin-type medications.

Physical Fitness

As people become older, they tend to exercise less and less. Some are afraid to leave their homes, unsure of their footing, and thus they stay indoors for long periods of time. This sedentary existence reduces aerobic and cardiovascular activity. Older people should be encouraged to walk as much as possible because walking is an excellent form of exercise. Some cities with senior citizen centers have regular exercise groups and even supervised swim programs. Making these programs and activities known and accessible to elderly people is a positive step in health promotion.

Sexual Activity

Older people have the same needs for intimacy and sexual expression as younger people. Griggs (1978) states: "Sexual needs and interest continue into the later years of an individual's life and deserve respect and accommodation if one is to provide total care for the older person. The drive for sexual fulfillment does not diminish with age, particularly if the person has led an active sex life in the past.

Masters and Johnson (1966) have done a great deal of research on the physiological sexual response cycles in both men and women. In aging women, the most common change is in the ability of the vagina to lubricate adequately. As the vagina ages and hormone production decreases, the vagina becomes shorter and narrower, less elastic, and dry. All these changes may cause discomfort during intercourse, but the problem can be remedied with topical application of lubricating creams. Women who remain sexually active have less difficulty than those whose sexual activity ceases completely. For women who are widowed or alone, relationships outside of marriage and sexual activity through methods other than intercourse may be a healthful outlet. Any sexual expression, including masturbation, may be appropriate for some women. If facts are presented in an objective manner without a proposal of compromise of any religious or moral values, it will be easier for women to decide for themselves what seems most comfortable.

The aging man has different sorts of problems, none of which is insurmountable. It takes the average man longer to achieve an erection, to ejaculate, and to become aroused again. The erection might not be as firm as it was when he was younger, and it might take some manual stimulation on the part of his partner to make his penis more erect. The reason for this is that the blood vessels serving the penis, which become engorged during an erection, are not as elastic as they once were. There is also a reduction in the amount of ejaculate, thus leading to a less forceful orgasm (Shearer and Shearer, 1977).

Elderly people who are concerned about their sexual functioning need to know that sexuality encompasses more than an orgasm. It is the essence of intimacy, warmth, and closeness, which might be as important as the sexual act itself. The elderly need to understand that performance is not the most important consideration, for there is nothing that will cause stress and eventual dysfunction faster than the notion that one has to meet some performance standard. What has to be learned are the physiological changes that occur in both men and women, how each can accommodate to meet the partner's needs, and perhaps most important, that sexual activity can continue as long as the people involved want it too. It may well be different, but it is the continuity that is important.

Some older people will think that it is not proper to be interested in sex after the age of 60, and some grown "children" are upset and astounded when they realize that their parents are not only still interested in sexual activity but are, in fact, still sexually active. Elderly patients should feel free to discuss sexual issues and be reassured of their right to feel sexual desire and to continue to engage in sexual activity.

Finally, there is one aspect of sexuality that should be addressed. In all of life, to work is considered separate from having fun. For many, the work ethic holds sway and fun becomes a guilt-ridden activity. "Fun and enjoyment," as Shearer and Shearer state, "are not luxuries; they are necessities to mental health." Depending on the individual's value system, a person's fun may or may not include sexual activity, a natural body function. Our society has grossly distorted the meaning of sexual activity, especially with the older generation.

Drug Usage

Drug overdose and misuse are common problems in the elderly. Often, there is confusion on the part of the patient, combined with the failure of physicians to reduce drug doses as the aging patient develops reduced kidney and liver functioning. Medication labels that all look the same with directions for used typed in small letters add to the confusion when patients try to remember which drug to take and at what intervals. Charts with colored pictures of the drugs to be taken along with large, clearly printed directions for the times when the medications are to be taken are helpful. Patients should rehearse the prescription directions with medical personnel. Prescriptions should contain minimal doses, not only to prevent overuse, but also to ensure that the patient is monitored frequently while on the drug. Dispensers with time and days of the week written clearly or with perforations through which one pill at a time can be removed would also help in keeping track of medications.

Because older patients often take more than one drug at a time, there is a danger of pharmacological interactions and reactions. Frequently, the alert geriatric physician will recognize that what appears to be senile confusion or lethargy is simply a drug reaction or overdose. Eliminating or reducing the dosage sometimes has the remarkable effect of restoring the confused patient to a state of clear thinking. For this reason, all medical personnel working with the elderly should be alert to the possibility of drug-induced problems and report their suspicions to the physician in charge.

Death and Dying

An understanding of death and dying has particular importance for health professionals working with the elderly. As people become older, infirm, and possibly ill, they have a tendency to start to "prepare" for death. It is useful to understand how this preparation may progress and impact on medical personnel. Using the familiar stages of dying as a frame of reference, Esberger (1980) discusses the process.

Stages of Dying

Denial. The previous lifestyle of a person has a direct bearing on how denial of potentially stressful experiences is expressed. This denial may make it difficult for an aged, ill person to accept any medical intervention or help from relatives or health care workers. It is important that time be available to acknowledge the possibility of death gradually.

Anger. Anger is frequently expressed in all directions and may be projected onto those who care for, love, and support the patient. The targets of the anger often are not the cause of the anger. Many patients may feel ignored, neglected, and forgotten and become excessively demanding and childlike. Some may even express resentment and envy of those who are younger or healthier. Patience and a calm approach, as well as a "thick skin," on the part of the caretakers are essential.

Bargaining Stage. After the rage associated with the realization of impending death has passed, some patients may bargain as a way of negotiating a guarantee of continued life. They will be on their best behavior, become model patients, take all their medications, and may plead for a little more time to be alive for a particular event. For those who have been religious in the past, there may be a reawakening of religious convictions and an urge to reconnect with a clergyman. For many, making peace with their deity is of upmost importance and should be respected.

Depression/Preparatory Grief. This stage may be the most difficult one for medical personnel to deal with. With the patient withdrawn and sad, this expression of impending loss and leavetaking may arouse a sense of futility and helplessness in health care personnel. The natural urge is for a caretaker to insist that there is still hope, not despair. But grieving is essential and must be accepted. Sitting quietly while holding a patient's hand can let the patient know that someone is available for comfort and support. It should not be assumed that the quiet patient wants to be alone. The assumption becomes an easy way of avoiding contact because the possibility of death makes everyone feel vulnerable. A depressed patient should not be left alone. The caretaker can marshal the help of family, volunteers, clergy, and friends to visit and maintain an active relationship.

Acceptance. Tired and weak, but peaceful with a quiet expectation, can best describe a patient at this stage, which is one that all dying elderly hopefully experience. Throughout, the nurse or other health care professional becomes an advocate, acting as a liaison between the patient, the physician, and the family, to make sure that this last passage is one of dignity, peaceful and pain-free. It is also important to realize that loss affects all people, that it is appropriate for a health care worker to express emotion, to hug, and to grieve. As Chow (1980) states: "A tenacious spirit, deep concerns, and pervasive sense of responsibility all have a primary place in the field of gerontology."

Geriatric Suicide

According to Shulman (1978) "Old people kill themselves at a higher rate than any other age group." Although many studies have been made regarding suicide among adolescents and others, very little attention has been paid to the numbers of elderly who commit suicide or try and fail. Statistics indicate that although 10 to 15 per cent of the population is over 65 years of age, the suicide rate among this age group is 25 to 30 per cent of all known suicides. We do not have accurate statistics on the actual numbers, however, since the cause of death is frequently given as one of the many diseases with which the person may have been plagued.

Shulman (1978) summarizes the high-risk ractors in suicide specific to the elderly as follows:

1. Being an older white man.

2. Suffering from a mild to moderately severe mental disturbance associated with a sleep disorder.

3. Living alone.

4. Having a physical illness.
5. Recently losing a spouse or important family member.
6. Attempting suicide within the previous 2 to 3 years.
7. Having an available way to commit suicide.

Medical personnel have to be alert to the possibility of suicide and can help marshal the needed community resources for the suicide-prone patient. People who have "given up," who have a great sense of desolution and isolation, and who are physically ill will need support and assistance.

There are those in our society who feel that the elderly, particularly, have the right to end their lives when and how they wish. Indeed, there seem to be more and more printed accounts of older couples who have terminated their lives together. The right of an individual to end his or her own life will be a topic that is likely to receive more attention as time passes.

THE ROLE OF THE HEALTH CARE WORKER IN GERIATRICS

In geriatrics, it is the quality of life that matters, not the quantity of years. Many older people do not want to live endless years of isolation and increasing debilitation or to endure heroic means of prolonging life. Geriatrics will certainly grow as populations continue to age and tax our health resources. Social workers, family, and community agencies will have to work together closely to provide assistance and advocacy for elders. The urge to cure, a basic motivation among health care professionals, will have to become one of sustaining, with multidisciplinary teams cooperating to provide a meaningful existence for the elderly. Being a health care professional bestows a privilege and a responsibility that few in our society can experience. The medical professional is a participant in life's progression, in contact with people from all walks of life in a manner that is both intimate and influential.

The medical worker has the responsibility to be instrumental in altering the quality of that life. The caregiver must be observant; must respond instinctively and immediately in a crisis and also to know when it is appropriate to watch and wait; must be listeners, advocates, and educators making decisions that may have profound implications.

Throughout the activity of giving medical support, the health care professional must maintain a sense of self in an often stressful and demanding environment, remembering that the will to survive is a potent one, and that humans are resilient, with the ability to enter into the healing process. When offered the power to act in their own behalf, few will fail to do so.

REFERENCES

Boland, M., Murray, R., Zentner, J.: Assessment and health promotion for the person in later maturity. In Murray, R., Zentner, J. (eds.): *Nursing Assessment through the Life Span*. Prentice-Hall, Englewood Cliffs, N.J., 1979.

Butler, R.: The tragedy of old age in America. In *Why Survive? Being Old in America*. New York: Harper & Row, 1975.

Chow, R.: Quality of care: A present and future challenge for all nurses, editorial. *Journal of Gerontological Nursing*, 6(5), 1980.

Esberger, K.: Dying and the aged. *Journal of Gerontological Nursing*, 6:11–15, 1980.

Ford, J., Roth, W.: Do cognitive abilities decline with age? *Geriatrics*, 32(9):59–62, 1977.

Griggs, W.: Sex and the elderly. *American Journal of Nursing*, 29(8):1352–1354, 1978.

Grills, N.: Nutritional needs of elderly women. *Clinical Obstetrics and Gynecology*, 20(1):138–143, 1977.

Jowsey, J.: Osteoporosis: Dealing with a crippling bone disease. *Geriatrics*, 32(7):41–50, 1977.

Lynne-Davis, P.: Influence of age on the respiratory system. *Geriatrics*, 32(8):57–60, 1977.

Masters, W., Johnson, V.: *Human Sexual Response*. Boston: Little, Brown & Company, 1966.

Nejat, M., Grief, E.: The aging heart. *Medical Clinics of North America*, 60:1059–1071, 1976.

New York Times, Meals on wheels feeds elderly. August 9, 1981.

Powers, J., Powers, E.: Hearing problems of elderly persons. *Journal of the American Speech Hearing and Language Association,* 20(2)79–83, 1978.

Ryan, J. G.: Periodic health examination of the elderly. *Australian Family Physician,* 7:285–290, 1978.

Shearer, M., Shearer, M.: Sexuality and sexual counseling in the elderly. *Clinical Obstetrics and Gynecology,* 20:197–208, 1977.

Shulman, K.: Suicide and parasuicide in old age: A review. *Age and Aging,* 7:201–209, 1978.

Stenbach, A., et al.: Illness and health behavior in septuagenarians. *Journal of Gerontology,* 33(1):57–61, 1978.

Toku, S., Smith, E.: Age, immunity and the skin. *Cutis,* 18(9):456–458, 1976.

Williams, G.: The elderly in family practice: An evaluation of the geriatric visiting nurse. *The Journal of Family Practice,* 5(3):369–373, 1977.

Wuest, F. C., et al.: The aging eye. *Minnesota Medicine,* 59(8):540–546, 1976.

List of photographers for chapter opening pages:

Chapter		
	1	Judith Kruger Michalik
	2	Judith Kruger Michalik
	3	Judith Kruger Michalik
	4	Judith Kruger Michalik
	5	Judith Kruger Michalik
	6	Judith Kruger Michalik
	7	H. Armstrong Roberts
	8	Judith Kruger Michalik
	9	Judith Kruger Michalik
	10	Judith Kruger Michalik
	11	H. Armstrong Roberts
	12	Judith Kruger Michalik
	13	Judith Kruger Michalik
	14	Kathy Pitcoff
	15	Judith Kruger Michalik
	16	Jim Tackett

INDEX